# TREATMENT PLANS AND INTERVENTIONS FOR INSOMNIA

## TREATMENT PLANS AND INTERVENTIONS
## FOR EVIDENCE-BASED PSYCHOTHERAPY
Robert L. Leahy, Series Editor
*www.guilford.com/TPI*

This series provides psychotherapy practitioners with a wealth of practical tools for treating clients with a range of presenting problems. Each volume synthesizes current information on a particular disorder or clinical population; demonstrates how to develop specific, tailored treatment plans; and describes interventions proven to reduce distress and alleviate symptoms. Step-by-step guidelines for planning and implementing treatment are illustrated with rich case examples. User-friendly features include reproducible self-report forms, handouts, and symptom checklists, all in a convenient large-size format. Specific strategies for handling treatment roadblocks are also detailed. Emphasizing a collaborative approach to treatment, books in this series enable therapists to offer their clients the very best in evidence-based practice.

TREATMENT PLANS AND INTERVENTIONS FOR DEPRESSION
AND ANXIETY DISORDERS, SECOND EDITION
*Robert L. Leahy, Stephen J. F. Holland, and Lata K. McGinn*

TREATMENT PLANS AND INTERVENTIONS FOR BULIMIA
AND BINGE-EATING DISORDER
*Rene D. Zweig and Robert L. Leahy*

TREATMENT PLANS AND INTERVENTIONS FOR INSOMNIA:
A CASE FORMULATION APPROACH
*Rachel Manber and Colleen E. Carney*

# Treatment Plans and Interventions for Insomnia

## A Case Formulation Approach

Rachel Manber

Colleen E. Carney

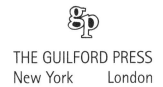

THE GUILFORD PRESS

New York    London

The authors have checked with sources believed to be reliable in their efforts to provide
information that is complete and generally in accord with the standards of practice that are
accepted at the time of publication. However, in view of the possibility of human error or
changes in behavioral, mental health, or medical sciences, neither the authors, nor the editor
and publisher, nor any other party who has been involved in the preparation or publication
of this work warrants that the information contained herein is in every respect accurate or
complete, and they are not responsible for any errors or omissions or the results obtained from
the use of such information. Readers are encouraged to confirm the information contained in
this book with other sources.

**Library of Congress Cataloging-in-Publication Data**

Manber, Rachel, author.
    Treatment plans and interventions for insomnia : a case formulation approach / Rachel
Manber, Colleen E. Carney.
        p. ;   cm. — (Treatment plans and interventions for evidence-based psychotherapy)
    Includes bibliographical references and index.
    ISBN 978-1-4625-2008-4 (pbk.)
    I. Carney, Colleen, author.   II. Title.   III. Series: Treatment plans and interventions
for evidence-based psychotherapy.
    [DNLM: 1. Sleep Initiation and Maintenance Disorders—therapy.   2. Cognitive
Therapy—methods.   3. Patient Care Planning.   WM 188]
    RC548
    616.8'4982—dc23
                                                                                        2014048114

*In memory of Richard Bootzin, a mentor, friend,*
*and founding father of behavioral interventions for insomnia*

# About the Authors

**Rachel Manber, PhD,** is Professor in the Department of Psychiatry and Behavioral Sciences and Director of the Insomnia and Behavioral Sleep Medicine Training Program at Stanford University. She is a clinical psychologist and has been certified by the American Board of Sleep Medicine in the practice of behavioral sleep medicine. Dr. Manber has trained many clinicians to deliver cognitive-behavioral therapy for insomnia (CBT-I) and has led the development and implementation of a nationwide CBT-I training initiative by the Department of Veterans Affairs. She has conducted sleep and depression research for 20 years and has published many articles in medical and psychiatric journals; numerous book chapters; and insomnia self-help books, including *Quiet Your Mind and Get to Sleep: Solutions to Insomnia for Those with Depression, Anxiety, or Chronic Pain,* coauthored with Colleen E. Carney.

**Colleen E. Carney, PhD,** is Associate Professor in the Department of Psychology and Director of the Sleep and Depression Laboratory at Ryerson University in Toronto. She is certified as a cognitive-behavioral therapist by the Canadian Association for Cognitive and Behavioural Therapies, is President of the Behavioral Sleep Medicine Special Interest Group of the Association for Behavioral and Cognitive Therapies, and is a Fellow of the Canadian Psychological Association. Dr. Carney's areas of research include CBT-I; insomnia in the context of other health conditions, notably depression and chronic pain; evidence-based fatigue management strategies; rumination and sleep; fear of the dark in adults; and improving access to CBT. The author of over 100 publications, including seven books, Dr. Carney is a recipient of the Early Researcher Award from the Canadian Ministry of Research and Innovation and the Pickwick Fellowship from the National Sleep Foundation.

# Preface

Almost everyone can relate to the experience of a fitful night and the unpleasant next-day consequences. Most people, however, experience sleepless nights as isolated or time-limited unpleasant occurrences during unsettling or distressing periods. They usually find it easy to understand why they lost sleep. For them, sleeping well after having lost sleep for a night or two feels refreshing and energizing, and represents a return to normality. People with insomnia have trouble sleeping almost every night. They may experience occasional nights of good sleep, but they rarely understand why they slept well. As a result, an occasional good night is not a trusted sign of the resolution of insomnia. In other words, the experiences of a good sleeper who occasionally sleeps poorly and a person with chronically poor sleep who occasionally sleeps well are psychological mirror images, yet fundamentally different sets of experiences.

It is gratifying to help people who experience poor sleep on most nights for months or years to sleep well. To do this, a therapist must understand the fundamental differences between these two types of experience, and must carefully listen with an open mind to the very personal ways each patient experiences insomnia. A therapist also needs to understand the physiological and psychological factors involved in the transition into and out of sleep. To help promote behaviors and thought habits that support good sleep, clinicians also need to be familiar with principles of behavioral change and cognitive therapy.

Cognitive-behavioral therapy (CBT) is an effective and brief treatment for insomnia. It combines behavioral and cognitive interventions that target behaviors, thoughts, and emotions affecting sleep regulation. CBT protocols for treating insomnia that have been researched have consisted of two to eight sessions, with five- to six-session protocols being the most common. Although the majority of patients improve quickly, some may need more sessions. The use of these CBT protocols is empirically supported across myriad populations. Empirical evaluation began with the study of carefully selected samples of individuals who had no comorbidities, and later included samples with specific comorbidities as well as heterogeneous samples. The results across populations are consistent: These CBT approaches are effective.

This book was shaped by our experience delivering and teaching others to deliver a form of CBT that targets insomnia, referred to as CBT-I. Our insights were gained from both successes and failures in our roles as teachers and therapists. We have translated these insights into a structured case formulation approach that guides the planning and treatment of insomnia. We have taught CBT-I to students and clinicians from multiple disciplines (psychologists, clinical social workers, mental health nurses, psychiatrists, counselors, nurses, pharmacists, and physicians). Mental health providers often begin CBT-I training with at least some knowledge and experience of helping patients change their behaviors, but little knowledge about sleep science. Medical practitioners often begin CBT-I training with some knowledge about sleep and its disorders, but little training in psychotherapeutic processes and tools to help patients mobilize their resources to make behavioral changes that can lead to better sleep. This book is geared toward the former group, in that it assumes some familiarity with psychotherapy process and with principles of CBT in general, as these apply to other disorders.

A prerequisite for meaningful case formation is understanding how sleep is regulated, how various factors promote and hinder optimal sleep, and how comorbidities affect sleep. Therefore, the first portion of the book is dedicated to these topics and culminates in suggestions for a structured sleep assessment. We then introduce specific components of CBT-I and discuss when and how to adapt standard treatment components to meet individual clients' needs. The last portion of the book is dedicated to case conceptualization and treatment planning, including illustration of the full course of treatment for two cases that are introduced in Chapter 1. The cases describe fictitious characters created from a fusion of several real cases. The cases highlight a few clinical features and implementation challenges. Throughout the book, we also provide vignettes that illustrate ways to address additional challenges to the implementation of CBT-I.

In training both licensed clinicians and students, we have observed the importance of in-depth understanding of the rationale for specific CBT-I recommendations. Absence of such understanding hinders the delivery of treatment in terms of both specific and nonspecific therapeutic elements. A clinician's failure to understand the scientific rationale will inevitably have an impact on patients' buy-in, and therefore adherence, which will then compromise outcome. A clinician who does not fully understand the scientific basis of CBT-I will also be less effective in case formulation and therefore may fail to offer a treatment component that might be essential for a given patient. Equally important, clinicians who are not comfortable with certain components of treatment may avoid using them, and in so doing dilute the efficacy of the treatment.

It is equally important that in the process of learning specific CBT-I techniques, clinicians do not neglect nonspecific therapeutic elements, such as forming a working alliance, providing understanding and support, and promoting self-efficacy and hope. Self-help CBT-based interventions for insomnia (books and, increasingly, Internet and mobile apps) have been created and tested. Research is showing that self-help interventions augmented with clinicians' structured involvement are more effective than those without such augmentation; these findings further highlight the importance of both specific and nonspecific factors in delivering CBT-I.

This book is not another treatment manual. Rather than offering a rigid session-by-session protocol, the book provides a framework for tailoring treatment to the specific presentation of each patient. Although individualizing therapy is an attractive notion, clinicians with minimal prior exposure to CBT-I may initially find this case formulation approach challenging. For this reason, we have also included a "typical" session-by-session treatment progression. However, the primary intent of the book is to promote flexible administration of CBT-I. We offer ideas on how to adapt the standard components to patients with specific comorbidities. We believe that the flexible approach to CBT-I and specific adaptations of its components will maximize the clinical relevance of the book and will make it useful even to clinicians with prior CBT-I experience.

# Acknowledgments

We wish to thank those who have helped shape this book. The list includes the many patients we have treated and the numerous individuals we have trained to provide the treatment. In writing this book, we have benefited from input from a few colleagues, and we thank them for their help and encouragement: Britney Blaire and Norah Simpson for their assistance in shaping the case examples, Christopher Fairholme for numerous theoretical discussions about hyperarousal that have influenced the writing of Chapter 3, and Leah Freedman and Donn Posner for their feedback on other sections. Special thanks go to Margaret St. John, a therapist naïve to CBT-I, who was willing to serve as its first user. We would also like to thank a few students who pilot-tested and provided feedback on the Case Conceptualization Form, especially Andy Harris, Taryn Moss Atlin, Angela Lachowski, and Dora Zalai. At The Guilford Press, we thank Jim Nageotte, Jane Keislar, Anna Brackett, and, most importantly, copy editor Marie Sprayberry. We also thank Robert Leahy for his valuable suggestions. Lastly, we want to thank our families for their constructive feedback and support.

# Contents

# List of Figures, Tables, and Forms

## FIGURES

## TABLES

## FORMS

# CHAPTER 1

# Introduction

Patients seeking treatment for insomnia describe difficulties falling or staying asleep at night and stress the impact that their poor sleep has on their lives, often citing it as the reason for seeking help. Consistent with patients' experiences, the clinical entity *insomnia disorder* (American Psychiatric Association, 2013) is considered a 24-hour condition, consisting of disturbed sleep at night and associated distress or impaired functioning during the day. Cognitive-behavioral therapy for insomnia (CBT-I) is a brief and effective sleep-focused treatment that is anchored in the science of sleep and utilizes principles of general cognitive-behavioral therapy (CBT) to address both nocturnal and daytime symptoms of insomnia disorder. Despite strong empirical support, CBT-I is not available to most patients who could benefit from it. To a large extent, this is because there is a shortage of therapists trained to deliver it.

This book aims to guide therapists in helping their adult patients, including those with comorbidities, to sleep better. The goal is to allow therapists to apply CBT-I in a flexible, patient-tailored manner. To enable this flexible approach, and based on our extensive experiences of training clinicians to deliver CBT-I, we have decided to devote the first part of the book (Chapters 1–5) to background information about the nature of sleep and insomnia. We believe that information about how normal sleep is organized and regulated, how behaviors influence the sleep regulation process, and how comorbidities affect sleep and its regulation is essential for effective delivery of CBT-I. The second portion of the book (Chapters 6–13) is about the treatment itself. After discussing a sleep-focused assessment, we introduce the treatment components, and then discuss how to select the most relevant component, in what order to introduce them, and when to alter the standard guidelines to the unique needs of each patient.

We provide a case conceptualization framework for making these important clinical decisions, and we discuss cautions and contraindications. Comorbidities and consumptions of sleep medications are carefully considered, but they are not contraindications. This book discusses specific effects of the comorbidities and the use of sleep medications on insomnia, and when and how to modify the standard CBT-I guidelines accordingly. Also in the spirit of promoting implementation of CBT-I that meets the unique needs of patients, we do not present a rigid session-by-session protocol in this book. Nonetheless, to aid therapists as they learn to use this treatment, we do include a template for a six-session treatment plan (an insomnia assessment session plus five treatment sessions), and we demonstrate a full course of treatment for two cases, both of which are introduced at the end of this chapter.

# DIAGNOSIS OF INSOMNIA DISORDER

The term *insomnia,* as it is often used colloquially in reference to poor sleep, is not the same as the clinical entity called *insomnia disorder.* According to the *Diagnostic and Statistical Manual of Mental Disorders,* fifth edition (DSM-5; American Psychiatric Association, 2013), the diagnosis of insomnia disorder includes the following two core criteria: (1) difficulties falling asleep or staying asleep (nighttime symptoms), and (2) associated distress and/or perceived negative impact on daytime functions and mood (daytime symptoms). In other words, as is the case with other disorders, a clinical diagnosis is not made unless symptoms are associated with clinically significant consequences.

## Operationalizing Insomnia Disorder Criteria

The diagnosis of insomnia disorder is based entirely on the patient's report and the clinician's judgment. Objective sleep measurements, such as staying overnight in a sleep laboratory while being physiologically monitored, are not required or even recommended for the diagnosis. The core clinical criteria for insomnia disorder are not well operationalized. For instance, the DSM-5 criteria for poor sleep do not specify a cutoff for time to fall asleep or for time awake in the middle of the night. Quantitative criteria that operationalize sleep difficulties have been proposed (Lichstein, Durrence, Taylor, Bush, & Riedel, 2003) and used in research. Specifically, the proposed quantitative criterion for poor sleep is having sleep onset latency or time awake after sleep onset greater than 30 minutes at least three nights a week for at least 6 months. However, there is evidence that morbidity can be similar in cases with less frequent but more severe sleep disruption (in term of number of minutes with unwanted wakefulness) and in cases with more frequent but milder sleep loss (Lineberger, Carney, Edinger, & Means, 2006). DSM-5 does provide a little more guidance on what is meant by *clinically significant* consequences of poor sleep, by listing examples of specific domains of daytime impairment; these are similar to those specified in the Research Diagnostic Criteria for insomnia (Edinger et al., 2004). The consequences of poor sleep include the following domains:

- Fatigue/ malaise
- Attention, concentration, or memory impairment
- Social/vocational dysfunction or poor school performance
- Mood disturbance /irritability
- Daytime sleepiness
- Motivation/energy/initiative reduction
- Proneness to errors/accidents at work or while driving
- Physical symptoms such as tension headaches and gastrointestinal symptoms
- Concerns or worries about sleep

DSM-5 includes a minimum frequency criterion (at least three nights a week), which was not present in DSM-IV-TR (American Psychiatric Association, 2000), and a minimum duration of 3 months, which is longer than was indicated in DSM-IV-TR. Another, and more major, revision to the definitions of sleep–wake disorders in DSM-5 relative to DSM-IV-TR is the elimination of the distinction between primary insomnia and insomnia related to a medical or psychiatric condition, which was made in the earlier version. DSM-5 defines a single condition: insomnia disorder. The elimination of the distinction between primary insomnia and insomnia related to other disorders is based on the notion that the presence of comorbidities is a dimension, rather than a defining feature, of the disorder. This change reflects the growing recognition that, even when poor sleep emerges as a symptom of another disorder, it may develop into a separate comorbid disorder that is not ameliorated by the treatment of the comorbid condition. For example, in the context of depression, insomnia is a common, unresolved residual symptom among patients whose depression remits following antidepressant therapy (Nierenberg et al., 1999, 2010). The implication is that a diagnosis of insomnia disorder can be made when sleep disturbances emerge in the context of another psychiatric or medical condition, as long as the complaint of poor sleep is accompanied by clinically meaningful consequences, such as distress and perceived impairment in function.

## AGREEMENT BETWEEN OBJECTIVE AND SUBJECTIVE SLEEP IN INSOMNIA

The "gold standard" objective measure of sleep is *polysomnography* (PSG). PSG is a method for studying brain waves and other physiological parameters, such as eye movements, muscle activity, respiration, and heart rate. Using such methods, research shows that compared to non-symptomatic control participants, individuals with insomnia take longer to fall asleep; they are awake for a longer time in the middle of the night; and their sleep efficiency (percentage of time asleep relative to time allotted for sleep) is lower. However, average differences between people with and without insomnia disorder are modest and of questionable clinical significance. For example, Perlis, Smith, Andrews, Orff, and Giles (2001) report that individuals with insomnia disorder sleep 25 minutes less and take 12 minutes longer to fall asleep than good sleeper controls.

In general, people with insomnia or insomnia disorder underestimate the time they sleep and overestimate the time it takes them to fall asleep, compared to their PSG sleep results (Carskadon et al., 1976; Perlis, Giles, Mendelson, Bootzin, & Wyatt, 1997). Also, compared to people without insomnia (symptoms or disorder), those with insomnia are more likely to identify themselves as having been awake when awakened from PSG-defined sleep (Carskadon et al., 1976; Perlis, Giles, Mendelson, et al., 1997).

There are, however, individual differences in the extent of sleep state misperception among people with insomnia disorder. At the extreme is a group of people (about 5–9% of people with sleep disorders; American Academy of Sleep Medicine, 2005; Coleman et al., 1982) for whom there is a profound mismatch between subjective and objective sleep estimates. The *International Classification of Sleep Disorders*, second edition (ICSD-2; American Academy of Sleep Medicine, 2005), which is distinct from the DSM classification system, classifies this extreme group as having *paradoxical insomnia*. Clinically, people with paradoxical insomnia report a chronic pattern of little or no sleep on most nights; although their self-reported levels of daytime impairment are similar to those of other people with insomnia disorder, their reported impairment appears much less severe than would be expected from the extreme level of sleep deprivation they report.

## PREVALENCE AND COURSE

Estimates of *point prevalence* (i.e., the proportion of people in a population who have a disorder at a particular time) depend on the operational definition of insomnia or insomnia disorder, the population studied, and the method of assessment. Epidemiological studies estimate the point prevalence of poor sleep that is associated with daytime distress or impairment and lasts at least 1 month as 5–10% (Mai & Buysse, 2008; Morin, LeBlanc, Daley, Gregoire, & Merette, 2006; Ohayon, 2002; Ohayon & Roth, 2001). As expected, the prevalence decreases as the criteria become more restrictive. For instance, 25.3% of 2,001 individuals sampled in a Canadian epidemiological study were dissatisfied with their sleep, but only 17.2% also had difficulty initiating or maintaining sleep (Morin, LeBlanc, et al., 2006). Most (78.2%) of those with insomnia complaints (dissatisfaction with sleep and difficulty with falling or staying asleep) had the problem for over a month, and 38.3% also experienced negative daytime consequences, resulting in a 9.6% prevalence estimate of insomnia disorder in this study (Morin, LeBlanc, et al., 2006). The *incidence* (rate of new cases) of insomnia per year is between 3 and 6% (Ford & Kamerow, 1989; Jansson-Frojmark & Linton, 2008; LeBlanc et al., 2009). There is roughly a 2:1 ratio of women to men (e.g., Mai & Buysse, 2008; Ohayon & Roth, 2001), and an increased prevalence with advancing age (Bixler, Kales, Soldatos, Kales, & Healey, 1979). The prevalence of insomnia is higher among people with comorbid medical and psychiatric conditions; the most prominent among these comorbidities are depressive disorders (Ford & Kamerow, 1989) and chronic pain conditions (Ohayon, 2005).

There is a large body of retrospective and prospective studies (summarized by Jansson-Frojmark & Linton, 2008) suggesting that poor sleep tends to be a chronic problem. The retrospective studies report that most individuals complaining of poor sleep (insomnia symptoms) have had the problem for more than 1 year, and approximately 40% have had it for more than 5 years. The longitudinal prospective studies have similarly found that roughly half of individuals with insomnia symptoms continue to experience poor sleep at least 1 year later. There is less research about the course of insomnia disorder. Two population-based studies that did examine the course of insomnia as a disorder found that over the course of 1 year, insomnia disorder was persistent for 31–44% of the baseline cases (reviewed in Jansson-Frojmark & Linton, 2008). One of the two studies further reported that 11% of individuals whose insomnia disorder remitted eventually experienced a relapse of insomnia disorder during the 3-year follow-up period (Morin et al., 2009). These two naturalistic studies included a mix of individuals with treated (usually over-the-counter or prescription medications) and untreated insomnia disorder. It is possible that rates of persistence of insomnia disorder are even higher among individuals with untreated insomnia disorder. Interestingly, although poor sleep tends to be persistent or recurrent, in most cases it does not develop into insomnia disorder. It is estimated that only 10–14% of people with poor sleep who do not meet all diagnostic criteria for insomnia disorder end up meeting these criteria at some assessment point during a 3-year follow-up (Morin et al., 2009).

## COST

Poor sleep and insomnia disorder are frequently encountered by mental health professionals and primary care physicians in their practices (Canals, Domenech, Carbajo, & Blade, 1997; Ford & Kamerow, 1989). Insomnia disorder carries significant personal costs, being associated with increased risk for other health conditions and mood disturbances, including a twofold increase in risk for depression (Baglioni et al., 2011; Ford & Kamerow, 1989). It also has a marked economic impact, which, when both direct and indirect costs are accounted for, is estimated at $100 billion annually in the United States (Rosekind & Gregory, 2010; Stoller, 1994). Compared to a healthy sleeper, a person with insomnia incurs roughly $4,500 more in costs per year, considering the costs of health care, absenteeism from work, disability, prescription medications, and over-the-counter medications (Daley, Morin, LeBlanc, Gregoire, & Savard, 2009).

## HELP–SEEKING BEHAVIORS

Although psychological distress is one of the main determinants prompting individuals with insomnia to seek treatment, only 6% of people with insomnia consult with a psychologist; most consult with a medical professional, primarily a primary care physician (Morin, LeBlanc, et al., 2006). In general, fewer than half of individuals with insomnia symptoms seek help over their lifetimes (Ancoli-Israel & Roth, 1999; Morin, LeBlanc, et al., 2006), and only 20% make an appointment to see a physician specifically about their sleep (Bartlett, Marshall, Williams, & Grunstein, 2008; Shochat, Umphress, Israel, & Ancoli-Israel, 1999). In addition to psychological distress, predictors of help-seeking behaviors for insomnia include insomnia severity (both poor sleep and perceived daytime impairment), short sleep duration (less than 6.5 hours), older age, poorer health, and higher income (Bartlett et al., 2008). Little is known about cross-referrals between medicine and psychology for the treatment of insomnia, or about help seeking for insomnia in the context of psychotherapy for other mental disorders.

## EMPIRICAL SUPPORT FOR CBT-I

A large and consistent body of literature provides strong empirical support for the efficacy of CBT-I. The evidence is based on studies that compare CBT-I to a control therapy (Edinger, Wohlgemuth, Radtke, Marsh, & Quillian, 2001; Manber et al., 2008) and to delayed-treatment controls (Edinger et al., 2001; Lichstein, Riedel, Wilson, Lester, & Aguillard, 2001; Morin, Kowatch, Barry, & Walton, 1993). Direct comparison with hypnotic medications demonstrates equivalence of CBT-I to sleep medications, such as temazepam (Morin, Colecchi, Stone, Sood, & Brink, 1999), zolpidem (Jacobs, Pace-Schott, Stickgold, & Otto, 2004), and zopiclone (Sivertsen et al., 2006). There is also evidence that the effects of CBT-I are durable, lasting 1–2 years following discontinuation of treatment, and in that way are superior to the effects of medication treatments (Morin, Colecchi, et al., 1999; Sivertsen et al., 2006). The weight of evidence supporting CBT-I has led to its recognition as a first-line treatment for insomnia in a National Institutes of Health Consensus Statement (2005). The British Association of Psychopharmacology has also recognized the importance of CBT-I in the management of insomnia and has issued a statement recommending CBT-I as a front-line treatment for insomnia (Wilson et al., 2010).

## CBT-I Is Effective for Insomnia Comorbid with Other Disorders

Sleep difficulties are common among those with psychiatric comorbidities and are diagnostic symptoms of depressive and anxiety disorders. However, sleep problems often do not resolve with general psychotherapy (Kopta, Howard, Lowry, & Beutler, 1994), pharmacotherapy (McClintock et al., 2011; Nierenberg et al., 1999, 2010), or psychotherapy for the comorbid disorders (Manber et al., 2003; Thase et al., 2002; Zayfert & DeViva, 2004). In the past, it was assumed that sleep difficulties experienced by individuals with mental illnesses were symptoms of psychiatric disorders that would resolve when the underlying disorders were successfully treated. This belief led clinicians to ignore sleep difficulties. A similar state of neglect is present for people with medical comorbidities, including sleep disorders other than insomnia disorder. As a result, poor sleep has rarely received special psychotherapeutic attention. This is unfortunate, because poor sleep among people with psychiatric and medical conditions contributes to the severity of the comorbid conditions and hinders response to treatment of these conditions (Buysse et al., 1999; Thase, Simons, & Reynolds, 1996). Several clinical trials have indicated that CBT-I is indeed effective for people with depression (Lancee, van den Bout, van Straten, & Spoormaker, 2013; Manber et al., 2008; Morawetz, 2003), posttraumatic stress disorder (PTSD) (Germain, Shear, Hall, & Buysse, 2007; Zayfert & DeViva, 2004), and pain (Currie, Wilson, & Curran, 2002; Edinger, Wohlgemuth, Krystal, & Rice, 2005; Rybarczyk et al., 2005). Evidence also suggests that in the case of depression, simultaneous treatment of depression and insomnia with a hypnotic (Fava et al., 2006) or CBT-I (Manber et al., 2008) enhances depression outcomes. Thus, psychotherapists could improve care of their patients who present with comorbid insomnia disorder by treating the insomnia disorder with this brief, empirically validated, insomnia-focused therapy.

## Can CBT-I Be Used When Hypnotic Medications Are Concomitantly Used?

Individuals with insomnia who take hypnotic medications but nonetheless have difficulty sleeping can benefit from CBT-I. Whereas randomized controlled trials of CBT-I usually exclude participants who use hypnotic medications, uncontrolled case series reports from clinic samples and studies that combine CBT-I with a medication taper protocol suggest that CBT-I is not less effective for hypnotic users than for nonusers (Morin et al., 2004; Rosen, Lewin, Goldberg, & Woolfolk, 2000).

Patients who meet criteria for insomnia disorder even though they use hypnotics may have developed tolerance to the medications or psychological dependence on them. *Tolerance* to a drug is a decrease in susceptibility to the effects of the drug, due to its continued administration; it results from cellular adaptation to the active substance in the drug, so that increasingly larger doses are required to produce the same physiological or psychological effect obtained earlier with smaller doses. *Psychological dependence* on a hypnotic medication is present when a patient does not believe that sleep can be attained without the use of the hypnotic medication. Abrupt discontinuation of a hypnotic medication is often associated with transient sleep difficulty immediately after discontinuation. Patients who interpret the experience of poor sleep immediately after discontinuation as evidence that they cannot sleep well without the medication develop psychological dependence. Patients with insomnia disorder who use hypnotics regularly and have developed tolerance to or psychological dependence on hypnotic medications are classified in ICSD-2 as having *hypnotic-dependent insomnia* (American Academy of Sleep Medicine, 2005). Among patients receiving CBT-I at the Stanford School of Medicine, about half indicated worry that they would not be able to sleep if they did not take medications, that they had "become too dependent on the medication," or that they had tried to stop taking medications and failed (Adler, Carde, Kuo, Ong, & Manber, 2008).

Some patients with hypnotic-dependent insomnia include hypnotic discontinuation as a treatment goal and others do not. In Chapter 12 we outline a treatment for Sam, introduced at the end of this chapter. Sam had been using a hypnotic medication for 20 years, and his physician who referred him to CBT-I described him as having hypnotic-dependent insomnia. Sam did not include hypnotic taper as a treatment goal. After five sessions of CBT-I, encouraged by the improvement in his sleep and daytime functioning, Sam spontaneously discontinued the sleep medication. Many patients with hypnotic-dependent insomnia who state that their goal is to sleep well without sleep medications express fear of not being able to sleep without the drugs. Psychologists in collaboration with physicians have developed and tested slow-taper protocols for patients with hypnotic-dependent insomnia, usually combining such protocols with CBT-I (Kirmil-Gray, Eagleston, Thoresen, & Zarcone, 1985). In Chapter 13, where we discuss collaboration between a CBT-I therapist and a prescribing clinician, we also briefly describe a few of these protocols.

### Patient Preference

Most people seeking help for insomnia are treated with a sleep medication; few know about CBT-I as a treatment option. However, when provided a description of CBT-I, patients with insomnia rate it more favorably than they do descriptions of pharmacological treatments (Azad, Byszewski, Sarazin, McLean, & Koziarz, 2003; Morin, Gaulier, Barry, & Kowatch, 1992). Vincent and Lionberg (2001) further reported that psychological treatment was judged to be more acceptable than pharmacological treatment, more effective in the long term, more likely to improve daytime functioning, and less likely to produce negative side effects (Vincent & Lionberg, 2001). Among middle-aged and older adults with insomnia symptoms, predictors of interest in CBT-I were reporting greater negative impact of poor sleep in terms of interference with daily functioning and daytime fatigue, and reporting more mood problems and physical symptoms (Cahn et al., 2005).

## Sleep Hygiene Alone Is Rarely Effective

*Sleep hygiene* is a set of popular recommendations for good sleep practices. A few examples are that patients should not drink coffee too late, should limit alcohol, should keep the bedroom at a comfortable temperature, and should always go to bed at the same time. However, sleep hygiene recommendations have limited efficacy and have often been used as control therapy in randomized controlled trials demonstrating the efficacy of CBT-I. Our experience has been that by the time patients seek our help, they have already tried these common recommendations. In such cases, it is best to emphasize that CBT-I involves much more than sleep hygiene recommendations.

## USING THIS BOOK

This book prepares therapists to deliver CBT-I effectively and flexibly, tailoring it to individual presentations (including those with comorbid conditions). This flexible approach to CBT-I requires readers to understand sleep regulation, presented in Chapters 2 and 3; to be familiar with models of insomnia, discussed in Chapter 3; and to be mindful of the impact of comorbid conditions on insomnia, the focus of Chapters 4 and 5. Thus Chapters 2–5 build a foundation for the assessment and effective implementation of CBT-I. Chapter 6 is devoted to the assessment of insomnia, and Chapters 7–9 present the behavioral and cognitive treatment components, including suggestions for when and how to alter these components to promote adherence and efficacy. In Chapter 10, we describe a treatment planning process that guides clinicians in how to select and sequence CBT-I components for each individual patient. Inherently, truly customized treatment is incongruent with a fixed session-by-session description of treatment. Nonetheless, we describe a general structure for a six-session treatment protocol, consisting of a comprehensive sleep assessment and five treatment sessions; we then demonstrate the full course of treatment with two case examples in Chapters 11 and 12. Chapter 13 discusses implementation and professional issues.

Below, we introduce the two case examples. We encourage our readers to keep these two cases in mind as they read the rest of the book, and to be curious about how the information being discussed applies to these cases.

## CASE EXAMPLES

### Sophie

Sophie was a 42-year-old unmarried woman who was having difficulty initiating sleep; she was also waking in the night and unable to fall back to sleep for hours. Sophie was an attorney specializing in corporate law. Her job was intermittently stressful when she was nearing project deadlines. She did not have a bed partner and lived alone. Sophie was very healthy and active; she loved to hike, swim, and ride her bicycle. She had regular wellness visits with her primary care physician and had never had any major health problems. She did not snore or have other symptoms of sleep apnea or other sleep disorders. She had never had a sleep study. Prior to the onset of her insomnia, she used to enjoy 1–2 cups of coffee in the morning, but now she did not drink any caffeinated drinks because she was concerned that they would negatively affect her sleep.

This was the first time Sophie had experienced problems sleeping for so long. Before the previous year, she had never had trouble sleeping. She said, "I used to love going to sleep and looked forward to it. I used to fall asleep when my head hit the pillow, and I never woke up until I had to in the morning." Her typical sleep schedule was 10:30 P.M. to 6:30 A.M., but she would sometimes sleep in a couple of hours on the weekends or stay up later to work if she had a deadline.

Roughly 1 year ago, Sophie had gone through a very painful breakup. She remembered an incident that had happened around the time of the breakup: As she was drifting off to sleep, she woke up feeling that it was hard to breathe and fearing she might be having a heart attack. She went to the bathroom, splashed water on her face, and felt a little better, but went to the emergency room to make sure she was OK. Sophie was medically cleared and told that she had probably had a panic attack. After this memorable night, Sophie started having difficulties falling asleep. She found herself lying in bed for hours trying to fall asleep, "fighting with" her sleep, and growing more and more frustrated the longer she was awake. She would eventually fall asleep, but then awaken with a start about 4 hours later and would again have difficulty returning to sleep. Sophie had never experienced a second panic attack. Although initially she was afraid it would happen again, she said that now she had no concerns about having a panic attack; her concern now was about sleep.

Sophie estimated that she was getting approximately 4 hours of sleep per night. After dinner, she surfed the Internet and watched TV. She got into bed around 9:30 P.M., because she wanted to have "plenty of time to fall asleep." She used to read in bed, but after she read somewhere that she should not do this, she stopped doing it; now she turned off the light right away. It took her 1–3 hours to fall asleep. She stayed in bed tossing and turning, checking the clock. She was not worried about anything in particular, but her mind skipped around aimlessly ("My mind is definitely not quiet"). She woke at around 2:00 A.M. and 4:00 A.M., and sometimes again around 5:00 A.M. When she woke up at 4, her mind would get going about what she needed to do, and she would start getting anxious that she was awake and only had a few hours left before she had to get up. She set an alarm for 7:00 A.M. on weekdays, but usually woke up a few minutes before it sounded. She did not set an alarm on the weekends, but she still woke up at about the same time. She estimated that she was awake for a total of about 30–90 minutes each night. Sophie had a very difficult time getting out of bed in the mornings, and as a result, she had discontinued her morning workout routine. On weekdays, Sophie "forced" herself out of bed by 7:30 A.M. so she could make it to work on time. On the weekends, she allowed herself to stay in bed until 9:00 A.M.; she found it "nice" to rest in bed, and she was occasionally able to fall back to sleep. On most days, Sophie would lie down for a nap when she got home from work, but she was usually unable to quiet her mind and would not actually fall asleep. On the weekends, she sometimes did sleep on the couch while watching a movie in the living room during the early afternoon.

Sophie reported feeling miserable during the day, finding it difficult to concentrate in meetings, and losing track of important work. Just last week, she had been arguing a case in front of a judge and completely lost her train of thought. She was also concerned that she was becoming more irritable with colleagues and with friends. She no longer went out much with friends in the evenings, because she did not feel that she had enough energy to do much, and she was concerned that if she went out in the evenings she would have problems sleeping at night.

When she first experienced difficulty with sleep, Sophie tried taking sleep medications. Eszopiclone was "not that helpful," and clonazepam left her feeling "fuzzy and groggy" in the morning, so she stopped taking either drug. She then experimented with drinking a glass of wine before going to bed. This helped her fall asleep a little faster, but she would wake more often at night—so she did it only rarely, when she felt particularly "wired" at bedtime. Sophie expressed skepticism that anything would help her sleep well again, but stated that she would "give anything to go back to sleeping like I did before."

## Sam

Sam was a 60-year-old accountant. He had recently been having a very hard time falling asleep and was waking up many times in the middle of the night. He also had a diagnosis of sleep apnea that was not fully treated. He would wake up in the middle of the night noticing that the mask used to treat his sleep apnea (see Chapter 4) was off, but he often would not put it back on. For the past 6 months, he had been out of work on disability for chronic pain and fatigue related to a diagnosis of fibromyalgia. Sam lived with his wife and an adult daughter, with both of whom he enjoyed positive relationships. His second daughter lived nearby with her husband and their two young children. Sam enjoyed interacting with his grandkids and had been spending 2 days a week with them until recently, in part because his insomnia had worsened and his energy "to keep up with toddlers" was diminished.

Sam had suffered intermittent insomnia for the past 25 years. At first he did not recall any specific trigger, but upon further reflection he remembered that he had first experienced insomnia around the time his second daughter was born. His doctor prescribed zolpidem, and he had been taking it every night for the past 18 years. He would like to stop, but although he did not feel it helped that much, he was worried that his sleep would "be even worse" if he stopped. He was also taking gabapentin and duloxetine for chronic neuropathic pain and fibromyalgia, and his doctor had said that these medications might also help him sleep better.

Sam estimated that most nights he slept around 5 hours, but noted that about once a month he was "up for 20 hours straight" and had no idea why. He believed that this long-standing battle with sleep was having a great impact on him. During the day, Sam was experiencing pain, fatigue, depressed mood, difficulty concentrating, irritability, and memory impairment, all of which he attributed to his sleep difficulties. He had also stopped driving more than 3 miles from home, because he feared he would fall asleep at the wheel. He and his wife slept separately, because he felt that her soft snoring made it difficult for him to sleep.

Over the years, Sam had seen many doctors and therapists to help him sleep better. He had been keeping notes about his sleep and the advice he had received. He brought these notes to his initial appointment, along with a three-ring binder with medical records related to his sleep problems. The notes in the binder included details about when and how long he was awake in the middle of the night, what time he woke up in the morning, and how he felt throughout the following day.

When asked to describe a typical night, Sam reported that he got into bed around 10:30 P.M. It took him about 2 hours to fall asleep. He usually slept 4 or 5 hours and then woke up. He said that the rest of the night he was in and out of sleep, sleeping in chunks of half an hour or less. He woke up sometimes between 5:00 A.M. and 6:00 A.M., but continued to try to sleep until 7:30 to 8:30 A.M., when he would get up to start the day. He said that he sometimes dozed off during the period before he got up, but did not feel that this was "real sleep." When he got out of bed in the morning, he felt as if he had been "fighting with sleep for hours." After breakfast, he would lie on the couch watching TV for a couple of hours. He thought that sometimes he dozed off during these periods, because he sometimes realized he had missed a short segment of the show he was watching. He would try to do things out of the house in the afternoons, but often stayed at home because of pain. If he did not go out of the house, he would lie down again in the afternoon to "rest from the pain" until his wife got home from work. He spent the evenings with his wife. They often watched a television program or a movie. He reported sometimes dozing off while watching television; when he did, his wife would wake him. Asked to describe his prior sleep schedule, Sam said that when he was still working, he used to sleep in on the weekends and on days off until 11:00 A.M.; he added that he used to be a bit of a "night owl" then, and on weekends he would go to bed after midnight.

Sam's goals were to sleep more, get rid of his pain, and not feel sleepy during the day so that he could spend more time with his grandchildren.

We will revisit the cases of Sophie and Sam throughout the book, and we present their treatment plans in Chapters 11 and 12, respectively.

## KEY PRACTICE IDEAS

- Insomnia disorder is a 24-hour disorder.

- People with insomnia tend to underestimate how long they sleep and overestimate how long it takes them to fall asleep.

- People with insomnia disorder comorbid with another physical or mental disorder can benefit from CBT-I.

- Hypnotic use is not a contraindication for using CBT-I.

# CHAPTER 2

# Sleep and Its Regulation

In this chapter, we discuss the structure of sleep and the two-process model of sleep regulation. Familiarity with the structure of sleep is important for understanding patients' insomnia experiences and for assessing sleep disorders other than insomnia disorder (see Chapter 4). Even more important is therapists' understanding of the regulation of normal sleep, because it can guide case formulation and treatment planning. A therapist can carefully select which specific information about sleep regulation is relevant for which patient, and can help all patients understand how their behaviors affect and/or are affected by the sleep regulatory system. Such information can enhance patients' commitment to and engagement in necessary behavior changes that, in the absence of a scientifically grounded explanation, may seem counterintuitive. Therefore, education about the regulation of sleep is essential to therapists and relevant to almost all of their patients with insomnia disorder.

## THE STRUCTURE OF SLEEP (SLEEP ARCHITECTURE)

As noted in Chapter 1, the predominant objective tool used to study the nature and organization of sleep is polysomnography (PSG). PSG is used to measure electrical activity in the brain, from which several sleep parameters can be derived. Important among these parameters are the time it takes to fall asleep (sleep onset latency, or SOL); the number and duration of awakenings after initially falling asleep (wakefulness after sleep onset, or WASO); the total sleep time (TST); and sleep efficiency (SE, defined as the percentage of time asleep relative to the time allotted for sleep. In addition to these gross measures, PSG provides information about the distribution of the different sleep states and stages (sleep architecture), which are described below. PSG involves attachment of electrodes to specific regions of the scalp (to measure electrical brain activity), face (to measure facial muscle tone and eye movement), and legs (to measure leg muscle activity). Other physiological parameters, such as respiration, are also included and are discussed in the context of diagnosing other sleep disorders (Chapter 4). PSG is not used as a clinical diagnostic tool to confirm a diagnosis of insomnia disorder, in part because this is a subjective disorder and in part because the aspects of sleep that are most relevant to insomnia, such as SOL and WASO, are often different in an artificial lab than at home. PSG is, however, used clinically for ruling out other sleep disorders (see Chapter 4); in research, it is used, among other things, to study objective sleep in relation to patients' subjective experience.

Research examining brain waves during sleep reveals that sleep is an active process that can be divided into two distinct *states*: rapid-eye-movement (REM) sleep and non-rapid-eye-movement (NREM) sleep. "Typical" young, healthy adults spend most (75–80%) of their sleep period in NREM. NREM sleep consists of several *stages*, defined by special brain–body activity patterns.

## NREM Sleep

Normal sleep begins with NREM sleep. The three stages of NREM sleep stages are labeled N1, N2, and N3. Prior to the publication of scoring guidelines by the American Academy of Sleep Medicine (Iber, Ancoli-Israel, Chesson, & Quan, 2007), NREM sleep was divided into four stages labeled stages 1–4. In the new scoring guidelines, stages 3 and 4 were merged into what is now labeled as stage N3. The brain wave form of stage N1 is characterized by a mix of brain activities with high frequencies, in the range characteristic of wakefulness, and slower frequencies, which occupy at least 50% of a 30-second time segment. (PSG data are scored in 30-second segments.) People's perceptions of the depth of the three NREM sleep stages also differ. Stage N1 is experienced as very light. It is easy to wake a sleeper from stage N1 sleep; when awakened from N1 sleep, many individuals do not think they have been asleep. Nonetheless, stage N1 is an essential part of normal sleep and serves as a "path" or "bridge" from wakefulness to deeper sleep, at the beginning or middle of the night. In young adults with no sleep problems, stage N1 occupies about 5% of total sleep time. Educating patients about the nature of stage N1 helps in discussing the possibility that the extended period of wakefulness they are describing may include some sleep. Patients who report no significant daytime impact of poor sleep on their daytime well-being, but are nonetheless worried about negative effects of sleep loss, are often relieved to learn they may be sleeping more than they think. Patients with sleep state misperception (see Chapter 1) may be willing to consider a suggestion that they are in fact sleeping more than they think when they learn that stage N1 is shallow sleep and that 50% of people awakened from it will, like them, not think they were asleep.

NREM stage N2 occupies about 40–55% of the total time a young adult with no sleep problems sleeps. Stage N2 is deeper than stage N1; it is harder to wake a person from this stage than from stage N1, and if awakened after spending several minutes in stage N2, most people report that they have been asleep. Stage N2 is characterized by two specific brain wave forms, sleep spindles and K-complexes; the significance of these brain wave forms remains beyond the scope of this book (for further reading, see De Gennaro & Ferrara, 2003).

NREM sleep stage N3 occupies about 10–20% of a night's sleep for young healthy adults. The percentage of time spent in stage N3 gradually declines with age. The brain activity during this stage is characterized by slow, distinctive waves called *delta waves*, which is why stage N3 is also called *slow-wave sleep* or *delta sleep*. Slow-wave sleep (stage N3) is perceived as the deepest sleep, in that it takes more stimulation to wake a person from this type of sleep than it does from any other sleep stage. Stage N3 is also viewed as the stage of sleep most sensitive to prior wakefulness; people tend to have increased stage N3 sleep on nights following prolonged wakefulness.

Moreover, slow-wave sleep is highest during the first third of the night and declines across the night as sleep depth decreases.

## REM Sleep

The brain wave form of REM sleep is similar to that of stage N1, with the exception of the occasional presence of patterns that resemble "saw teeth." To some degree, the brain wave form of REM sleep is also similar to quiet wakefulness. In most other aspects, REM sleep is different from state N1 and other NREM sleep stages. A salient feature of REM sleep is the occurrence of bursts of rapid eye movements, for which this sleep state is named. These eye movements are usually associated with dreaming. Most dreams occur during REM sleep in association with eye movements. Another salient feature of REM sleep is the relative paralysis (*atonia*) of the body's skeletal muscles, which prevents an individual from "acting out" dreams. REM sleep has been also referred to as *paradoxical sleep*—both because the brain wave form during REM sleep is a bit similar to quiet wakefulness, and because many of the body systems operate at a level that is more similar to wakefulness than to NREM sleep. Heart and breathing rates become less regular, and there is increased blood flow to the brain. REM sleep deprivation creates so-called "REM pressure," which means that in subsequent sleep, REM sleep may occur earlier and be longer. Education about REM and REM pressure may help patients with nightmares realize that postponing bedtime is not an effective strategy for averting nightmares. In fact, the reverse is true: Sleep deprivation increases REM pressure, which means that more REM sleep will occur when a patient is finally asleep—thus increasing the likelihood of dreams, including nightmares.

## The Organization of Sleep across the Night

When good sleepers go to sleep at night, they usually experience a period of relaxed wakefulness. The length of this period of relaxed wakefulness varies from one person to the next, but it is typically less than 30 minutes. During a typical night of sleep, NREM and REM sleep states and stages occur in consistent and predictable cycles, each beginning with NREM sleep (usually stage N1) and ending with REM sleep. A schematic illustration of the sleep cycles can be found in Figure 2.1. The first cycle lasts an average of 70 minutes, and the first REM period is relatively short. Subsequent sleep cycles last an average of 90 minutes. As can be seen in Figure 2.1, deep sleep (N3) occurs mostly early in the sleep period, and most REM sleep occurs in the second half of the sleep period.

A close look at Figure 2.1 shows that some wakefulness is a normal part of the night's sleep even in good sleepers. These awakenings become more frequent closer to an individual's morning wake-up time. A few brief awakenings are normal and need not be a cause for concern. Figure 2.1 also shows other interesting trends. First, most deep sleep (stage N3) occurs during the first half of the night. The second half of the night is composed of somewhat lighter sleep. This explains why most people are more easily awakened in the later part of the nocturnal sleep period. This also means that even when patients sleep poorly, they are unlikely to be totally deprived of the deepest, most restorative stage of sleep. Second, REM periods become longer toward the morning rising time. This is why people are more likely to awake from a dream during the second half of the night, which also applies to nightmares.

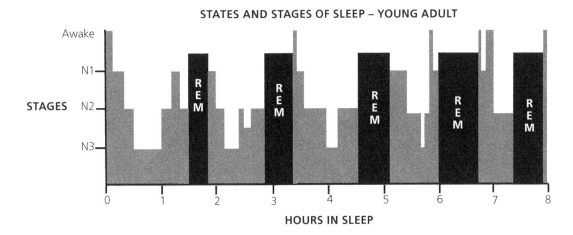

**FIGURE 2.1.** Distribution of sleep states and stages across the night in a healthy young adult.

## Sleep in Older Adults

The literature on sleep on older adults lacks a consensus definition of a cutoff age, with cutoffs usually ranging between 55 and 65 years. Regardless of the exact cutoff used, older adults seem to report more frequent awakenings, and to spend more time in light (N1) sleep and less time in deep (N3) sleep (Ohayon, Carskadon, Guilleminault, & Vitiello, 2004). Older adults also tend to go to bed and wake up earlier than younger adults (Buysse et al., 1992). Reasons for the observed lightening of sleep and shift to an earlier sleep schedule include behaviors and psychological factors associated with role transition, increased medical and psychiatric illness, and alterations in sleep regulatory processes (Buysse, Monk, Carrier, & Begley, 2005; Duffy, Dijk, Klerman, & Czeisler, 1998). Although the percentages of time spent in the different sleep stages are affected by aging, the relative distribution of sleep stages remains unaffected; that is, the relative order of sleep stages and states within a sleep cycle and across the night is the same in the young and old.

## THE FUNCTION OF SLEEP

There is no unified theory about the function of sleep. The current consensus is that sleep probably has more than one function; possible functions include energy conservation, nervous system recuperation (including memory consolidation), brain plasticity, and emotional regulation (Siegel, 2005). An evolution-based theory suggests that sleep confers benefits for survival by reducing risk of detection by predators, injury, and consumption of resources, but opponents argue that the same benefits could have been derived simply from inactivity (Siegel, 2009).

We know that sleep is needed, because when people do not get an adequate amount of sleep, they suffer negative consequences during the day (e.g., reduced alertness, compromised immune function) and also sleep longer than usual the following night (sleep rebound). People often ask, "How much sleep do I need?" From the current state of the science, the answer is not clear. Moreover, the construct of *sleep need* does not have an agreed-upon definition, in part because there is no clear understanding of the function(s) of sleep. If we all agreed about the function or functions of sleep, we would define sleep need as the amount of sleep needed to fulfill these functions. Broadly speaking, our position in this book is that how much sleep each person needs is defined subjectively by the minimum amount of sleep that does not produce impairment in functioning the next day. In other words, we generally consider sleep to be adequate when there is no daytime sleepiness or dysfunction the next day. There is an accumulation of data suggesting that large individual differences exist in the amount of sleep needed for optimal alertness and functioning, and that these differences have a genetic basis. We return to this definition of sleep need in Chapter 7.

## THE REGULATION OF SLEEP

In this section, we discuss the *two-process model of sleep* (Borbely, 1982). The two-process model describes the regulation of normal sleep as a balance between two processes, *Process S* (sleep drive) and *Process C* (the circadian clock). We first describe the two processes, pointing to scientific findings about each one and highlighting their clinical relevance. We then describe how Process S and Process C interact to determine when and how much people sleep. The discussion of sleep regulation we provide in this section lays the ground for the discussion of case formulation in Chapter 10, where we provide more examples of how to tailor sleep education to patients' presentations, as well as sample scripts.

### The Homeostatic Sleep Process (Process S)

Process S represents *sleep drive* or *pressure to sleep*, and as such it is an index of a biological need for sleep at a given moment. The sleep drive is lowest in the morning when people wake up; it gradually increases as the day progresses, and diminishes during sleep, as energy reserves are recharged. The more time that passes after an individual wakes up for the day, the greater the sleep debt, and hence the greater the sleep drive. In addition to the length of time awake since the last sleep episode, the intensity of Process S depends on the duration of previous sleep (Webb & Agnew, 1971). In other words, Process S is more intense or stronger when a person is more sleep-deprived.

The physiological marker of Process S is the amount of slow-wave brain activity during NREM sleep. Early research on sleep revealed that sleep deprivation leads to more slow-wave brain activity. The longer a person is awake, the greater the amount of slow-wave brain activity in the sleep period that follows (Borbely, Baumann, Brandeis, Strauch, & Lehmann, 1981; Webb & Agnew, 1971). Recall that in adults, stage N3, which is characterized by slow-wave brain activity, predominates during the first third of the night. Later in the night there is less Stage N3 and less slow-wave brain activity, because sleeping reduces the sleep drive, and slow-wave brain activity is a physiological marker of the sleep drive. For the same reason, persons who nap in the evening have less slow-wave brain activity during their subsequent sleep (Werth, Achermann, & Borbely, 1996)—and, by definition, a weaker sleep drive when they go to bed for the night. Consistent with the idea that prior wakefulness increases the intensity of the sleep drive is the finding that naps taken early in the day contain less slow-wave sleep than naps taken later in the day, after more time has been spent awake and the sleep drive has become stronger (Knowles, MacLean, Salem, Vetere, & Coulter, 1986). In sum, both the sleep drive and the amount of slow-wave brain activity increase under conditions of sleep deprivation and decrease after sleep. Because sleep is perceived as deeper when more slow-wave brain activity is present, we can also say that a stronger, more intense sleep drive leads to deeper, more intense sleep.

The exact mechanism by which sleep deprivation leads to increased slow-wave sleep during a subsequent sleep episode is not known. It is likely that several neurotransmitters and neuropeptides are involved. Among these neuropeptides, adenosine (a byproduct of energy expenditure in cells) has received much attention as a sleep-inducing factor. It is an inhibitory neurotransmitter, believed to play a role in promoting sleep and suppressing arousal. Levels of adenosine increase with each hour of wakefulness. (For additional reading about adenosine, see Basheer, Strecker, Thakkar, & McCarley, 2004.)

## What Behaviors Weaken the Sleep Drive?

Process S is an automatic process that operates in the background, governed by the normal accumulation of sleep debt as the day goes on. A person needs to do little to promote it except to avoid interfering with it. Most people with insomnia do not obtain sufficient sleep, and therefore one would expect that they would have a strong sleep drive when they go to bed. However, some people may engage in behaviors that weaken their sleep drive and/or interfere with the natural buildup of the sleep drive. These behaviors include extending sleep (by napping or sleeping longer than usual on a given night) and consuming caffeine (because caffeine interferes with adenosine buildup).

### THE IMPACT OF NAPS AND LONG SLEEP ON PROCESS S

As stated earlier, the sleep drive is more intense (or stronger) after a person has been awake longer and decreases after a person sleeps. Because naps involve sleep, additional time awake after the nap is required in order to build up the sleep drive to be strong enough to support sleep. Naps taken early in the day are therefore less detrimental to subsequent sleep, simply because there is more time for the sleep drive to increase sufficiently and promote sleep at night. Indeed, using slow-wave brain activity as a physiological marker of the sleep drive, research shows that naps in the late afternoon or early evening lead to weaker sleep drive at bedtime, or, equivalently, a reduction of slow-wave activity in the subsequent nocturnal sleep (Werth et al., 1996). Short naps lead to smaller decrements in the sleep drive and are also less detrimental to subsequent sleep at night. However, a short evening nap—even just dozing while watching TV in the evening—can be detrimental to nocturnal sleep. This is because, even though dozing only decreases the sleep drive slightly, the remaining period of wakefulness may be too short for the sleep drive to increase again to a level needed for supporting sleep. In some ways, sleep drive is similar to hunger: Napping or dozing close to bedtime is like snacking before supper.

Sleeping longer than usual, particularly oversleeping in the morning, may also diminish sleep drive. This is because sleep drive is lower upon waking from an extended sleep episode than it is following a shorter sleep episode; when sleep extension is associated with a later than habitual rise time, less time is available for building up the sleep drive before the next habitual bedtime. In Chapter 7, we discuss behavioral components of CBT-I that strengthen the sleep drive and harness it to aid sleep.

THE IMPACT OF CAFFEINE CONSUMPTION ON PROCESS S

Most people know that caffeine interferes with sleep. Fewer know why. Briefly, caffeine is an adenosine antagonist—and, as noted above, adenosine promotes sleep and suppresses arousal. Adenosine is most strongly related to the amount of slow-wave brain activity, and hence to the sleep drive. By suppressing adenosine, caffeine consumption reduces the sleep drive and its physiological correlate, slow-wave brain activity in the subsequent sleep episode, in a manner that depends on how much and when it is consumed relative to when sleep is initiated (Landolt et al., 2004). The amount of caffeine and the timing of consumption relative to bedtime are relevant because both have an impact on the time needed (or remaining) for rebuilding the sleep drive to a level that supports sleep. In Chapter 8, we discuss additional facts about caffeine and make recommendations about how much and when caffeine can be consumed to minimize its negative impact on the sleep drive.

## The Circadian Process (Process C)

The circadian process (Process C) is governed by a biological clock, to which we refer here as the *circadian clock* and sometimes the *circadian rhythm*. This clock is a cyclic process whose rhythm is internally determined but is reset regularly by daylight, wakefulness, and other activities. The word *circadian* has its roots in two Latin words: *circa*, which means "around," and *dies*, which means "a day"; the combination is apt, because the clock cycle lasts about 24 hours. The prevailing theory about how the clock, which in biology is called an *oscillator*, contributes to the regulation of sleep is as follows: The clock generates alerting signals of varying magnitude across the 24-hour day. These alerting signals keep an individual awake throughout the day. They increase in magnitude as the day progresses and start diminishing a few hours after darkness, only to start increasing again 1–3 hours before the person naturally wakes up. This is depicted in Figure 2.2.

One physiological marker used in the study of the sleep–wake circadian clock is the rhythmic change in core body temperature across the 24-hour day. The biological study of Process C involves monitoring the core body temperature under well-controlled laboratory conditions, using an indwelling rectal thermometer. Findings from studies using such methodology show that approximately 1–3 hours before wakening, core body temperature starts rising from a nighttime low of approximately 36.5°C, keeps rising slowly during the day to a peak of 37.4°C in the evening, and then slowly falls during the night back to its lowest level of 36.5°C. Research has shown that the rise and fall in temperature parallel the rise and fall of the alerting signal from the clock, so that higher core body temperature corresponds to a higher alerting signal, and lower core body temperature corresponds to a lower alerting signal. People sleep best when they go to bed shortly after their core body temperatures start decreasing, which is also when the alerting signals from their biological clocks start declining; they naturally wake up about 1–3 hours after their core body temperatures reach minimum, a point at which the alerting signals from their biological clocks start increasing. The hypothetical person depicted in Figure 2.2 goes to sleep at 11:00 P.M., approximately 2 hours after the alerting signal begins to decline from its peak value, and gets up 3 hours after the alerting signal begins to rise from its lowest point. (Because the alerting signal is closely correlated with core body temperature, we could have labeled the vertical axis "core body temperature," but we have chosen to highlight the functional outcome of the circadian clock and avoid complicating the figure with technical methodological data.)

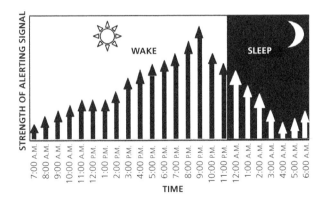

**FIGURE 2.2.** Alerting signals from the clock across the 24-hour cycle. The dark shaded section of the figure is the period of sleep, and the white section is the period of wakefulness. The time stamping on the horizontal axis is somewhat arbitrary. The general pattern also applies to people with different sleep–wake habits (e.g., those who regularly sleep between 2:00 A.M. and 9:00 A.M.), but the labels on the horizontal axis will be different (e.g., starting at 10:00 A.M., with the dark period beginning at 2:00 A.M.).

The propensity for sleep at any given moment is governed by the balance between the magnitude of the pressure for sleep (Process S) and the magnitude of the alerting signal generated by the circadian clock (Process C).

### The Circadian Clock and Behavior

Here we discuss two issues related to the circadian sleep–wake rhythm that can contribute to sleep difficulty. The first issue results from attempting to sleep at a time that is not compatible with the internal circadian clock (i.e., a person's internal clock and the earth's clock are misaligned). The second issue arises when the alerting signals from the circadian clock are not robust. We discuss each of these two issues below.

#### WHEN THE INTERNAL CLOCK AND THE EARTH'S CLOCK ARE MISALIGNED

People sleep according to their own circadian rhythms. Most people have circadian clocks that are well aligned with the societal (the earth's) clock, but some have earlier or later circadian clocks. Misalignment between a person's internal circadian clock and the earth's clock can create sleep disruptions in predictable ways. Someone with a late clock who tries to go to sleep at a conventional time may have difficulty falling asleep because at that time the person's internal circadian clock may be still sending strong alerting signals. Conversely, a person with an early clock may struggle to stay awake until a conventional bedtime, because the alerting signals from the internal circadian clock are weak and therefore cannot support wakefulness.

Knowing whether a person's circadian clock is running late, early, or in synchronization with the earth's clock involves complex laboratory procedures that are not feasible in most clinics, at least not at present. However, it is possible to determine people's chronotypes, which are well correlated with their physiological circadian clocks. *Chronotype* refers to a personal prefer-

## Scientific Facts about Circadian Rhythm

The field of circadian rhythm biology has made great strides in understanding the molecular and genetic bases of Process C. We highlight here a few clinically relevant findings from this rich field.

- Many aspects of human physiology and behavior have circadian rhythms (Czeisler & Khalsa, 2010). These include alertness, cognition, and endocrine function, among others (Dijk, Duffy, & Czeisler, 1992; Van Cauter & Turek, 1995).
- The circadian process (Process C) is, to a large extent, independent of sleep need (Process S). This is best shown when a person is placed in an environment without time cues (such as daylight, clocks, cell phones, computers, watches, and all other devices that indicate the time of day) and is kept awake for 36 hours. In this environment, the person continues to show a 24- to 25-hour temperature rhythm and sleep–wake pattern. Even when the sleep drive is strong, the person tends to sleep longer if he or she initiates sleep when the core body temperature is falling (after it reached its peak); the person's sleep is shortest if it is initiated 1–3 hours after the core body temperature starts rising.
- The circadian rhythm is a cyclic process that can be described by its *period* (time from minimum to minimum) and *amplitude* (half-distance from the maximum to the minimum).
- The average period of the clock is about 24.2 hours, with a range between 23.5 and 24.7 hours.
- The period of the circadian clock remains largely stable with age (Czeisler et al., 1999), though earlier studies proposed a shortening of the period of the circadian clock with older age.
- Light has a potent influence on the circadian clock. Depending on the time of exposure, light determines the timing of the minimum and maximum of the circadian rhythm (Chesson et al., 1999).
- Melatonin, a hormone secreted by the pineal gland, starts rising in the early evening and peaks around the time of the temperature minimum. It is suppressed by light. Melatonin is involved in the regulation of seasonal breeding in mammals by providing information about the length of the night (Arendt, 1998).
- Circadian rhythm sleep disorders (discussed in Chapter 4) occur as a result of abnormalities in Process C.

ence for when to sleep. Some people describe themselves as clearly being "morning persons" or "night persons." By this, they usually mean that they prefer to go to bed early and wake up early (if they are morning persons) or the opposite (if they are night people). Most people do not exhibit extremes of either tendency. An alternative term used by sleep and circadian researchers to describe these preferences is *morningness–eveningness*. We use these terms interchangeably in this book. It turns out that these sleep schedule preferences are related to the period of the circadian clock, as well as to the timing of the internal clock's minimum and maximum relative to the earth's clock. Both of these attributes are inherent and influenced by a set of clock genes (Duffy, Rimmer, & Czeisler, 2001). Below, we briefly describe the sleep of morning and evening people, because having one of these two chronotypes increases the likelihood of experiencing insomnia.

*Morning People (Morningness Chronotype).* People with a preference for earlier bedtimes and rise times than their peers describe themselves as "morning people." They tend to go to bed and wake up earlier than most people, and they may find it difficult to stay up late or to sleep late in the morning. Research shows that the minimum and maximum of a morning person's internal clock also occur earlier than average, and that this internal clock has a shorter period than average (Duffy et al., 2001); in other words, this circadian clock is advanced relative to the earth's clock. The core body temperature minimum of a morning person occurs near the middle rather than the end of his or her habitual sleep episode. As a result, when the person wakes up in the early morning hours, the alerting signals are already relatively high. This means that the person is feeling alert and likely to have a hard time extending sleep. When morning people reflect on their sleep during adolescence, they say that, compared to their peers, they were less able to sleep in on weekends and other school breaks. Their lifelong preference for earlier sleep schedules than those of others in their age group is consistent with having a genetic predisposition to morningness. It is not known whether there are sex differences in morningness. Patients with insomnia who have a morning chronotype rarely have difficulty failing asleep. They usually describe difficulties maintaining sleep, particularly in the second half of the night.

*Night People (Eveningness Chronotype).* People with a preference for later bedtimes and rise times than others describe themselves as "night people." They tend to go to bed later and wake up later, and they find it difficult to wake up in the morning (sometimes needing more than one alarm reminder). They also report that they take a while to feel fully alert after they wake up in the morning. Research shows that the minimum and maximum of an evening person's internal clock are also later than average, and that this internal clock has a longer period than average; that is, the clock is delayed relative to the earth's clock. The later than average core body temperature minimum of night people means that when most people are awake and getting ready for the day, the alerting signals from the internal clocks of night people have not yet started to rise. This makes it difficult for them to wake up at a conventional morning wake-up time, and they would much prefer to sleep in. When reflecting on their sleep during adolescence, they say they used to sleep in until late morning or early afternoon on weekends and other school breaks. Their lifelong preference for later sleep schedules than those of others in their age group is consistent with having a genetic predisposition to eveningness. Men are more likely than women to have night tendencies (Adan & Natale, 2002). Patients with insomnia who have an evening chronotype usually describe difficulty failing asleep and waking up, but may also have difficulties maintaining sleep, particularly in the first half of the night. Their sleep difficulties usually begin in adolescence or young adulthood with sleep initiation difficulties.

## WHEN THE ALERTING SIGNALS FROM THE CLOCK ARE UNSTABLE

The stability of the signals from the circadian clock is influenced by behavioral factors. An irregular wake-up time is particularly detrimental to the integrity of the circadian clock; the greater the irregularity, the more detrimental the effect. Extremely irregular sleep schedules, due to such things as jet lag and shift work, are associated with poor sleep in part because the sleep period is incongruent with the circadian clock, and in part because Process C is unstable, due to highly variable sleep schedule.

A regular wake time in the morning means regular exposure to light, which is a potent signal that helps stabilize the circadian clock and align it with the solar day. The implication is that irregular wake-up times should be avoided because such irregularity destabilizes the circadian sleep–wake clock (Process C) and therefore does not support optimal sleep. For example, more than 2 hours' difference between the sleep schedules on work (or school) nights and weekend nights, typically with later bedtimes and wake times on weekends, is a common form of sleep schedule irregularity. To understand the negative impact of this type of schedule irregularity, it may help to think about it as a social form of jet lag: Going to bed 2 hours later on weekends than on work days has the same effect on the body as traveling two time zones. The greater the variability in the sleep schedule, the greater its interference with the circadian clock. Later in the book, we discuss two behavioral components of CBT-I, stimulus control and sleep restriction, that help improve the robustness of Process C. That is, we recommend that the wake-up and out-of-bed times be kept the same every day, independent of the amount of sleep on the prior night.

## The Interaction between Process C and Process S

The interaction between Process C (the biological clock and generator of alerting signals) and Process S (the homeostatic sleep drive) affects the onset, duration, and quality of sleep. The propensity for sleep at any given moment is governed by the balance between the magnitude of the pressure for sleep (Process S) and the magnitude of the alerting signal generated by the circadian clock (Process C). When the sleep drive is strong and the alerting signal from the circadian clock is relatively lower, the balance is in favor of sleep. If sleep is initiated at this point, then sleep onset is likely to be short, and the ensuing sleep period is least likely to be interrupted and most likely to be of optimal duration. In contrast, when the sleep drive is weak (e.g., immediately after waking up from an evening nap) and the alerting signal from the circadian clock is relatively stronger, the balance is in favor of wakefulness. If sleep is initiated at this point, then it can be difficult to fall asleep; if sleep does occur, the ensuing sleep period is likely to be interrupted and/or short.

Under normal conditions, the ideal time to initiate sleep is when the sleep drive is high and the opposing alerting signal from the circadian clock is decreasing. Then during the rest of the night, sleep gradually replenishes energy reserves and reduces the drive for sleep (Process S); in parallel, the alerting signals generated by the circadian process (Process C) also progressively decrease, although the balance remains in favor of sleep. The net effect is that sleep is maintained at night. Then about 1–3 hours after the alerting signal reaches its lowest point, the balance tips toward wakefulness. During the day, the alerting signal from the circadian clock (Process C) and the sleep drive (Process S) gradually increase, but the balance stays in favor of the alerting signal until a little after the signal from the circadian clock starts increasing again (Dijk & Edgar, 1999). At that point, the balance flips back in favor of wakefulness, and a new cycle begins. In this roughly 24-hour dynamic process, the sleep drive (Process S) increases during the day and the alerting signal from the circadian clock (Process C) opposes it, so that wakefulness is maintained during the daytime (Mistlberger, 2005).

# EXPLAINING SLEEP REGULATION TO PATIENTS

Education about sleep regulation is integral to CBT-I and lays the ground for explaining the rationale for certain behavioral recommendations that are discussed in Chapters 7 and 8. Our flexible and individualized treatment protocol is different from the approach taken in clinical trials, in which education is standardized and scripted, so that all participants receive the same information. Examples of patient-friendly scripts for Sophie and Sam (who have been introduced in Chapter 1) can be found in Chapters 11 and 12, respectively. These two examples demonstrate how information about sleep regulation can be explained in simple language without too much scientific jargon. In each of these examples, the patient's therapist focused mainly on the relevant components of the case. For example, in Sophie's case, her therapist focused on explaining sleep drive and asked her to identify which of her behaviors might be diffusing the sleep drive. Her most detrimental behavior turned out to be spending an excessive amount of time in bed at night and during the day. The therapist did not spend time explaining the circadian clock to Sophie because it was less relevant to her case. In contrast, because Sam had an eveningness tendency, his therapist originally planned to spend time explaining the circadian clock and the negative impact of its misalignment with the earth's clock (although this plan was later discarded for other reasons).

A therapist needs to tailor the explanation to each specific patient by focusing on the aspects of sleep regulation that are most relevant to this patient, and the patient should be encouraged to be actively involved in the discussion. Because much of the information is likely to be new to most patients, the therapist will usually be talking more than the patient. Nonetheless, the therapist should pause periodically and ask how certain facts are relevant to the patient and how certain of the patient's behaviors might affect the two sleep processes. The therapist can also encourage the patient to ask clarifying questions and identify personal behaviors that may have positive and negative impacts on the sleep drive and the clock. An engaging educational process helps the patient internalize the information, allows the therapist to assess the patient's comprehension of concepts, and enhances the therapeutic relationship.

## KEY PRACTICE IDEAS

- The rationale for treatment recommendations is most effective when patient-relevant facts about sleep regulation are highlighted.

- The propensity for sleep is determined by the balance between the amount of built-up pressure for sleep (Process S) and the strength of the alerting signal generated by the circadian process (C). Conditions are optimal for sleep when the sleep pressure is high and the alerting signal is low.

- Behaviors that can have a negative impact on the circadian clock (Process C) include these:
  - Getting up at irregular times. This behavior causes the signal from the internal clock to become less robust.
  - Trying to sleep at a time that does not match the patient's chronotype; this usually also means trying to sleep at the wrong time relative to the internal clock.

- Behaviors that may weaken the homeostatic sleep system (Process S) at bedtime include these:

  - Going to bed earlier than usual, sleeping in, dozing, and napping. These behaviors shorten the time available to build sufficiently high sleep drive at bedtime.
  - Spending extended time in bed. Brief sleep episodes may be present during periods that are perceived as wakefulness. As a result, total time asleep may be longer than the individual estimates. Therefore, the sleep drive may be lower than what would be expected from the reported total sleep duration.
  - Caffeine consumption may affect sleep in a manner that depends on the dose and time of day. Caffeine reduces the homeostatic drive for sleep by binding to the adenosine receptors, thus reducing the levels of sleep-inducing adenosine.

- Patients with insomnia who have a morning chronotype rarely have difficulty falling asleep. They usually describe difficulties maintaining sleep, particularly in the second half of the night.

- Patients with insomnia who have an evening chronotype usually describe difficulty falling asleep and waking up, but may also have difficulties maintaining sleep, particularly in the first half of the night.

# CHAPTER 3

# Behavioral Regulation of Sleep

## *The Role of Arousal*

In Chapter 2, we have explained the two-process model of sleep: the sleep drive (Process S), which is directly related to the amount of prior sleep and the time since a person last slept; and the circadian clock (Process C), which opposes the sleep drive during the day and permits sleep at night. We have described these two physiological processes and their interaction, and have highlighted behaviors that affect them. In this chapter, we focus on a third process: arousal. Sleep naturally unfolds when the two processes optimally align (i.e., when it is initiated at a time that is congruent with the endogenous clock and a time when the sleep drive is strong), and when, in addition, the arousal (physical, emotional, and cognitive) associated with normal waking activities is sufficiently reduced. Arousal down-regulation is considered a third sleep regulatory process that is ancillary to the two-process model (Sewitch, 1987). Arousal down-regulation involves both physiological deactivation (e.g., decrease in muscle tone, a slowing of the heart and respiration rates, and reduction in blood pressure) and emotional and cognitive deactivation (e.g., decreasing goal-oriented processes, such as planning, problem solving, worry, and rumination). Espie (2002) argues that these deactivation processes are automatic and that the loss of automaticity is involved in the pathological state of insomnia—an idea we return to and elaborate later in this chapter. In general, people find it very difficult to sleep when they are in a state of high autonomic arousal (e.g., when feeling afraid or upset). This is evolutionarily adaptive. There is a survival advantage to being able to postpone sleep when the environment presents danger, even when the sleep drive is strong and the biological clock time is optimal for sleep. The arousal system is activated in reaction to perceived danger and does not permit sleep, so that the individual can stay alert and deal with the perceived danger.

Insomnia is associated with an overactive arousal process, which we refer to as *hyperarousal*. In this chapter, we review evidence for physiological arousal in insomnia and discuss the role of psychological and learned (conditioned) hyperarousal. We conclude with a discussion of theories about factors contributing to the development and maintenance of insomnia, with particular attention to cognitive and metacognitive factors. In Chapters 7 and 8, we discuss components of CBT-I that reduce different aspects and manifestations of hyperarousal.

# PHYSIOLOGICAL AROUSAL
# IN INSOMNIA

There is a convergence of evidence that individuals with insomnia have a more active sympathetic nervous system than healthy controls. Specifically, people with insomnia have greater sympathetic hyperactivity than controls, as evidenced by consistent findings of greater low-/high-frequency spectral power of heart rate (Bonnet & Arand, 1998; Lushington, Dawson, & Lack, 2000) and higher basal metabolic rates (i.e., whole-body oxygen use) during the day and night (Bonnet & Arand, 1995). Some, but not all, studies report increased levels of circulating catecholamines (Vgontzas et al., 1998) and nocturnal core body temperature (Lushington et al., 2000). There is also evidence for high cortical activation in insomnia. Specifically, individuals with insomnia have greater activation in brain regions involved in the regulation of sleep (Nofzinger et al., 2004), and their sleep electroencephalographic (EEG) patterns include more activity in frequency bands characteristic of wakefulness (Freedman & Sattler, 1982; Perlis, Merica, Smith, & Giles, 2001).

In a series of studies, Bonnet and Arand (1997) used the multiple sleep latency test (MSLT) to study arousal in insomnia disorder. MSLTs are conducted in a sleep laboratory. After a night's sleep, participants are provided five 20-minute opportunities to sleep during the day, while their brain activity is monitored with polysomnography (PSG). For each of the five nap opportunities, the experimenters use the PSG data to determine the time it takes to fall asleep, setting this value at 20 minutes if the participant did not fall asleep at all. The MSLT score is then computed as the average time to fall asleep across all five nap opportunities. Among good sleepers, sleep deprivation leads to low MSLT scores (i.e., on average, they fall asleep quickly across the naps), and the scores are significantly correlated with self-reported levels of sleepiness, fatigue, and vigor in the expected direction. In contrast, people with insomnia disorder, as well as healthy sleepers who ingest high doses of caffeine (400 mg three times a day for 7 days), have high MSLT scores despite the fact that they have not slept well at night and are therefore sleep-deprived (Bonnet & Arand, 1992, 1995). In both experiments, the investigators additionally found evidence for physiological hyperarousal (indexed by the resting metabolic rate) across the day and night. The difference is that in the case of caffeine the source of sleep-interfering hyperarousal is external, and in the case of insomnia disorder it is internal. The two studies have been interpreted as evidence that hyperactivity in the arousal system is causally linked to disrupted sleep in insomnia disorder (Bonnet & Arand, 1997). Concerned about causal inference from findings of association, these same investigators conducted a third study to examine the possibility that the high arousal evident in insomnia disorder is not simply the direct result of poor sleep. In this study they compared a group of individuals with insomnia disorder to a group of healthy sleepers whose sleep was manipulated in the laboratory to mirror the sleep disruption experienced by people with insomnia disorder. In this study, in which sleep disruptions were simulated without caffeine, the MSLT scores of the experimental group were lower than the scores of the insomnia group (Bonnet & Arand, 1996). The results from Bonnet and Arand's studies are consistent with the idea that high levels of physiological arousal are present in insomnia disorder and interfere with sleep at night as well as with the ability to take naps even after a night of poor sleep.

# PSYCHOLOGICAL AROUSAL
# IN INSOMNIA

Sleep is a naturally unfolding process, and it emerges effortlessly when the sleep drive is strong, the timing is congruent with one's circadian clock, and the mind is quiescent. When sleep is normal, the down-regulation of arousal is automatic and effortless (Espie, 2002). Individuals who sleep well do not *try* to sleep. They simply go to sleep. In contrast, people with insomnia often try to sleep, thus disrupting the automatic nature (or automaticity) of sleep. They try to "not think" (e.g., counting sheep) or to "think positive"; adopt rigid rules about sleep (e.g., no socializing past 8:00 P.M.); and engage in avoidance and safety behaviors (e.g., reducing/eliminating early morning obligations in order to increase sleep opportunity). Some people even start planning their lives around their sleep, avoiding previously enjoyed evening activities, canceling planned daytime activities, sleeping in a separate bed from a bed partner, and avoiding traveling because of concerns over poor sleep due to jet lag and/or sleeping in a new environment. These thoughts and behaviors are manifestations of putting effort into sleeping, and are referred to as *sleep effort*. The cases introduced in Chapter 1 included multiple indicators of sleep effort. In response to her sleep problem, Sophie began spending an average of 12 hours per night in bed, as well as attempting to nap, to try to produce more sleep. Sophie also reported decreased socialization out of fear that it would interfere with sleep. Sam had used sleep medications for almost two decades and spent excessive amounts of time in bed in a 24-hour period attempting to produce sleep. Additionally, even though Sam described himself as a bit of a "night owl" by nature, he went to bed hours before he could realistically fall asleep. Thus both Sophie and Sam believed they must exert effort to sleep, and this contributed to their hyperarousal. We discuss these cases in detail in Chapters 11 and 12, respectively.

Ironically, putting more effort into sleeping increases cognitive and emotional arousal during the time allotted for sleep, and hence is counterproductive. Indeed, asking good sleepers to try to fall asleep as fast as possible prolongs their latency to sleep onset (Ansfield, Wegner, & Bowser, 1996). Putting effort into sleeping is similar to trying to remove a Chinese finger cuff: The harder one tries to pull one's fingers out of the cuff (or to sleep), the more stuck the fingers become (the longer it takes to fall asleep). The solution is to let go of the effort and ease the fingers out. One way of letting go of sleep effort is engaging in a competing task. Engaging in mental exercises that distract attention from intrusive thoughts and sleep effort, such as repeatedly saying the word *the*, hasten sleep onset (Levey, Aldaz, Watts, & Coyle, 1991). Similarly, Haynes, Adams, and Franzen (1981) compared time to fall asleep among individuals with and without insomnia disorder on baseline nights and on nights when they were instructed to engage in moderately difficult arithmetic tasks before sleep. They found that whereas engagement in mental arithmetic increased sleep onset latency for participants without insomnia disorder, the opposite was the case for participants with insomnia disorder. For the participants with insomnia disorder, the task led to a decrease in sleep onset latency, presumably because it shifted attention away from sleep effort and/or from worries about catastrophic consequences of insufficient sleep. These studies support the utility of "counting sheep," a commonly used strategy for facilitating sleep onset that has become a universal graphic symbol of insomnia. To a large extent, CBT-I helps individuals abandon efforts to control sleep and return to reliance upon the involuntary sleep process (Espie, Broomfield, MacMahon, Macphee, & Taylor, 2006).

## Cognitive Arousal

Multiple lines of research suggest that insomnia disorder is associated with high cognitive arousal. Most individuals with insomnia disorder believe that cognitive factors alone (55%) or in combination with physiological factors (35%) contribute to their difficulties in sleeping (Lichstein & Rosenthal, 1980). People with insomnia report higher levels of presleep cognitive activity than controls do (Nicassio, Mendlowitz, Fussell, & Petras, 1985), and their thoughts tend to be associated with more negative emotional valence, both before sleep (Kuisk, Bertelson, & Walsh, 1989; Nicassio et al., 1985) and after being awakened 5 minutes into their first stage 2 sleep (Borkovec, Lane, & VanOot, 1981). Studies of people's presleep cognitions find that affect-laden cognitions are more likely to interfere with sleep than emotionally neutral thoughts are (Haynes et al., 1981; Kuisk et al., 1989; Van Egeren, Haynes, Franzen, & Hamilton, 1983). In contrast, people without insomnia disorder most frequently report thinking about "nothing in particular" (Harvey, 2000). In a content analysis of voice-activated audio recordings of spontaneous thoughts before sleep onset, general problem solving and thinking about sleep or the anticipated negative consequences of poor sleep were the strongest predictors of objectively determined time to sleep onset (Wicklow & Espie, 2000), probably because such thoughts tend to be associated with emotions of negative valence and high arousal.

When thoughts are characterized by worries about general life problems, individuals tend to describe their emotional state as anxious, and they often engage in behaviors aimed at reducing their anxiety, such as efforts to "not think" about the problem or to think about something else. Lundh and Broman (2000) refer to presleep worries and intrusive thoughts about life problems and events as *sleep-interfering thoughts*, and argue that the resulting negative emotional states and associated hyperarousal directly interfere with sleep. An inability to unwind from the day's activities and to disengage from the day's worries may increase the likelihood of experiencing sleep-interfering thoughts.

When the focus of thoughts is on sleep (e.g., thoughts about loss of control over sleep and the potential negative consequences of insufficient sleep), individuals tend to describe feeling "wired," and they engage in behaviors aimed at hastening sleep; in other words, they increase their sleep effort. Lundh and Broman (2000) refer to this class of thoughts as *maladaptive sleep-interpreting thoughts*. Such thoughts stem from unhelpful expectations and attributions concerning sleep, such as beliefs in catastrophic consequences of poor or insufficient sleep. These scholars argue that sleep-interpreting beliefs and attributions interfere with sleep indirectly.

Morin, Stone, Trinkle, Mercer, and Remsberg (1993) studied unhelpful expectations, beliefs, and attributions and found that compared to controls, people with insomnia (1) endorsed stronger beliefs about the negative consequences of insomnia (e.g., "When I do not sleep well, I make mistakes at work the next day," and "When I feel irritable, depressed, or anxious during the day, it is mostly because I did not sleep well the night before"); (2) expressed greater fear of losing control of their sleep ("I am worried that I may lose control over my ability to sleep"); and (3) reported greater feelings of helplessness about sleep and its unpredictability (e.g., "I have little ability to manage the negative consequences of disturbed sleep," and "I can't ever predict whether I'll have a good night's sleep"). These cognitions are examples of unhelpful beliefs and attitudes about sleep and functioning. Such unhelpful beliefs contribute to distress about poor or insufficient sleep, daytime preoccupation and nighttime rumination about sleep and increased effort to sleep. Some individuals with insomnia have unrealistic expectations about sleep. For example, Sophie's stated goal was to "fall asleep when my head hits the pillow and never [wake] up until the morning." However, normal sleep involves some brief awakenings and up to 30 minutes to fall asleep, so Sophie's sleep goal was probably unrealistic. Based on her sleep expectations, she would probably have been dissatisfied with her sleep even if she had normative sleep values. Her sleep expectations might have been particularly unrealistic, given that she was in her 40s.

Several scholars have described pathways by which beliefs about sleep interact in a reciprocal manner with presleep arousal and sleep difficulties. For example, Lundh (2005) describes a "vicious cycle of sleeplessness" in which detecting difficulties in falling asleep leads to thoughts about the negative consequences of insufficient sleep, which in turn increase negative emotional arousal; this increased arousal then interferes further with sleep, and subsequently reaffirms and strengthens negative beliefs about one's self-efficacy with regard to sleep. Carney, Harris, Falco, and Edinger (2013) describe how beliefs about negative consequences about poor sleep affect the interpretation of daytime experiences. They argue that when people with insomnia who hold such beliefs experience fatigue or concentration problems during the day, they tend to conclude that such problems are due to poor or insufficient sleep, and that in order to be less fatigued they need more sleep. Their sleep-related performance anxiety increases, and as a result, they approach sleep with apprehension and are likely to ruminate about anticipated, imagined, or real negative consequences of poor sleep. This apprehensive stance and active rumination lead to heightened arousal that directly interferes with sleep. These ideas are depicted in Figure 3.1.

Harvey (2002) has proposed a cognitive model of insomnia that explains how attention biases contribute to this vicious cycle. She argues that people with insomnia demonstrate attention bias toward sleep-related threat cues, such as deficits in their daytime performance. As they

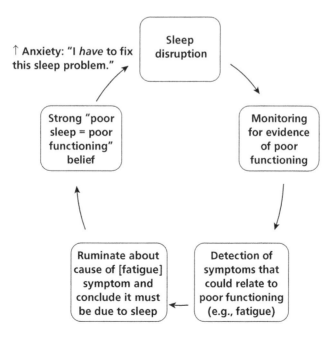

**FIGURE 3.1.** The relationship among beliefs about functioning, sleep loss, monitoring for daytime symptoms, and perception of/attribution for symptoms, and how this increases anxiety.

pay closer attention and monitor carefully for performance deficits, they are more likely to detect them and tend to attribute their cause to poor or insufficient sleep, even when the cause of the observed deficit may be unrelated to the quality or quantity of their sleep the previous night. This misattribution then intensifies their beliefs about catastrophic outcomes of poor sleep, and this increases their worry about not sleeping. Harvey (2002) extends this idea to explain how attention and monitoring for other sleep-related threats, such as bodily sensations, passage of time (clock watching), and environmental noises, contribute to the vicious cycle of insomnia; she also discusses counterproductive *safety behaviors* that people with insomnia tend to engage in when they detect threat cues.

*Safety behaviors* is a term psychologists use to refer to behaviors aimed at reducing and/or coping with fears. Calling in sick in order to avoid the feared consequence of poor performance following a night of poor sleep is an example of a safety behavior. Ironically, this safety behavior reduces the likelihood of experiencing a situation that could provide evidence to dispel the belief that poor sleep at night will inevitably lead to poor performance during the day. In this example, if, rather than calling in sick, the person goes to work despite the feared negative consequences, it is possible that high performance and a productive work day will ensue. By avoiding going to work, this person misses the opportunity to have such corrective experiences. As another example, consider a person who monitors mind sensations when in bed at night and notices a racing mind as a sign that "I am not going to get to sleep." In this case, the person might try to stop all thinking. Trying not to think is a safety behavior but not an effective strategy for falling asleep faster. Research shows that when individuals with insomnia are instructed to suppress thoughts they have previously identified as likely to preoccupy them when they go to bed at night, they take longer to fall asleep and sleep more poorly than individuals with insomnia who are not instructed to suppress their thoughts (Harvey & Greenall, 2003). This seemingly paradoxical effect is related to Wegner's famous "white bear" experiment, which concluded that attempts at suppression of thoughts tend to trigger a rebound in the occurrence of that thought (see, e.g., Becker, Rinck, Roth, & Margraf, 1998; Wegner, Schneider, Carter, & White, 1987). In Chapter 9, we discuss behavioral experiments that a therapist and a patient can design in order to test sleep-interfering beliefs and reduce the patient's engagement in safety behaviors.

*Metacognitive processes* may also play a role in insomnia (Lundh, 2005; Ong, Ulmer, & Manber, 2012). Metacognitive processes are distinct from the sleep-interfering and sleep-interpreting processes discussed above. This term refers to the ways people relate to their thoughts about sleep. One example of a metacognitive process is a strong attachment to a belief about sleep (i.e., difficulty in letting go of the belief), rather than to the content of the belief. Ong et al. (2012) argue that such metacognitive processes may contribute to the intensity and prolongation of insomnia, in part because they tend to amplify the negative emotional valence of sleep-related thoughts. For example, a rigid attachment to the belief "I need 8 hours of sleep to function well the next day" interferes with the ability to consider or accept alternative beliefs (such as "I can find other ways to cope if I get less than 8 hours"). In that way, the arousal that is directly triggered by thoughts stemming from a belief in needing 8 hours of sleep (e.g., thoughts about catastrophic consequences if one does not sleep for 8 hours) is amplified by the rigidity of attachment to this belief. Rigid beliefs may also have an impact on daytime behaviors. For example, a rigid belief that tiredness during the day is mostly due to insufficient sleep the night before may lead the believer to feel helpless and unable to cope.

In summary, sleep-related and non-sleep-related cognitive processes lead to emotional states that are incongruent with sleep. Worries about general life problems are sleep-interfering thoughts. They lead to anxious emotional states and behaviors aimed at trying not to think about the source of anxiety. Worries about sleep lead to states of high emotional arousal, which may or may not involve anxiety but nonetheless are incongruent with sleep, and to behaviors that reflect high sleep effort (trying harder to sleep). Table 3.1 summarizes this distinction. The discussion above also highlights the fact that daytime cognitive processes, such as attention biases to sleep-related threats, can also interfere with sleep and contribute to insomnia. In Chapter 9, we discuss cognitive therapy techniques that can be used to reduce cognitive hyperarousal.

## Conditioned Arousal

Richard Bootzin (1972) proposed that for people with insomnia, the bed is not a strong cue (stimulus) for sleep; instead, through repeated pairing of the bed with states of hyperarousal (e.g., frustration, fear, agitation, and anxiety), the bed and its surroundings (e.g., the bedroom) become cues for arousal (Bootzin, 1972; Bootzin & Epstein, 2000). In the language of learning theory, the bed has become a conditioned cue for arousal and wakefulness rather than for sleep. Whereas for good sleepers the bed is a cue for sleep, for people with insomnia the bed has become a cue for arousal, thus interfering with the automaticity of sleep. We refer to this process as *conditioned arousal*. Conditioned arousal is an example of hyperarousal that may be manifested even in the absence of clear signs of arousal-producing cognitions (although conditioned arousal and increased cognitive arousal may coexist and synergistically contribute to insomnia). As noted in Chapter 1, Sophie described the onset of her insomnia as following the breakup of a romantic relationship. She recalled that during the period after the breakup, she used to lie in bed at night upset about the breakup and "fighting with sleep." It is conceivable that in her

**TABLE 3.1. Cognitive Hyperarousal**

| Presleep thoughts | Emotional valence | Intensity of emotions | Associated responses |
|---|---|---|---|
| Worries about general life problems (sleep-interfering thoughts) | Anxious emotional states | Determined by metacognitive processes (e.g., personal meaning of thoughts in relation to personal value system) | Behaviors aimed at reducing anxiety (e.g., distraction from anxiety-producing thoughts, trying to "not think") |
| Worries about sleep (sleep-interpreting thoughts) | States of high emotional arousal | Determined by metacognitive processes (e.g., attachment to beliefs about sleep, personal meaning of thoughts in relation to personal value system) | Increased sleep effort and behaviors aimed at promoting sleep (e.g., extending time in bed, avoiding situations that are perceived as decreasing the chance to sleep) |

case, conditioned arousal developed through repeated pairing of the bed with being upset about the breakup. (Again, Chapter 11 provides further discussion of Sophie's case and her treatment.)

Because conditioned arousal occurs without awareness, clinical signs of conditioned arousal are inferred. For example, conditioned insomnia may be inferred when a patient with insomnia reports dozing off or struggling to stay awake in the living room in the evening, while reading or watching TV on the sofa, and then becoming fully alert when getting into bed. This was the case with Sam, also introduced in Chapter 1 (and later discussed in Chapter 12). At night he usually dozed off in front of the television, but when he retired to bed, he felt wide awake.

People with insomnia engage in behaviors that create opportunities for strengthening the association between the bed and wakefulness, and thus cause or intensify conditioned arousal. For example, they tend to stay in bed trying to attain sleep and becoming upset about their failure to do so. They also start going to bed earlier and/or waking up later than before they had insomnia, believing that this will result in more sleep. To use a fishing industry metaphor, they are "casting a wide net" for "catching" sleep. Unfortunately, this is not an effective strategy. Instead, extended time in bed creates more opportunities for being in bed in a state of hyperarousal (e.g., more time to worry about tomorrow's tasks or today's problems, and/or to become frustrated with difficulty falling asleep). As a result, the likelihood of a learned association between bed and arousal increases. Failure to unwind from the day's activities and disengage from the day's worries before going to bed at night may also strengthen the association between the bed and arousal. This is because arousal-producing intrusive thoughts and worries about the day are more likely to emerge when an individual turns off the light intending to go to sleep.

Historical events outside one's control can also contribute to conditioned arousal. These include past unpleasant experiences that occurred in bed or during sleep and were associated with high arousal. Examples include a history of trauma that occurred when a person was in bed or was awakened from sleep (such as sexual or physical abuse), and exposure to a sleep environment that required hypervigilance (such as a combat zone). In fact, any reexperiencing of a trauma while in bed, including nightmares, may strengthen the association between the bed and arousal. Another example can be seen in the case of Sophie: She experienced a panic attack in bed and subsequently found herself unable to readily initiate sleep. Although conditioned arousal often occurs with repeated pairing, a powerful association between the bed and wakefulness can sometimes form even after a single pairing of the bed with a stimulus, if the stimulus is very strong—such as a panic attack or a nightmare.

## AN ETIOLOGICAL MODEL OF INSOMNIA DISORDER

Arthur Spielman and his colleagues have provided a conceptual model for the development of insomnia disorder (Spielman, Caruso, & Glovinsky, 1987), to which we refer here as the *etiological model of insomnia disorder*. These scholars posit that *predisposing factors, precipitating events, and perpetuating mechanisms* are sequentially involved in the development of insomnia and insomnia disorder, as depicted in Figure 3.1. Predisposing factors are individual characteristics that explain individual differences in the likelihood to experience disturbed sleep during a time of stress. Some people may be more likely than others to lose sleep when stressed, and therefore have greater predisposition for developing insomnia and insomnia disorder. This may be because their biological sleep systems (the two processes discussed in Chapter 2) may be less robust and therefore more easily perturbed than the systems of other people, or because they are responding to stress with higher levels of arousal or are slower to return to their baseline levels after having been aroused. Precipitating events are events that people identify as the proximal causes of their difficulties sleeping. Roughly three-quarters of people with poor sleep identify a precipitating event (Healey et al., 1981), most commonly related to a stressful life event such as separation, divorce, death of a loved one, illness, birth of a child, or work/school stress (Bastien, Vallieres, & Morin, 2004). As noted in Chapter 1, Sam, after some difficulty recalling a cause, reported that his sleeping difficulties started around the time of his second child's birth.

Stress-induced sleep problems are usually transient and resolve when the original distress subsides. However, according to the etiological model of insomnia disorder proposed by Spielman and colleagues, some people become overly alarmed and focused on their sleep problems, and therefore experience high arousal in bed and engage in behaviors that *perpetuate* their sleep difficulties. They develop maladaptive strategies and practices that, although intended to improve sleep, actually worsen it. Some examples of maladaptive strategies include spending excessive time in bed, developing rigid sleep-related rituals, and avoidance behaviors (e.g., canceling planned activities during the day in anticipation that poor sleep at night may lead to being too tired for the activities). As we have discussed earlier in this chapter, cognitive processes (such as sleep-interfering, sleep-interpreting, and metacognitive processes) and conditioned arousal also perpetuate insomnia. In summary, this model posits that people's behavioral and cognitive responses to an acute sleep problem, and some of the practices they adopt for improving sleep or coping with the consequences of poor sleep, result instead in prolonging or exacerbating the very problems they are trying to solve. CBT-I targets these maladaptive coping behaviors (see Chapters 7–9).

Figure 3.2 depicts the etiological model of insomnia and insomnia disorder proposed by Spielman and colleagues. In this figure, an insomnia severity of 14 (the darker vertical line) represents a threshold for insomnia disorder. In the absence of precipitating events, individuals who are predisposed to develop insomnia remain in a premorbid state; they may experience occasional insomnia symptoms. When experiencing a precipitating stressful event, the predisposed individuals may cross the threshold of insomnia disorder and experience an acute episode of insomnia; they may experience difficulties falling or staying asleep almost every night, but usually they understand why they are not sleeping well and experience minimal distress. When a precipitating event becomes less relevant, either because it is no longer in the picture or because an individual has adjusted to it, perpetuating factors—which include maladaptive compensatory coping behaviors, arousal-producing cognitive processes, and conditioned arousal—lead to a transition to a chronic course and maintenance of insomnia disorder.

## KEY PRACTICE IDEAS

- Patients with high arousal can have sleep problems even when Process S and Process C are at the optimal inflection point.

- Patients often experience conditioned insomnia, in which their bed has lost its value as a stimulus for sleep and is instead a stimulus for wakefulness and arousal.

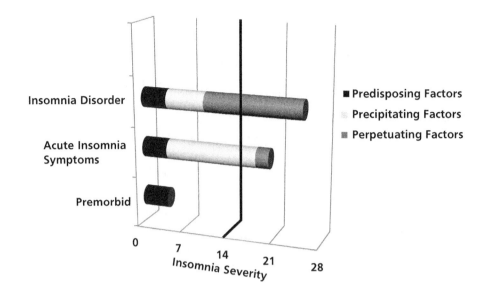

**FIGURE 3.2.** An etiological model of insomnia. The vertical axis represents the time course for insomnia. The horizontal axis is insomnia severity, with 14 as a threshold for insomnia disorder. During an acute episode of insomnia, predisposing factors and precipitants (stress) contribute to poor sleep and some distress (insomnia). The individual may start to engage in coping behaviors that are ineffective. Over time, as the precipitating stress decreases, the ineffective coping strategies intensify in magnitude and scope, and maladaptive cognitions may emerge. As the precipitating stress diminishes, the maladaptive processes perpetuate the presence of insomnia and often lead to worsening of symptoms, distress, and impairment (i.e., insomnia disorder). Based on Spielman, Caruso, and Glovinsky (1987).

- The belief that one must exert effort to sleep is an example of an insomnia-perpetuating belief.

- Patients are vulnerable to insomnia when there is evidence of the following:

  - Sleep-interfering thoughts (e.g., worries about life events and stressors).
  - Sleep-interpreting thoughts (e.g., beliefs about sleep and one's ability to cope with sleep loss).
  - Excessive monitoring for sleep threats (e.g., monitoring poor performance, which is perceived as evidence of the need for more sleep).
  - Engagement in safety behaviors (e.g., calling in sick after a night of poor sleep, to protect oneself from the anticipated poor performance that might follow).
  - Excessively high personal attachment to an unhelpful belief about sleep.

# CHAPTER 4

# Other Sleep Disorders

The *International Classification of Sleep Disorders*, second edition (ICSD-2; American Academy of Sleep Medicine, 2005) includes more than 80 sleep disorders; most remain beyond the scope of this book. Instead, we focus on discussing some of the most common sleep disorders that are relevant to the diagnosis of insomnia disorder (to aid in the differential diagnosis process, outlined in Chapter 6) and its treatment (to guide treatment planning and case conceptualization, discussed in Chapter 10). We focus on the most common sleep disorders whose presence complicates the diagnosis of insomnia disorder or necessitates alterations of the standard CBT-I protocol to promote its safe and effective application. Specifically, we discuss two circadian rhythm sleep–wake disorders (delayed and advanced sleep phase types), as well as obstructive sleep apnea hypopnea (OSAH), restless legs syndrome (RLS), and nightmare disorder (relevant to insomnia with comorbid PTSD). The diagnosis and treatment of most of these sleep disorders requires referral to and consultation with sleep disorder specialists, but do not necessarily preclude initiation of CBT-I. The sequencing of the treatments of insomnia disorder and other sleep disorders is discussed in Chapter 10.

## CIRCADIAN RHYTHM SLEEP–WAKE DISORDERS

As their name indicates, the circadian rhythm sleep–wake disorders are thought to stem from abnormal circadian rhythm or misalignment of the internal biological clock (see Chapter 2) with the timing of sleep opportunities. Clinically, this class of disorders is characterized by persistent sleep disturbances that are causing significant problems. Circadian rhythm sleep–wake disorders include four subtypes that are due primarily to alterations in the endogenous (i.e., intrinsic) circadian clock (delayed sleep phase type, advanced sleep phase type, irregular sleep–wake type, and non-24-hour sleep-wake type), and one subtype that is due primarily to changes in the physical environment in relation to the endogenous (i.e., extrinsic) clock (shift work type). We include a brief description of these sleep disorders here, because they are important for differential diagnosis. The diagnostic criteria for all can be found in DSM-5 (American Psychiatric Association, 2013). The treatments of these disorders require expertise that are beyond the scope of this book, and necessitate referral to a sleep disorder specialist. Interested readers are referred to articles that review the scientific literature on the evaluation and treatment of these disorders (Lu & Zee, 2006; Sack et al., 2007).

*Delayed sleep phase type* is characterized by difficulties in falling asleep and waking up at conventional clock times. It is also referred to as *delayed sleep phase syndrome* (DSPS). In a patient with an eveningness chronotype, the differential diagnosis between insomnia disorder and DSPS is not trivial. The key distinguishing feature is that unlike a patient with DSPS, a person with insomnia disorder has sleep difficulty even when going to sleep very late. Table 4.1 highlights the main distinctions between DSPS and insomnia disorder in a person with an eveningness chronotype. The following are clinical features of DSPS:

1. DSPS usually emerges during adolescence, but may be present in earlier childhood.
2. When the person is free to choose later than conventional bedtimes and rise times, sleep is of normal sleep quality and duration for age, and a stable delayed sleep–wake pattern can be maintained.
3. The problem usually starts with difficulty initiating sleep; however, over time, difficulties maintaining sleep may emerge, representing comorbid insomnia disorder.
4. People with DSPS (as well as those with mild eveningness tendencies who do not meet diagnostic criteria) often report that their best sleep occurs during the second half of the night.
5. People with DSPS (as well as those with mild eveningness tendencies who do not meet diagnostic criteria) tend to maintain irregular sleep–wake patterns, with later bedtimes and rise times when permitted by life demands. This tendency constitutes a predisposition to insomnia disorder (Chapter 2). They also tend to dislike regularity of other daily activities, such as eating meals (e.g., they often skip breakfast).
6. People with DSPS (as well as those with mild eveningness tendencies who do not meet diagnostic criteria) are more likely to be able to nap than people with insomnia disorder and normal circadian tendencies.
7. As discussed in Chapter 2, a longer than average circadian period is a predisposition for DSPS (Archer et al., 2003).

*Advanced sleep phase type* is characterized by difficulties in postponing bedtime and in remaining asleep until desired conventional times. It is also referred to as *advanced sleep phase syndrome* (ASPS). An individual with ASPS is likely to report having always been a morning person and to state that best sleep occurs in the first half of the night. The following are other clinical features of ASPS:

**TABLE 4.1. Main Diagnostic Distinction between DSPS and Insomnia Disorder Experienced by a Person with an Eveningness Chronotype**

| Sleep problem | Characteristic |
|---|---|
| DSPD | Sleep difficulty only when going to sleep earlier than biological tendency |
| Insomnia disorder with eveningness chronotype | Sleep difficulty *even* when going to sleep late, in sync with biological tendency |

1. When free to choose earlier than conventional bedtimes and rise times, an individual with ASPS experiences normal sleep quality and duration.
2. ASPS can make it difficult to socialize in the evening.
3. Waking up earlier than desired can be a symptom of depression, and this possibility needs to be considered in the differential diagnosis. However, in such cases the pattern is present only during depressive episodes.

*Irregular sleep–wake type* is present when sleep occurs in three or more short (less than 4-hour) bouts throughout the 24-hour period. Usually the longest bout occurs at night. This subtype is characterized by the absence of a clearly discernible rhythm to the sleep–wake pattern. It is also referred to as *irregular sleep–wake disorder* and is most often present in individuals with dementia, intellectual disability, brain injury, or other neurological disorders (McCurry & Ancoli-Israel, 2003). The disorder can be exacerbated by decreased exposure to environmental synchronizing factors, such as light (Shochat, Martin, Marler, & Ancoli-Israel, 2000).

*Non-24-hour sleep–wake type* is characterized by sleep onset and offset that are progressively delayed, often accompanied by difficulty in falling asleep or in awakening from sleep. At times during this progressive delay, there is complete reversal of night and day. This makes it difficult to maintain a stable 24-hour sleep–wake pattern. A person with this subtype will experience periods of good sleep when the endogenous and external clocks are aligned, and sleep difficulties when they are not. Non-24-hour sleep–wake type primarily afflicts blind people, and is present in approximately 50% of blind people (Sack, Lewy, Blood, Keith, & Nakagawa, 1992), with no known sex differences. The disorder is rare among sighted people, afflicting mostly males, and is usually due to living in environments with continuous low light levels and atypical sleep–wake schedules, such as among individuals with submarine duty (Naitoh, Beare, Biersner, & Englund, 1983). Traumatic brain injury can also trigger this type of circadian rhythm disorder (Ayalon, Borodkin, Dishon, Kanety, & Dagan, 2007).

*Shift work type* occurs when work hours are scheduled during the usual societal sleep period, most commonly night and early morning shifts. The complaints include difficulties initiating and/or maintaining sleep, sleepiness during the desired wake period (daytime equivalent), and impaired performance. People who travel across many time zones very frequently subject their body to similar circadian rhythm adjustment challenges, as do people working rotating shifts.

The treatments for all these subtypes of circadian rhythm sleep–wake disorders are primarily behavioral (e.g., sleep schedule manipulation and properly timed exposure to bright light and darkness); these go beyond the scope of this book and require referral to a sleep specialist. However, in Chapter 7 we describe strategies for helping people with insomnia disorder and mild evening and morning tendencies to maintain a conventional sleep schedule.

## OBSTRUCTIVE SLEEP APNEA HYPOPNEA

OSAH is a chronic respiratory sleep disorder caused by obstructions/narrowing at various sites along the upper airways, illustrated schematically in Figure 4.1. Obstructive breathing events are characterized by a complete or partial cessation of breathing (*hypoxemia*), caused by full or partial obstructions of the airways (referred to as obstructive *apnea* or *hypopnea* events, respectively); the

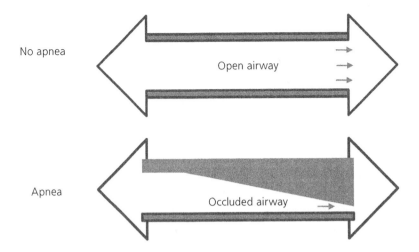

**FIGURE 4.1.** Occlusion of airways during the night in OSAH. The top panel depicts unrestricted airflow (i.e., air freely flows in and out during inhalation and exhalation). The bottom panel depicts an airway obstructed by loose muscle tissues in the throat that impinge on the airway, stopping or limiting airflow into the lungs.

hypoxemia is followed by a decrease in oxygen saturation of the blood and/or arousal from sleep. OSAH has a negative impact on mood, attention, and vigilance (believed to be mostly due to sleep fragmentation), and, to a lesser degree, on executive functioning, memory, and psychomotor performances (Aloia, Arnedt, Davis, Riggs, & Byrd, 2004). Untreated OSAH increases the risk for hypertension, heart disease and stroke, impaired immune function, insulin resistance, motor vehicle accidents, and lower productivity at school and work (Aloia et al., 2004). Common risks for OSAH include obesity, older age, male sex, and abnormal facial morphology. Because OSAH can cause hypertension, the presence of hypertension alone is often taken as indication that OSAH may be present and should be assessed (Chung et al., 2008). The sex difference in prevalence of OSAH decreases after menopause (Resta et al., 2003).

The most salient clinical sleep symptoms of OSAH include loud snoring, snorting, and gasping for air. An individual with OSAH may be aware of waking up gasping for air, but most commonly these patients lack awareness of snoring and are often urged to seek help by their bed partners. Clinical daytime symptoms of OSAH include feeling unrefreshed upon waking up in the morning and sleepy during the day. Other morning symptoms of OSAH include a headache (typically resolved shortly after rising) and a dry mouth. The diagnosis of OSAH requires an overnight sleep study. The severity of OSAH is measured by the *apnea–hypopnea index* (AHI), which is the average number of apneas and hypopneas (combined) per hour of sleep. OSAH is considered mild if the AHI is 5–15 events/hour, moderate if the AHI is 15–30 events/hour, and severe when the AHI is greater than 30 events/hour. The severity of hypoxemia is measured by the level of oxygen desaturation (minimum and mean oxygen saturation during sleep) and percentage of sleep time below a saturation threshold (80% or 90%). Patients' experiences of the diagnostic and treatment processes for OSAH vary, depending on their clinical presentation, the type of insurance they have, and the health care system where they receive care. Generally the first step is a visit with a clinician, who assesses signs and symptoms, performs a physical examination (including a detailed assessment of structural aspects of the airway system), and makes a referral for a diagnostic sleep study as needed. The diagnostic sleep study is performed in the sleep laboratory or, increasingly, in a patient's homes (ambulatory). Such a study consists of PSG (see Chapters 1–2) and also includes sensors to monitor blood oxygenation, respiration, heart rate, and brain and muscle activities. The next step is usually a return visit, during which treatment options are discussed.

The standard treatment for OSAH is the use of a continuous positive airway pressure (CPAP) machine, which delivers a stream of compressed air via a hose to a nose mask, nasal pillow, or full-face mask that facilitates breathing during sleep. Although CPAP is the most common and reliable method of treating OSAH, adherence can be a problem: One study found that 25–50% of patients with OSAH refused or could not tolerate CPAP therapy (Zozula & Rosen, 2001). Patients may discontinue use altogether or take the mask off in the middle of the night, with or without memory of the event. Many CPAP machines have a feature that enables objective assessment of use and efficacy. As mentioned in Chapter 1, Sam was prescribed CPAP a few years before he sought CBT-I. He reported that he used it on most nights. He also reported that when he woke up in the middle of the night, the mask often was no longer on his face. Sam (see Chapter 12 for more details) was advised to put the mask back on in the middle of the night; over time, his adherence to CPAP therapy improved.

In some cases, as in Sam's, simple encouragement and support of the patient's continued use are all that is necessary to improve adherence. In other cases, the solution may be more complex and may require addressing multiple factors, including discomfort with the mask, claustrophobia, increased difficulties with falling or staying asleep when trying to use the mask, an objection by a bed partner, and personal meaning (e.g., "I will look unattractive"). Close follow-up during the early stages of using CPAP is important, so that adherence issues can be addressed early. Sometimes it is necessary to make adjustments/modifications (e.g., trying a different mask, adding a humidifier to the CPAP system, changing pressure settings). Behavioral sleep specialists work with other sleep specialists, sleep technologists, and/or respiratory therapists to determine whether adjustments are needed and to assist in the process. Psychologists have also studied the use of motivational enhancement techniques (Aloia et al., 2007), desensitization (Aloia et al., 2001), and psychoeducation (e.g., Chervin, Theut, Bassetti, & Aldrich, 1997). Although behavioral sleep specialists can help patients adhere to CPAP, the protocols for doing so remain beyond the scope of this book. Second-line treatments for OSAH include a variety of surgical procedures and use of dental appliances to address upper-airway abnormalities; reducing supine sleep position (when the breathing events are mostly in the supine position) (Oksenberg, Silverberg, Offenbach, & Arons, 2006); and even didgeridoo playing, to tone the upper-airway muscles that control airway dilation (Puhan et al., 2006). Weight loss through dietary and lifestyle changes (and, in cases with refractory, medically complicated obesity, through bariatric surgery) have been studied and found to have some short-term effectiveness, although this tends to diminish over time when weight is regained (Morgenthaler et al., 2006).

## Insomnia Disorder Comorbid with OSAH

Breathing events fragment sleep by causing arousals, which, in the absence of insomnia disorder, tend to be brief. When patients with OSAH experience prolonged time awake in the middle of the night, they likely have a comorbid insomnia disorder. When OSAH and insomnia disorder coexist, both conditions need to be treated independently. It is important to recognize the effects of the two disorders and their treatments on each other. Insomnia disorder complicates adherence to CPAP therapy. Patients with OSAH and insomnia disorder tend to discontinue use of CPAP, in part because the mask (or nasal pillow) initially disrupts sleep even in people with no difficulties sleeping, and in part because people with insomnia mistakenly expect that CPAP therapy will resolve their insomnia. They discontinue CPAP use because they become disheartened by the worsening of insomnia during the adjustment period and/or by failure of the CPAP to help their insomnia. Conversely, as we discuss in Chapter 7, daytime sleepiness—a common symptom of severe untreated OSAH—is an important safety consideration when CBT-I is being implemented. The treatments of insomnia disorder and OSAH target different pathological processes and symptoms. CPAP aims to reduce the number of breathing events, which can be expected to result in feeling more refreshed in the morning and less sleepy during the day, but is not expected to affect the time it takes to fall asleep at the beginning of the night or the ease of returning to sleep in the middle of the night. The treatment of insomnia disorder with CBT-I, on the other hand, aims to help with falling and returning to sleep, but it does not affect the number of breathing events during sleep.

## RESTLESS LEGS SYNDROME

RLS is characterized by a very strong urge to move the legs that starts or gets worse during periods of rest or inactivity, particularly with reduced alertness. The urge begins or increases in the evening or night, and it is usually accompanied or caused by discomfort and disagreeable sensations in the legs that are partially or completely relieved by movement, such as walking (Allen et al., 2003). The urge is sometimes present without the uncomfortable sensations. The arms may also be involved, but arm involvement tends to emerge later in the course of the disorder (Michaud, Chabli, Lavigne, & Montplaisir, 2000; Winkelmann et al., 2000). The sensation is difficult to describe. It is not strictly pain, but rather a sensation deep in the leg described as burning, itching, tingling, tightness, grabbing, pulling, or other discomfort. In very severe cases, no activity provides relief and symptoms are present throughout the day, with no daily variations. RLS usually has an insidious onset and has a genetic basis (Desautels et al., 2001), with 60% of patients who have the disorder reporting a family history of RLS (Walters et al., 1996). However, it may also emerge in the context of other medical diseases, such as end-stage renal disease (Roger, Harris, & Stewart, 1991), peripheral neuropathy, and radiculopathy (Ondo & Jankovic, 1996); it may also emerge, or worsen, during pregnancy, in which case it resolves after delivery, or returns to pre-pregnancy severity (Goodman, Brodie, & Ayida, 1988). Restless legs sensations are distinct from discomfort caused by positions, leg cramps, or habitual foot tapping. RLS is diagnosed when the leg symptoms are associated with clinically meaningful distress or impaired functioning. Its severity is determined by the frequency of the leg symptoms and the extent to which they interfere with sleep. The diagnosis of RLS is based on clinical symptoms and does not require an overnight sleep study. Treatment includes iron supplements and medications, most commonly dopaminergic drugs, which unfortunately can be activating and may disrupt sleep (Trenkwalder et al., 2008).

CBT-I can be safely administered to those with RLS, and we have experienced success in implementing it. Although the leg sensations are not likely to diminish with CBT-I, it is reasonable to expect that CBT-I will reduce prolonged wakefulness for reasons unrelated to RLS. However, we are not aware of empirical studies of the efficacy of CBT for insomnia disorder comorbid with RLS.

The symptoms of RLS are experienced during waking hours, but the discomfort can interfere with the ability to fall or return to sleep. It is unclear in what percentage of people with RLS the symptoms lead to sleep disturbance (Allen et al., 2003). Approximately 80% individuals with RLS also have a sleep disorder called periodic limb movement disorder (PLMD) (Montplaisir et al., 1997), characterized by arrhythmic extension of the big toe and dorsiflexion of the ankle, which last 0.5–5 seconds and occur in series (at least 4) with a periodic pattern. The periodic leg movement (PLM) events may cause arousal from sleep, but afflicted individuals are oblivious to these events, though a bed partner may notice leg kicks or jerks. The leg movements are identified by using electromyography of the anterior tibialis during an overnight sleep study. The PLM index is the average number of leg movements per hour of sleep, and the PLM arousal index is the average number of leg movements that are associated with arousal per hour of sleep, which may be of greater clinical significance than the overall PLM index. The diagnosis of PLMD requires an overall index that is greater than or equal to 5 events per hour of sleep (American Academy of Sleep Medicine, 2005). The treatment of PLMD is the same as the treatment for RLS (i.e., pharmacotherapy).

## NIGHTMARE DISORDER

A *nightmare* is a dream that elicits a strong emotional response, such as fear or horror, accompanied by an awakening. In other words, a nightmare involves negative feelings, negative images, and awakening. The dream content is remembered and usually involves threats to one's survival or integrity. The presence of a nightmare cannot be inferred solely from a bed partner's report of observed thrashing during sleep, because the clinical definition of a nightmare requires the patient to remember waking up and having negative imagery or emotions. Nightmares most frequently occur during the second half of the night, when REM sleep is most predominant. Nightmares are relevant to insomnia because they cause awakenings that can become prolonged. Prolonged awakenings, particularly when accompanied by a high degree of distress, can lead to conditioned arousal. A formal diagnosis of nightmare disorder requires repeatedly occurring nightmares that cause clinically distress or impaired functioning in important areas (American Psychiatric Association, 2013).

Nightmare disorder can be treated with prazosin (Raskind et al., 2003, 2007; Taylor, Freeman, & Cates, 2008), an alpha agonist, and/or imagery rehearsal therapy (Krakow et al., 2001). Imagery rehearsal therapy involves instructing a patient to change the content of a nightmare so that it includes more acceptable features that are neither unpleasant nor distressing, or to create an alternative dream and then to rehearse the revised or new dream by means of imagery during the daytime. Some, but not all, imagery rehearsal protocols recommend focusing on repetitive nightmares (Forbes et al., 2003). To minimize occurrences of intrusive, unpleasant images during practice, some protocols recommend not focusing on nightmares that represent replays of real-life events, and instead rehearsing a new, pleasant dream (Germain & Nielsen, 2003a). At this writing, it is not yet clear whether exposure to dreams representing replay of traumatic experience, such as those experienced by people with combat-related PTSD, is detrimental or beneficial (the latter would be consistent with exposure-based theories and treatments of PTSD). In Chapter 9, we describe how to use behavioral and cognitive therapy techniques to help reduce time awake after an awakening caused by a nightmare. We also note that CBT for PTSD reduces nightmares experienced when nightmares occur in the context of PTSD (Zayfert & DeViva, 2004).

## KEY PRACTICE IDEAS

This chapter has focused on providing background and clinical features of sleep disorders that are most common among patients with insomnia disorder. The assessment of these sleep disorders is covered in Chapter 6. Related considerations for treatment planning and implementation of CBT-I are discussed in Chapter 10. Below, we summarize key features of the sleep disorders covered in this chapter.

- Circadian rhythm sleep–wake disorders are associated with a mismatch between the timing of the sleep opportunity window and the internal biological circadian clock or abnormalities in the circadian clock. Their treatment requires referral to a sleep specialist.

- The diagnosis and treatment of OSAH also require referral to a sleep specialist. Definitive diagnosis of OSAH is based on an overnight study (PSG). CPAP therapy is the standard treatment for OSAH. Adjustment and adherence to CPAP treatment can be problematic.

- OSAH can be associated with daytime sleepiness, which, when severe, is a contraindication for certain components of CBT-I.

- RLS is diagnosed via self-report. It is treated pharmacologically and requires referral to a sleep specialist.

- When the primary sleep complaint is waking up with a nightmare and having difficulty returning to sleep, nightmare disorder is a likely differential diagnosis.

# CHAPTER 5

# The Impact of Comorbid Disorders on Sleep and Insomnia

Most commonly, insomnia presents not on its own, but along with another condition. In Chapter 4, we have discussed comorbid sleep disorders; in this chapter, we discuss other comorbidities. Poor sleep may be present before a psychiatric condition develops, or it may emerge at the same time or after the condition develops. For example, among those with a first major depressive episode and insomnia, insomnia symptoms emerged before major depressive disorder (MDD) in 41%, at the same time as the MDD in 29%, and after the depressive episode in 29% (Ohayon & Roth, 2003). In contrast, in the vast majority of cases with an anxiety disorder, insomnia emerged at the same time as or after the anxiety disorder (Ohayon & Roth, 2003). The presence of comorbidities requires considerations about sequencing CBT-I and the treatment of the comorbid condition, as well as about the relative emphasis on and presentation order of CBT-I components. We address these considerations in Chapter 9. The purpose of this chapter is to familiarize clinicians with sleep features of common comorbidities that will help in the assessment, planning, and implementation of CBT-I for insomnia disorder that is comorbid with other disorders. As discussed in Chapter 1, evidence for the efficacy of CBT-I in insomnia disorder with comorbidities is accumulating.

We have elected to focus on the conditions that have received most research attention as comorbid with insomnia disorder: MDD, bipolar disorder (I and II), panic disorder (PD), generalized anxiety disorder (GAD), posttraumatic stress disorder (PTSD), obsessive–compulsive disorder (OCD), and chronic pain. We do not discuss social anxiety disorder and specific phobia because of the paucity of research on sleep in these two disorders. Because the connection between eating and sleeping behaviors has received much attention recently and adds to patients' distress about poor sleep, we have also included a brief discussion of feeding and eating disorders.

## MAJOR DEPRESSIVE DISORDER

Poor sleep is a diagnostic symptom of depressive disorders. Until recently, it has been assumed that poor sleep will improve when depression remits. It is now understood that the relationship is not unidirectional. Poor sleep predicts future depressive episodes (Ford & Kamerow, 1989; Perlis,

Giles, Buysse, Tu, & Kupfer, 1997), is not fully resolved after remission from depression (Carney, Segal, Edinger, & Krystal, 2007; Nierenberg et al., 2010), and predicts poorer response to treatment and recurrence (Buysse et al., 1999; Thase et al., 1996).

Sleep difficulties are very common among patients with depression and often remain unresolved with general psychotherapy or antidepressant medications (Carney, Segal, et al., 2007; Kopta et al., 1994; Manber et al., 2003). In general, individuals with co-occurring MDD and insomnia tend to have poorer depression outcomes than those without insomnia (Dew et al., 1997), and are at increased risk for suicide and are more vulnerable to recurrence of depression (Agargun, Kara, & Solmaz, 1997; Fawcett et al., 1990; Pigeon et al., 2008). It is therefore important to diagnose and treat insomnia when it is comorbid with depression.

Patients with comorbid depression who present for treatment of insomnia may be more likely to discontinue CBT-I (Ong, Kuo, & Manber, 2008), but those who stay with the treatment derive levels of benefit equal to those for patients with insomnia but without depression (Manber et al., 2011). Moreover, CBT-I appears to have positive effects on depression as well. A randomized pilot study provides an initial indication that when patients with depression and insomnia received CBT-I in conjunction with medication management for depression, they had significantly better response to the antidepressant medication (Manber et al., 2008). There is no reason to believe that the same will not hold true for a combination of CBT for depression and CBT-I.

To treat insomnia effectively in those with depression, therapists can benefit from knowledge about aspects of sleep that are particularly relevant to individuals with depression. Some of these factors may compromise the ability of patients with depression to make behavioral and cognitive changes that even nondepressed patients often find difficult to implement. Table 5.1 provides a summary of these factors.

Sam's initial case description (Chapter 1) suggests that he may have had depression. Sam reported that during the past year, he had experienced a worsening in his fatigue, pain, depressed mood, memory problems, and concentration problems. During his initial assessment, the therapist asked about depressed mood and anhedonia, and found that neither symptom was present at or above threshold (i.e., Sam did not experience either every day for most of the day). In the absence of at least one of these two core symptoms, Sam did not meet full diagnostic criteria for MDD. Nonetheless, his depression might impair his ability to engage in treatment, and the therapist therefore needed to consider this when conceptualizing his case and planning his treatment. For example, Sam (who is further discussed in Chapter 12) had several of the features outlined in Table 5.1. He held very strongly to unhelpful beliefs about sleep and had a very irregular sleep schedule. He also had sleep apnea and took duloxetine, which can cause sleep disruptions.

## BIPOLAR DISORDERS

Most of the research on sleep in bipolar disorders has been conducted with bipolar I disorder. Sleep alterations are present in both the manic/hypomanic and the depressive states in bipolar I disorder. During depressive episodes, sleep alterations are largely similar to profiles of patients with MDD. During a manic or hypomanic state, most patients with bipolar disorders report disturbed or shorter than usual sleep (Harvey, 2008; Riemann, Voderholzer, & Berger, 2002). Table 5.2 summarizes findings relevant to insomnia in bipolar disorders.

**TABLE 5.1. Features of Depression, and Sleep- and Mood-Related Consequences**

| Clinical feature | Sleep- and mood-related consequences |
|---|---|
| A patient with depression may use the bed as an escape from emotional suffering or a way to cope with anhedonia. | These behaviors increase the time spent in bed. Some of the extra time in bed will be spent asleep, thus weakening the sleep drive, and some of the extra time in bed may be spent trying to sleep or ruminating, thus increasing conditioned arousal. Both the weaker sleep drive and the increased arousal contribute to poor sleep. This may also be an example of sleep effort (trying to get more sleep) as a strategy for dealing with low mood or managing fatigue. Given Sam's increased time in bed and depression symptoms, this was something his therapist asked him about during assessment. |
| Patients with both insomnia and depression have stronger levels of unhelpful beliefs than people with insomnia who do not experience depression (Carney, Edinger, Manber, Garson, & Segal, 2007), as well as greater proneness to rumination. | Rumination is common in both those with depression and those with insomnia. Rumination that occurs at bedtime and the middle of the night can interfere with sleep. Because both dysfunctional beliefs about sleep and nocturnal rumination can be prominent among people with depression and insomnia, it may be particularly important for therapists treating such patients to address cognitive hyperarousal. As discussed in Chapter 3, daytime rumination about the perceived consequences of insomnia can intensify the focus on the sleep problem and increase the pressure to "fix" the sleep problems. Sam had a considerable number of sleep-effort-related beliefs. He kept a binder of sleep-related information and engaged in behaviors such as sleeping alone to help him sleep better. |
| People with both insomnia and depression have more irregular sleep schedules than people with insomnia but without depression (Suh et al., 2012). | Sleeping in, not setting an alarm, going to bed early, and in general having less of a routine all render people with depression at risk for having less robust circadian clocks. Additionally, irregular schedules can limit the possibility of social engagement. It may also be difficult to be socially engaged if a person is not up for the day until the afternoon. This also shortens the amount of sunlight exposure needed to regulate the clock. Sam was at risk for circadian dysfunction, because he was in bed for up to 12 hours per day, not including the time he spent falling asleep on the couch in the evening; thus the amount of light exposure Sam received in a 24-hour period was limited. |
| Waking up earlier than desired is more common among individuals with than without depression (Gillin, Duncan, Pettigrew, Frankel, & Snyder, 1979). | The mechanism of early morning awakenings is unclear and may vary from patient to patient. Mood worsening, fatigue, and/ or anhedonia all increase the likelihood that someone with insomnia and depression will respond to such awakenings by staying in bed and "trying" to sleep. This limits the amount of homeostatic pressure that can accumulate during the day, sends irregular input to the clock, and increases the possibility for conditioned arousal. It is also an example of sleep effort that requires targeting. |

*(cont.)*

**TABLE 5.1** (*cont.*)

| Clinical feature | Sleep- and mood-related consequences |
|---|---|
| Sleep apnea may be more prevalent among patients with insomnia and depression (Ong, Gress, San Pedro-Salcedo, & Manber, 2009), possibly because of depression-associated inactivity and weight gain. The precise mechanism is not known. | Sleep apnea will fragment sleep further. Sleep apnea increases sleepiness during the day and will exacerbate fatigue and mood disturbance. Moreover, the increased malaise may not be correctly attributed to untreated apnea, and may instead be interpreted by the patient as due to insomnia or depression; this can increase helplessness about the situation. The sleepiness will make it less likely that the patient can remain active, which will increase fatigue further and decrease exposure to reinforcing experiences in the environment. Sleep apnea also makes it more likely that the patient will gain weight. These processes can be seen in Sam, who had sleep apnea, insomnia, and many features of depression. |
| Medical treatment of depression may disrupt sleep in several ways. | Disturbed sleep is a side effect of some antidepressants, such as fluoxetine and other selective serotonin reuptake inhibitors (SSRIs) (Wilson & Argyropoulos, 2005). Most antidepressant medications suppress REM sleep, and some interfere with sleep by exacerbating sleep apnea or causing periodic limb movements during sleep. Sam was taking duloxetine for fibromyalgia, which can have insomnia as a side effect. |

# ANXIETY DISORDERS

The reader should keep in mind that the literature reviewed below was published before the publication of DSM-5 (American Psychiatric Association, 2013), when PTSD and OCD were still considered anxiety disorders. For the same reason, and given that this book was written during the period of transition to the new classification, we have used the heading "Anxiety Disorders" above, even though this section also covers two disorders that DSM-5 no longer classifies as anxiety disorders (PTSD and OCD). Compared to depressive disorders, fewer studies have examined sleep disturbances in anxiety disorders. There is a high lifetime association between DSM-IV anxiety disorders and insomnia, with 24–36% of individuals endorsing difficulty in initiating or maintaining sleep having a DSM-IV-defined anxiety disorder (Breslau, Roth, Rosenthal, & Andreski, 1996; Ford & Kamerow, 1989; Ohayon & Roth, 2003). A history of disturbed sleep also increases the risk for developing a DSM-III/IV-defined anxiety disorder, compared to having no prior history of disturbed sleep (Breslau et al., 1996; Ford & Kamerow, 1989; Ohayon & Roth, 2003). Conversely, individuals with these disorders take longer time to fall asleep, have lower sleep efficiencies, and have shorter sleep duration (Benca, Obermeyer, Thisted, & Gillin, 1992).

## Panic Disorder

Sleep symptoms in PD are generally characterized by difficulties in falling asleep, difficulties in staying asleep, and nocturnal panic attacks. A nocturnal panic attack is a spontaneous awakening (without a recognizable trigger) in sudden fear and other symptoms of panic attack, such as heart palpitations and increased breathing rate. The symptoms are generally similar in quality, severity, and duration to waking-state panic attacks. Nocturnal panic attacks tend to occur within 3 hours of sleep onset (Uhde, 2000). Breathlessness may be more common in nocturnal than in waking panic attacks, but it should not be confused with the choking sensation upon awakening from an apnea event, in that an awakening from an apnea event is not associated with fear. A nocturnal panic attack is also distinct from a nightmare, in that there is no memory of an upsetting narrative upon awakening.

Retrospective estimates of the lifetime prevalence of nocturnal panic attacks among people with PD range between 45 and 71% (Craske & Barlow, 1989; Craske & Tsao, 2005; Krystal, Woods, Hill, & Charney, 1991; Mellman & Uhde, 1989; Stein, Chartier, & Walker, 1993). Patients with nocturnal panic attacks have more frequent daytime panic attacks than patients with only daytime panic attacks have, and their panic attacks are associated with more somatic sensations (Sloan et al., 1999). Nocturnal panic is the predominant symptom among some patients with PD (Mellman & Uhde, 1989) and may represent a subtype of PD, characterized by fearful associations with sleep and sleep-like states (Craske et al., 2002). Craske and colleagues propose an interoceptive conditioning model to explain nocturnal panic attacks (Craske et al., 2002; Craske & Tsao, 2005). They suggest that individuals with PD may preferentially attend to somatic stimuli during sleep. They further suggest that normal internal events such as changes in respiration and heart rate, to which those with PD may be attuned, trigger a panic attack. Consistent with the interoceptive conditioning theory of nocturnal panic is the fact that noc-

## TABLE 5.2. Features of Sleep in Bipolar Disorders

- The number of wake periods and the duration of early morning awakening are higher during a bipolar depressive episode than during a unipolar depressive episode (Riemann et al., 2002).

- During a bipolar depressive phase, sleep duration over the 24 hours is longer than during euthymic states (Bowden, 2005; Detre et al., 1972). However, the frequency of daytime sleepiness in these two phases is similar (Nofzinger et al., 1991).

- The majority (44–77%) of patients with bipolar I disorder identify sleep disturbance as a prodromal symptom to a manic episode (Jackson, Cavanagh, & Scott, 2003). Patients with rapid cycling between manic and depressive states may be particularly likely to experience sleep loss as a prodromal symptom of a manic episode.

- Sleep deprivation causes a temporary elevation of mood among people with unipolar depression (Colombo, Benedetti, Barbini, Campori, & Smeraldi, 1999). It has therefore been theorized that, enjoying the mood elevation caused by sleep loss, some patients with bipolar disorders further restrict their sleep. This increases their euphoric mood even more, until it reaches hypomanic or manic intensity.

    However, although increased vulnerability to elevated mood after sleep deprivation has been reported, a relatively small proportion of patients with bipolar I disorder experience a switch to a manic phase following experimentally induced sleep deprivation (Colombo et al., 1999). It is thus possible that poor sleep before a manic episode is an early symptom of the impending hypomania/mania, rather than the cause of a manic episode per se. In other words, poor sleep is likely to be a prodrome of (hypo)manic episode in bipolar disorder.

turnal panic attacks tend to arise during the transition from stage 2 to stage 3 sleep as respiration slows and becomes more regular (Hauri, Friedman, & Ravaris, 1989; Mellman & Uhde, 1989). Tsao and Craske (2003) suggest that in some cases, nocturnal panic may relate to fear of loss of vigilance.

## Generalized Anxiety Disorder

Being in a worried state is not conducive to sleep. An experiment in which participants were told they must give a speech the next morning found that worries about the next day's performance led to prolonged latency to sleep onset (Gross & Borkovec, 1982). It is therefore not surprising that most individuals with GAD, a disorder characterized by excessive worry, report insomnia symptoms (Arriaga, Lara, Matos-Pires, Cavaglia, & Bastos, 1995; Belanger, Morin, Langlois, & Ladouceur, 2004; Benca et al., 1992; Monti & Monti, 2000). These symptoms include decreased sleep duration and efficiency and increased sleep latency. Objective measures of sleep similarly document more disturbed sleep among those with GAD than controls (Monti & Monti, 2000). However, despite the fact that there is a strong relationship between worry and sleep disruption in general (e.g., Watts, Coyle, & East, 1994), insomnia symptom severity is not correlated with GAD severity (Belanger et al., 2004). This is most likely because presleep worries are more relevant to sleep difficulties than daytime worries. As discussed in Chapter 3, even in the absence of a GAD diagnosis, individuals with insomnia disorder report that presleep worries about life's problems and about sleep contribute to their sleep difficulties. We are not aware of research comparing the content of presleep worries of people with insomnia disorder with and without comorbid GAD. Even though insomnia severity does not appear to contribute to anxiety severity, when the two disorders co-occur, treating both at the same time leads to greater improvements in anxiety than treating only the anxiety does (Pollack et al., 2008).

## Posttraumatic Stress Disorder

Complaints about sleep disruption are common among people suffering from PTSD (Maher, Rego, & Asnis, 2006) and include sleep continuity disturbances and nightmares. Other sleep symptoms in PTSD include unusual behaviors during sleep, such as bursts of arm and leg muscle twitches and vocalizations during sleep (Germain & Nielsen, 2003b; Lavie, 2001; Ross et al., 1994), and dream enactment behavior resulting from the maintenance of muscle tone during REM sleep (i.e., loss of muscle atonia). Poor sleep and anger are the two most common residual symptoms after treatment of PTSD (Zayfert & DeViva, 2004). Zayfert and DeViva found that 48% of patients with PTSD who were successfully treated with a form of CBT tailored to this disorder continued to experience insomnia symptoms even after their nightmares remitted. This is a remarkably similar figure to the estimated prevalence (44%) of residual sleep disturbance among patients in remission from MDD (Nierenberg et al., 1999).

PSG studies of patients with PTSD yield findings that are consistent with the clinical presentation. Consistent with heightened hyperarousal in PTSD, PSG studies comparing patients with PTSD to control patients find more frequent brief awakenings (lasting less than 1 minute) and lighter sleep (more stage N1 sleep, less slow-wave sleep) among the patients with PTSD (Breslau et al., 2004; Kobayashi, Boarts, & Delahanty, 2007). Consistent with the increased frequency of nightmares among patients with PTSD, research shows a greater number of rapid eye movements during REM sleep among such patients compared with controls (Kobayashi et al., 2007). Other aspects of sleep that are particularly relevant to individuals with PTSD are presented in Table 5.3.

## Obsessive–Compulsive Disorder

Some, but not all, individuals with OCD report difficulties initiating and/or maintaining sleep (Uhde, 2000), often associated with obsessional worries during the night and with checking behaviors. Compulsive behaviors/nighttime rituals may delay sleep onset, particularly if presleep rituals are detailed and have to be repeated if interrupted (Smith et al., 2005). In general, those with OCD tend to have stronger inaccurate and unhelpful beliefs (Mogg & Bradley, 1998); thus assessing cognitions relating to sleep may be of particular importance. To our knowledge, no studies to date have examined the impact of sleep-specific treatments on OCD symptoms.

# CHRONIC PAIN

More than 50% of patients with chronic pain conditions complain of sleep disturbances, particularly insomnia (Morin, Gibson, & Wade, 1998; Smith, Perlis, Smith, Giles, & Carmody, 2000). The type and severity of sleep disturbance may vary by type of pain condition. (For a review, see Menefee et al., 2000.) In general, acute uncontrolled pain and bursts of increased pain, such as muscle spasms, may awaken a sleeper and prolong the return to sleep following awakenings. In contrast, chronic moderate pain, although it may cause brief arousals, does not usually cause full awakenings. Chronic pain may, however, "lighten" sleep so that a person's waking threshold is lower (Harman et al., 2002). Experimental studies document that sleep deprivation in healthy individuals can increase next-day pain sensitivity and experience (Edwards, Almeida, Klick, Haythornthwaite, & Smith, 2008). It has also been documented that among those with chronic pain, disturbed sleep is associated with an increase in self-reported pain the following day (Affleck, Urrows, Tennen, Higgins, & Abeles, 1996; Drewes et al., 2000). Understandably, an individual with chronic pain responds to having experienced more daytime pain following nights of poor sleep by increasing effort to optimize sleep. As discussed in Chapter 3, increased effort to sleep leads to heightened arousal, which interferes with sleep and contributes to the insomnia experience.

Patients with chronic pain often use resting as a pain relief strategy. If rest during the day takes place in the bed used for sleep at night, the sleeping bed gets paired with pain, thus heightening conditioned arousal (see Chapter 3). Moreover, daytime rest may lead to dozing and associated weakening of the sleep drive (see Chapter 2). As in the case of insomnia comorbid with depression, some individuals with insomnia and chronic pain try to sleep during the day—often in the nighttime sleeping bed—as a means for coping with (escaping from) pain, but are often unable to sleep. This too can contribute to conditioned arousal. As noted in Chapter 1, Sam had fibromyalgia and used his sleeping bed for resting during the day. He sometimes slept during these rest periods—resulting in a lower sleep drive at bedtime than would be optimal for good sleep. Again, see Chapter 12 for a description of Sam's treatment planning and course.

**TABLE 5.3. Features of Sleep in PTSD, and Mood-Related Consequences**

| Clinical feature | Sleep- and mood-related consequences |
| --- | --- |
| Patients with PTSD often exhibit increased hypervigilance at bedtime. | Examples of sleep-related hyperarousal include lying in bed listening for signs of danger (e.g., noises outside) and performing "perimeter checks" (checking locks on the doors and windows) at bedtime and/or upon awakening in the middle of the night. Some veterans with PTSD keep a loaded weapon or gun accessible next to the bed. |
| Some people with PTSD report fear of sleep (Inman, Silver, & Doghrarnji, 1990). | Fear of sleep can occur in response to having experienced a trauma that occurred in bed or when a person was asleep (e.g., rape, natural disaster, or an attack in the line of combat). Other reasons for fear of sleep include fear of losing vigilance (i.e., not being able to respond to urgent situations that might arise) or fear of having a nightmare. Sometimes these fears are associated with avoidance behaviors, such as delaying bedtime and sleeping in locations other than the bedroom (e.g., the living room), which may feel safer. When sleep avoidance is associated with sleep loss, the homeostatic sleep drive increases, and with it the arousal thresholds. These diminish the ability to respond when urgent situations arise, and increase the probability of being confused when suddenly awakened from sleep. Research has found that patients with PTSD have higher auditory arousal/awakening thresholds at night than controls (Lavie, Katz, Pillar, & Zinger, 1998). |
| PTSD is associated with increased prevalence of some sleep disorders in addition to insomnia. | Common comorbid sleep disorders include OSAH (see Chapter 4; Krakow et al., 2002; Sharafkhaneh, Giray, Richardson, Young, & Hirshkowitz, 2005), periodic leg movements (Brown & Boudewyns, 1996), REM behavior disorder (i.e., dream enactment due to loss of muscle atonia), sleep paralysis (i.e., waking up with transient paralysis), and confusional arousal (cf. Ohayon & Shapiro, 2000). |
| Patients with PTSD often experience discomfort with silence. | Patients may sleep with music or the television on. However, changes in volume can cause sleep to be shallow and potentially fragmented, and can lead to negative consequences similar to those of sleep deprivation. |
| Nightmares are reported by approximately 20% of those with PTSD in the general population (Ohayon & Shapiro, 2000) and by about half of Vietnam veterans with PTSD (Neylan et al., 1998). | Systematic investigation of the content of the nightmares experienced by people with PTSD reveal that they tend to be threatening, but not always exact replicas of traumatic experiences. Posttraumatic nightmares seem to initially replicate the traumas, but tend to change over time to include threatening themes that are not directly trauma-related. In Chapter 4, we have discussed nightmare disorder and briefly reviewed treatments to reduce nightmares. In Chapter 9, we discuss strategies for dealing with postnightmare awakenings. |

Medications used for pain management can have an impact on sleep as well. Some are sedating, others disrupt sleep, and still others have mixed effects. For example, antidepressants are commonly used in the management of chronic pain—and, as discussed earlier in this chapter, some have sedating side effects and others cause sleep disruptions. Drowsiness is a common side effect of some pain medications. For example, two-thirds of people who take high doses of gabapentin, used for management of chronic pain (e.g., fibromyalgia and chronic neuropathic pain), experience *carryover sedation effects* (Moore, Wiffen, Derry, & McQuay, 2011). That is, the sedating effects of the pain medication extend to the morning, resulting in grogginess, difficulty getting out of bed, and extended time in bed. Moreover, waking up feeling drowsy is often interpreted as an indication that last night's sleep was of poor quality or insufficient, and that therefore one should try to get more sleep (i.e., should increase sleep effort).

## FEEDING AND EATING DISORDERS

Relatively little is known about sleep in patients with eating disorders. With respect to anorexia nervosa, it has been reported that severely underweight patients report poor sleep quality and reduced total sleep time, and that these symptoms improve with weight gain (Pieters, Theys, Vandereycken, Leroy, & Peuskens, 2004). With respect to bulimia nervosa, research suggests that patients report later bedtimes (Latzer, Tzischinsky, Epstein, Klein, & Peretz, 1999), potentially related to late evening binges (Benca & Schenck, 2005).

Night eating syndrome is classified in DSM-5 under other specified feeding or eating disorder. It is characterized by eating large amounts of food during the night with full awareness, or consuming large amounts of food after the evening meal. When awakened in the middle of the night, such patients often have difficulty returning to sleep unless they eat. Having been fully awake when they eat in the middle of the night, they remember having done so. They tend to have little appetite for breakfast and consume more than half of their daily calories after dinner. Their unusual eating habits can affect their sleep–wake circadian rhythm—as discussed in Chapter 2. Indeed, patients with night eating syndrome appear to have a 1- to 3-hour delay in their internal circadian clocks relative to controls (Goel et al., 2009).

ICSD-2 (American Academy of Sleep Medicine, 2005) includes a sleep-related eating disorder that is not included in DSM-5: nocturnal sleep-related eating disorder. This disorder involves consuming abnormal quantities of food while asleep. It belongs to a class of sleep disorders called *parasomnias*, which, as discussed in Chapter 4, includes a variety of abnormal or unwanted sleep-related behaviors, dreams, or autonomic changes manifested during sleep. Patients with nocturnal sleep-related eating disorder usually do not remember in the morning that they ate during the night and infer the presence of a nocturnal eating episode from evidence in their environment, such as empty food containers. The treatment of nocturnal sleep-related eating disorder and other parasomnias requires referral to a sleep specialist.

Both nocturnal sleep-related eating disorder and night eating syndrome are more common among women. These two disorders are understudied. We have included brief discussions of the two disorders because a mental health clinician may encounter patients with these behaviors, as they are more common among patients with eating disorders than in the population at large. At the time of this writing, empirically supported standard treatments for night eating syndrome have not been established (Howell, Schenck, & Crow, 2009). Proposed treatment for this syndrome is based on cognitive-behavioral principles (Allison, Stunkard, & Thier, 2004). As hybrids of eating and sleep disorders, these disorders may be best managed through collaboration between specialists in these two types of disorders.

## KEY PRACTICE IDEAS

- Insomnia disorder comorbid with other disorders warrants separate treatment attention, even when the comorbid disorders have an impact on sleep (e.g., chronic pain and depression).

- CBT-I has proven efficacy across the range of disorders, including MDD, bipolar, anxiety disorders, and pain syndromes, but there may be unique challenges in delivering CBT-I to these patients. Such challenges are not limited to, but include, the following:

  - Asking people with depression to limit their time in bed, when the bed is used as a coping strategy for emotional pain.
  - Asking those with PTSD to go to bed when sleepy, when they may be avoiding the bed/bedroom because they feel unsafe, vulnerable, or afraid of having a nightmare.
  - Asking individuals with pain to get out of bed at night, when they may be physically uncomfortable doing so.

- In subsequent chapters (Chapters 7 and 8), we provide specific advice on how to address these potential barriers to adherence.

# CHAPTER 6

# Assessment of Insomnia

The two primary clinical tools for the initial assessment in CBT-I are the insomnia intake interview and the sleep diary. Tools to track progress are the sleep diary (essential) and the Insomnia Severity Index (ISI; Morin, 1993; Morin, Belleville, Belanger, & Ivers, 2011; see Appendix B). The insomnia intake interview should be considered a complement to, rather than a substitute for, a full psychiatric intake interview. The insomnia interview we discuss here is also not a comprehensive sleep disorders intake, because it does not cover the full range of existing sleep disorders. Instead, the insomnia intake is focused on factors relevant to the patient's insomnia, which may include limited assessment of psychiatric, sleep, and other medical disorders. Specifically, the insomnia intake interview covers: the nature of the presenting sleep problem (i.e., history, current sleep habits, and daytime effects); unhealthy sleep practices, including evidence of sleep effort, substances, and other behaviors that disrupt sleep; underlying circadian tendency and circadian factors relevant to the presenting problem; evidence of hyperarousal, including conditioned arousal; presence of comorbidities (i.e., psychiatric, medical, and sleep disorders) and their impact on sleep; and treatment goals. The sleep diary provides prospective daily information about sleep that is more accurate than retrospective reports obtained during the insomnia intake interview. It is to be completed each morning throughout treatment and is used to guide treatment decisions, such as recommendations about the time in bed (discussed in Chapter 7). The sleep diary is also incorporated into behavioral experiments and cognitive components of treatment (discussed in Chapter 9).

## THE INSOMNIA INTAKE INTERVIEW

Creating a structure to the insomnia intake interview helps the clinician collect pertinent information with sufficient detail to permit a valid case conceptualization and treatment planning. People with insomnia are often relieved to have someone to talk to about their problem, because most of the time no one else expresses that much interest in or understanding of the nature of their sleep problem and its effects on their lives. When insomnia has lasted for years, the amount of information a patient wishes to convey may be overwhelming and difficult to sort through. The challenge is to balance empathy and active listening with a structure that permits efficiency and clarity. Creating structure and focus to the session can be done in a warm, empathic manner that does not interfere with the therapeutic alliance—which is essential to CBT-I, as it is to all forms of therapy.

An example of a form that can help structure the interview is the Insomnia Intake Form in Appendix A; it was adapted from the Insomnia Intake Form created by one of us (Rachel Manber) for the Insomnia and Behavioral Sleep Medicine Program at Stanford University. Using this or a similar form helps keep clinicians on track and promotes a comprehensive intake. When a patient volunteers information out of order, a therapist can find the right place on the form and note the information as it provided. This becomes easier with experience.

## Nature of the Current Sleep Problem

The intake interview usually begins with an open-ended question about the nature of the presenting problem(s), such as "Tell me about your problems with sleep." A patient will typically describe problems with initiating and/or maintaining sleep. If the patient has difficulty falling asleep initially and is also up in the middle of the night, the therapist should clarify which of the two is more problematic. This should be followed by a series of questions to gather details about the frequency, onset, course, precipitant(s), and past treatment(s). Later in the session, the clinician will gather detailed information about a typical night in a structured way, but at this point it is best simply to listen carefully to how the patient describes the problems and his or her level of distress about them. The following are sample questions for obtaining this information:

"How many nights a week do you have these problems?"
"When did the problems start?"
"What happened in your life around the time the problems started?"
"Has the nature of the problems changed since they started? How?"
"What have you tried to help the problems? How helpful were the treatments you received?"

Some patients may spontaneously describe the effects that their sleep difficulties have on their lives, but if they do not, then the clinician should ask about it: "What impact do your problems with sleep have on your life?" Patients most commonly describe the impact on their mood (e.g., irritability), energy level (e.g., mental and/or physical fatigue), and/or performance (e.g., cognitive or physical ability to perform their work or home roles). It is a good idea to ask about the impact of the problem on these and other specific domains that may be relevant to the patient—for instance, "Does poor sleep have an impact on your mood or concentration the next day?" It is important to clarify whether the patient is more distressed about the experience of not sleeping well or the specific negative consequences the next day: "Which is a bigger problem for you—not sleeping well at night, or the impact it has on you during the day?"

This initial discussion of the symptoms and their impact on the patient should provide sufficient information to determine whether the patient meets the main criteria for insomnia disorder (i.e., difficulty falling or staying asleep, occurring at least three times a week, associated with distress and impairment, and lasting at least 3 months). The rest of the interview is dedicated to gathering information to understand the nature of the sleep problem in more depth; assessing factors that affect each of the three aspects of sleep regulation (i.e., sleep drive, circadian factors, and arousal); and evaluating other factors that may be contributing to the sleep problem (e.g., comorbidities, substances, sleep environment, and sleep-incompatible behaviors).

## History of the Present Problem

The therapist should ask about when insomnia first emerged and about event(s) or life circumstances that may have precipitated insomnia. Sometimes there is no clear precipitant for the current insomnia episode, but there was one for a previous episode. Knowledge about precipitants of previous episodes will later help the therapist tailor the explanation of the etiological model of insomnia and conditioned arousal (Chapter 3) to the patient. Also relevant is the history of treatment. A patient may have already read self-help books and tried a variety of recommendations, with disappointing results. Knowledge about past failures may help prevent future failures. For example, the patient may have tried to always go to bed at the same time, but may still have had problems falling asleep because the issue of high cognitive arousal (Chapter 3) has not been addressed. Another patient may have been disappointed because he or she got out of bed when unable to sleep one night and still did not sleep well that night; this patient may have failed to understand that to be effective, this particular recommendation has to be followed consistently.

## Current Sleep Habits

A daily sleep diary, discussed later in this chapter, is an essential tool for the assessment of current sleep patterns, but diary data are not always available at the initial assessment interview. Chapter 11 describes the case of Sophie, to whom blank copies of the sleep diary form and instructions on how to complete the form were mailed ahead of the insomnia intake appointment; Chapter 12 provides another case example, in which copies of the sleep diary form were provided at the end of the insomnia intake appointment, and therefore diary data were not available at the time of initial assessment. Which of these two options for introducing the sleep diary is used depends on a therapist's preferences; on whether the therapist has already been seeing the patient for another problem (in which case the therapist can introduce the diary when the focus of therapy shifts to addressing insomnia); and on the availability of resources to mail or otherwise provide copies of the diary form ahead of the initial insomnia intake interview (which may depend on the type of practice setting). In this section, we discuss how to collect detailed information on sleep habits during the insomnia intake interview. Later in this chapter, we discuss how to use the diary data when these data become available.

During the interview, the therapist assesses specific domains; these are presented below chronologically, starting with bedtime and ending with rise time. For each of the domains, the key is to focus on the past week. For cases in which the past week was atypical, the therapist should focus on the most recent typical week and periodically remind the patient that the focus is on the past week. People with insomnia tend to describe night-to-night variability in sleep schedule and sleep difficulties, and thus when they are asked question about their sleep habits, they will preface their responses with the statement "It depends." The structured Insomnia Intake Form in Appendix A provides space to indicate the lower and upper ends of ranges in responses. One source of variability in sleep–wake schedules is related to the day of the week. Some people have a different bedtimes and rise times on weekdays (or workdays) versus weekends (or off-work days), which should also be probed and documented. When a patient answers, "It depends," the therapist can explore the sources of variability. For patients who have difficulty focusing on the past week or articulating the source of variability, the therapist can ask the following:

1. Ask about last night.
2. Ask about the worst night in the past week.
3. Ask about the number of times in the past week that a given pattern was present.

### Beginning of the Sleep Period

A good starting point is to ask about the time when the patient gets into bed and, separately, the time when the lights are turned out with the intention to sleep; these are often not the same time. For example, the patient may go to bed at 9:00 P.M. to read or watch a favorite TV program, and turn off the light when feeling drowsy or when the program ends. Sam's sleep diary (Chapter 12) revealed several nights in which he retired to bed early and did not attempt to sleep until much later. For most patients, turning the lights out signifies the intent to start sleeping now, but this is not always the case. Some patients may intentionally leave the lights on, or they may fall asleep in the middle of reading or listening to music. Others may turn off the light when they get into bed and lie in bed in the dark watching TV. In such a case, there may or may not be a specific time at which the patient intended to start sleeping; this is a point worth clarifying, because the answer can provide information about how the patient copes with difficulties in initiating sleep.

At this point it is often good to explore whether time is taken to unwind before bedtime by asking about activities during the 2 hours before going to bed. This is important, because failure to unwind before bedtime can lead to being too activated, which interferes with the natural, effortless unfolding of sleep. This is also a good time for the therapist to ask if the patient nods off to sleep in the evening when doing relaxing activities, such as watching TV. This is important because, as discussed in Chapter 2, brief sleep episodes close to bedtime can compromise the sleep drive at bedtime.

It is helpful to be curious about what determines when the patient goes to bed. Is it the clock? That is, does the person habitually go to bed at the same time because it is a reasonable "bedtime"? Does bedtime depend on when the bed partner goes to bed? Does it depend on how well the patient slept on previous nights or when he or she has to wake up the next morning? Does it depend on the schedule for the next day? Is the patient postponing bedtime due to fears of letting go of vigilance or of having negative experiences during sleep (e.g., nightmares or sleeplessness?)

Another aspect to explore with regard to bedtime is whether the patient feels sleepy at bedtime. It may be helpful to distinguish between being sleepy and being tired; patients with insomnia tend to use the terms interchangeably. As mentioned in Chapter 2, *sleepiness* refers to the propensity to fall asleep when given the opportunity, and *tiredness* refers to a low energy level that does not necessarily reflect the propensity to fall asleep. Thus, whereas tiredness signals the need for rest, sleepiness signals the need to sleep. Many patients with difficulties falling asleep are not sleepy at bedtime; they may be "tired, but wired."

Next, the therapist turns attention to how long it usually takes to fall asleep. If the patient has difficulty falling asleep, what does the patient do when unable to fall asleep quickly? For example, is the patient staying in bed *trying* to sleep? Ideally the therapist is attuned to subtle indications of "trying to sleep." Even trying to be still or not think of anything is a "trying to sleep" behavior. It is best to start with an open-ended inquiry and follow up with clarifications as needed. The short excerpt from an interview below demonstrates the assessment of the early night sleep habits and behaviors.

THERAPIST: When do you typically go to bed?

PATIENT: I am not sure I have a bedtime. Maybe 9 or 10 P.M.?

THERAPIST: It may help if we focus on the past week. Would it be accurate to say that in the past week you went to sleep between 9 and 10 P.M.?

PATIENT: Hmmm, I think so. Maybe it is closer to 10 P.M. on the weekend and closer to 9 or 9:30 P.M. during the week.

THERAPIST: OK, great. So you get into bed around 9 or 9:30 P.M. during the week and closer to 10 P.M. on weekends. Do you intend to fall asleep at those times, or do you do something in bed before you shut your eyes, such as watching television or reading?

PATIENT: It depends.

THERAPIST: Let's focus on last week again. Can you answer the question just about last week?

PATIENT: During the week, I get into bed and turn out the lights right away. I am tired and I have to get up for work, so I am trying to start sleeping early. But on the weekend, for some reason, I like to relax in bed before I turn out the light. I used to read in bed, but I heard that's not a good idea. I try and relax, maybe breathe. Unfortunately, I think about work, even though it is the weekend—particularly on Friday night.

THERAPIST: So during the week, your bedtime is pretty much the time at which you try to fall asleep, but on the weekend, you spend a little time in bed, awake and trying to relax before turning out the lights to attempt to sleep?

PATIENT: Yes. On weeknights I don't want to do anything that will make me sleep less.

THERAPIST: I see; you are concerned your wind-down period could cut into your sleep period. Is the relaxation helpful?

PATIENT: Not really. Nothing seems helpful any more.

### Middle of the Night

The following are examples of questions for gathering details about middle-of-the-night awakenings:

"Do you wake up in the middle of the night? If so, how many times? When?"
"How long does it take you to fall back asleep?"
"Is one of these awakenings long? If so, how long is it? When does it tend to occur?"
"In total, how long are you awake in the middle of the night (counting across all awakenings)?"

If the patient experiences prolonged middle-of-the-night awakening(s), the therapist needs to find out what the patient does when awake in the middle of the night:

> "Do you get out of bed? If so, what do you do when you get out of bed?"
> "How do you decide when to get back into bed?"

### End of the Night

To explore end-of-the-night experiences, the therapist asks about morning wake-up time and about when the patient gets out of bed. These may not be the same times. Also, how do these times vary from day to day and between weekend days and weekdays? And is awakening spontaneous, or does the patient use an alarm or rely on another external source (e.g., bed partner, pet)? For example, the therapist can ask, "Do you set an alarm? If so, do you wake up before the alarm sounds?" If the patient does not use an alarm, it is important to ask, "Do you wake up earlier than you wish?" And explore "how much earlier?" If the patient wakes up too early relative to the desired wake time, the therapist will later use the assessment guidelines below to ascertain whether this is related to having a morningness tendency (first discussed in Chapter 2). Because people with depression can have greater problems with waking up too early than people who are not depressed, the possibility of depression will need to be explored.

Some patients have difficulty waking up in the morning. This possibility needs to be asked about and further explored. Examples of questions to explore this issue are as follows:

> "Do you use the snooze button several times before finally getting out of bed?"
> "When you finally get up, how long does it take you to become fully awake?"

If the patient has difficulty waking up in the morning, the therapist should later use the assessment guidelines below to ascertain whether this is related to having an eveningness tendency (again, first discussed in Chapter 2).

### Estimated Total Nocturnal Sleep Time

The therapist can compute the patient's total time asleep from information about total time in bed and reported unwanted wakefulness. However, it is also clinically informative to find out the patient's estimate of sleep duration, on average or on a typical night, because it allows the therapist to assess potential reporting biases. People with insomnia often underestimate the time they spend asleep. It is too soon at this very early phase of treatment to discuss a discrepancy between computed and reported total time asleep. Such discussion, which requires time and needs to be approached delicately, is best postponed until the patient is ready and as relevant to treatment (see Chapter 7). At this point, the therapist should simply obtain the estimate(s).

## Premorbid Sleep Schedule

The next task is to determine whether the patient's premorbid sleep schedule is different from the current one. A good first question for this is "When did you go to bed and wake up before you had problems sleeping?" If the patient's premorbid sleep schedule is different from the current schedule, the therapist may want to ask about reasons for the schedule change. Most commonly, when patients alter their times into and out of bed, they do so in order to cope with insufficient sleep; the end result is an extension of the time they are in bed relative to the premorbid time. Knowing the patient's premorbid sleep schedule and, if different, why it was changed can later assist in tailoring the behavioral interventions to the patient's current presentation and explaining its rationale (Chapter 7). Less commonly, when fear of sleep is present, the change in sleep schedule results in reduction in total time in bed. These issues are discussed in Chapters 7 and 9, and illustrated in the two case examples in Chapters 11 and 12. Regardless, knowing about changes to sleep schedule relative to times before insomnia started provides insight into the patient's response to insomnia and associated maladaptive cognitions that will be targeted later during treatment.

## Medications for Sleep

When asking about all medications taken to help with sleep, the therapist should inquire about both prescribed and over-the-counter drugs, including herbal preparations: "Do you take medications to help you sleep? If so, what medications do you take?" "What about health food formulas?" For a prescribed medication, it is important to know:

"Who is prescribing this medication?"
"What is the dose?"
"When did you start taking the medication?"
"How many nights per week do you take it?"
"Do you take the medication before or at bedtime? Do you take sleep medication in the middle of the night?"
"Do you take it just when you go to bed or do you take it after you first try to sleep without it?"

The answer to the last question above can be particularly informative, because clinicians may prescribe a sleep aid to be taken when needed (i.e., p.r.n.). This means that a patient may be attempting to sleep without the medication, and then taking it only if experiencing problems falling asleep. When taking hypnotics nightly in this fashion (e.g., contingent upon an initial sleep failure), the patient may come to view the medication as a "rescue" and may therefore be at risk for developing psychological dependence. In Table 6.1, we list current sleep medications approved by the U.S. Food and Drug Administration (FDA), as well as typical dosages.

The therapist should also pay attention to the time of ingestion and the half-life of each medication taken to promote sleep. The *half-life* of a medication is the time it takes for it to reach half its potency. Sleep medications with a long half-life have the advantage of helping with sleep maintenance, but can have carryover effects in the morning (making it difficult for the patient to wake up), and in some cases can have effects later in the day. This can create anxiety, because the sluggishness can be misattributed to the sleep problem instead of the medication, and this increases the pressure to fix the sleep problem. The problem with such carryover effects is most pronounced when a medication that is taken in the middle of the night has a half-life that is lon-

**TABLE 6.1. FDA–Approved Sleep Medications**

| Name[a] | Lowest recommended dose | Half-life |
|---|---|---|
| Estazolam (Prosom) | 1 mg | 10–24 hours |
| Triazolam (Halcion) | 0.125 mg | 2–6 hours |
| Temazepam (Restoril) | 15 mg | 8–20 hours |
| Flurazepam (Dalmane) | 15 mg | 48–120 hours |
| Quazepam (Doral) | 7.5 | 39–73 hours |
| Eszopiclone (Lunesta) | 1 mg | 6 hours |
| Zaleplon (Sonata) | 5 mg | 1 hour |
| Zolpidem (Ambien) | 5 mg | 1.5–2.4 hours |
| Zolpidem-ER | 6.25 mg | 1.6–4.5 hours |
| Ramelteon (Rozerem) | 8 mg | 0.8–2 hours |
| Doxepin (Silenor) | 3 mg | 17 hours |

[a]Trade names are given in parentheses.

ger than the time between its ingestion and the planned wake-up time. In such cases, the patient may experience sluggishness and impaired judgment, and may therefore be at increased risk for accidents. This issue may also be relevant to safe implementation of certain CBT-I instructions, such as the recommendation to get out of bed at the same time each morning (see Chapter 7). A different problem is that sleep medications with a short half-life may not be helpful for end-of-night sleep disruptions. This problem is most pronounced when a medication with a short half-life is taken earlier than bedtime. The issues discussed above also apply to other substances taken by patients to help them sleep—not only over-the-counter sleep aids and herbal supplements, but alcohol (additionally discussed below) and marijuana.

## Napping Behaviors

*Napping* refers to actually falling asleep at a time other than the main nocturnal sleep episode and is distinct from resting. Recall from Chapter 3 that people with insomnia have high scores on the multiple sleep latency test (MSLT), which means that they are not physiologically sleepy. Therefore, for most people with insomnia, the relevant clinical question is whether they are able to nap—for example, "If you had the right opportunity and conditions, and you lay down for a nap, would you be able to fall asleep?" If a patient is able to nap, the therapist needs to inquire about the frequency, length, and timing of daytime naps. Separate questions should be asked about resting while lying down during the day, in order to assess the presence of dozing (brief sleep episodes). Naps and/or frequent dozing, particularly in the evening, can diminish an individual's sleep drive and compromise nocturnal sleep. Both Sophie and Sam (introduced in Chapter 1 and further discussed in Chapters 11 and 12) tried to nap/rest. Sophie regularly attempted to nap in order to make up for lost sleep at night. Her resting behavior represented high sleep effort (Chapter 3), and on occasions when she dozed off, her sleep drive at bedtime was compromised. Moreover, since she rested with the intent to sleep, she created opportunities for strengthening the bed as a cue for wakefulness rather than sleep (conditioned arousal, discussed in Chapter 3). Sam lay down to rest several times a day, in part because of chronic fibromyalgia pain and in part because he hoped to get some sleep. His resting often included periods of dozing and even some short naps, thus (as in Sophie's case) compromising his sleep drive and strengthening conditioned arousal.

## Sleep Environment

It is important to know if the sleep environment is conducive to sleep. Specifically, the environment needs to be safe, dark, quiet, comfortable, and not too warm. Is the bed shared? If so, does the bed partner interfere with the patient's sleep (for example by snoring)? Do pets interfere with sleep? Are there caregiving issues?

## Other Behaviors That Can Affect Sleep

### Substance Use

The therapist needs to assess whether substances that impact sleep are used, and, if so, which ones are used and when they are consumed. These include stimulants, such as caffeine, nicotine, prescription and nonprescription medications with stimulating side effects, and some illicit drugs, as well as alcohol, which is a central nervous system depressant. It is also important to ask about "energy" drinks, as the caffeine content in these beverages can be extremely high. Asking about "energy" drinks is particularly important when assessing young adults. In the context of a sleep assessment, it is particularly important to know the proximity of ingestion relative to bedtime, in order to assess the possibility that the substance interferes with sleep; again, the substance's half-life must be taken into account.

Because caffeine, nicotine, and alcohol are widely used, we provide information about their impact on sleep and factors that may moderate this impact.

Caffeine is a relatively long-acting stimulant, with a somewhat unpredictable half-life (4.5 hours on average). Caffeine has a longer half-life when consumed in conjunction with oral contraceptives, hormone replacement therapy, and SSRIs, and a shorter half-life when consumed in conjunction with nicotine. Caffeine's negative effects on sleep—namely, longer sleep onset, less stage N3 sleep, and/or more fragmented sleep—depend on the amount consumed and are related to reducing the homeostatic sleep drive by binding to the adenosine receptors (Fredholm, Battig, Holmen, Nehlig, & Zvartau, 1999). See Chapter 2 for a discussion of the role of adenosine in sleep regulation. Individual sensitivity to the effects of caffeine on sleep may be related to genetic factors (Retey et al., 2007) and aging (Drapeau et al., 2006). Whereas Sophie had stopped caffeine consumption altogether, Sam's insomnia intake interview revealed that he drank as many as four caffeinated beverages per day, and did so as late as 9:00 P.M.

Nicotine is a stimulant with a short half-life (i.e., approximately 2 hours). It causes sleep fragmentation and sleep initiation difficulties. Nicotine withdrawal is associated with significant sleep disturbance, but nicotine replacement treatment (e.g., a nicotine patch) is associated with better sleep than during smoking (Wetter, Fiore, Baker, & Young, 1995). Despite its being classified as a stimulant, people often report that nicotine is "relaxing." This is likely because each dose of nicotine relaxes the tension and agitation that were produced by withdrawal from the previous nicotine consumption.

Alcohol may be consumed socially in the evening or at bedtime, as a form of self-medication (Ancoli-Israel & Roth, 1999). Its effects on sleep are dose- and time-dependent, with higher dose and closer proximity to the sleep period having greater impact on sleep. Alcohol facilitates sleep onset at the beginning of the night, but later in the night, elimination of alcohol from the bloodstream causes wakefulness (Landolt, Roth, Dijk, & Borbely, 1996; Roehrs, Zwyghuizen-Doorenbos, & Roth, 1993). There are individual differences in the metabolism of alcohol and its central effects, including on sleep disruptions in the middle of the night and REM suppression. The clinician is advised to take a conservative approach. In our experience, in some sensitive individuals, drinking two glasses of wine with dinner 4 hours before bedtime can have detrimental effects on sleep. When consumed at bedtime, alcohol leads to suppression of REM sleep in the first half of the night, with a rebound (longer REM episodes) in the second half. Alcohol also increases sleep apnea severity (Taasan, Block, Boysen, & Wynne, 1981). When consumed in the middle of the night, alcohol may have carryover sedating effects the next morning.

## Exercise and Daytime Activity Levels

It is important to assess the timing of physical activities relative to bedtime, because vigorous exercise less than 4 hours before sleep is thought to interfere with sleep (see Buxton, Lee, L'Hermite-Baleriaux, Turek, & Van Cauter, 2003). The therapist can start by asking, "When do you exercise?" If the answer is a time that is within or close to the start of the 4-hour window, the therapist should find out how vigorous it is by asking, "What type of exercise do you do at that time?"

Intellectual and social stimulation during the day should also be assessed. Earlier in the insomnia intake interview, the therapist will have asked about unwinding routines, which are particularly relevant to an overstimulated person who is busy and on the go until close to bedtime. It is also important to find out whether the patient is understimulated, including whether there have been changes in level of stimulation—such as a shift from an active to a less active life (e.g., in association with retirement or children leaving the home), or a change in response to having insomnia. Being understimulated or socially isolated can lead to spending prolonged time in bed; as discussed in Chapter 3, this can lead to conditioned arousal.

## Eating at Night

Certain eating behaviors can disturb sleep. For example, eating a heavy meal close to bedtime, or grazing on high-calorie snacks all evening, may lead to indigestion and gastrointestinal reflux during the night and may cause wakefulness. Some patients eat in the middle of the night when unable to sleep. This may be a habit they acquired, or it may be related to a belief that certain foods will help them sleep. In either case, this is not a good habit, because engaging in any wake activity can destabilize the circadian clock.

## Cognitive and Emotional Hyperarousal

In Chapter 3, we have discussed the role of cognitive arousal in insomnia disorder and provided a few examples of sleep-interfering beliefs and cognitions. Such cognitions often emerge spontaneously during the insomnia intake interview. As the patient describes his or her sleeping problems and their impact on the patient's life, the therapist is advised to stay attuned to expressions of distress about and preoccupation with sleep, the personal meaning of having insomnia, beliefs about sleep, and fears about the consequences of poor sleep. The patient may also describe behaviors providing indirect evidence that unhelpful beliefs about sleep may be present. These behaviors may constitute manifestations of sleep effort. For example, following rigid rules and rituals concerning sleep is usually motivated by a belief that sleep is very fragile and one should be careful to set the stage right for sleep (a safety behavior). As the insomnia intake interview unfolds, the therapist should write down direct statements and indirect evidence of cognitive arousal, so that they can be later addressed during treatment. Table 6.2 lists questions that can be used to assess sleep-related cognitions, as well as the cognitive domains (all previously discussed in Chapter 3) that responses are likely to fall into.

A validated questionnaire that assesses cognitions about sleep, such as the 16-item version of the Dysfunctional Beliefs and Attitudes about Sleep (DBAS-16; Morin, Vallieres, & Ivers, 2007), can assist in evaluating beliefs and cognitions about sleep. Patients are asked to rate the extent to which each of 16 statements listed is true for them on a 10-point Likert scale. These 16 statements are listed in Table 6.3; the DBAS-16 itself is provided in Appendix B. Each statement falls into one of four categories: (1) catastrophic worries about the consequences of sleep loss, (2) misattribution about causes of insomnia and insomnia symptoms, (3) unrealistic beliefs about sleep needs, and (4) viewing sleep as unpredictable and out of one's control. The DBAS-16 is scored by adding the score on each item that was rated, and dividing by the number of items rated. Total scores above 3.8 are suggestive of an unhelpful degree of beliefs about sleep (Carney et al., 2010). The therapist can note items that are endorsed higher than 5 and use cognitive therapy techniques to address them. (Again, cognitive techniques are discussed in Chapter 9.)

The therapist can also assess emotions and the emotional intensity associated with specific thoughts by directly asking how a thought makes the patient feel, as well as general emotional arousal. For example, the therapist can ask, "How do you feel when you are in bed trying to sleep? Are you anxious? Are you frustrated? Is your mind still?"

## Chronotype (Morningness–Eveningness)

In Chapter 2, we have discussed the circadian clock and its relevance to the regulation of sleep. We have also discussed circadian preferences (chronotype) for morningness or eveningness, and their relationship to the period of the internal circadian clock. Clinicians cannot directly assess the circadian clock, because research procedures for such assessments are not clinically feasible, but they can and should assess chronotype (morningness–eveningness tendencies). Such assessment is based on clinical features, such as lifelong sleep–wake schedule preferences, particularly during periods of few or no environmental constraints on the sleep–wake schedule. Patients' current sleep habits provide some indication about circadian tendencies. However, a current

**TABLE 6.2. Examples of Questions to Assess Sleep-Related Beliefs and Cognitions That Could Interfere with Sleep**

| Assessment question | Cognitive domain |
|---|---|
| "What do you tend to think about while lying awake in bed?" | Sleep-interfering thoughts (worries about general life stressors) or sleep-interpreting thoughts (beliefs and worries about sleep) |
| "You told me that your sleep problem makes it is difficult [to do your work]. What are you aware of during your day when you are [trying to work]?"<br><br>"You told me that it is difficult to sleep when you notice [a noise]. What are you aware of when you are trying to sleep?" | Excessive monitoring for sleep threats (e.g., monitoring poor performance during the day, monitoring the sleep environment for suboptimal conditions such as noise or an internal symptom) |
| "What do you do after a particularly poor night of sleep?"<br><br>"What do you do in the evening to increase the likelihood that you will sleep well?" | Engagement in safety behaviors (e.g., calling in sick after a night of poor sleep to protect from anticipated poor performance that might follow) |
| "What do you worry will happen if you sleep poorly?"<br><br>"How much sleep do you think you need? Why?"<br><br>"What do you see as the primary cause of your insomnia?" | Beliefs, expectations about sleep, and personal meaning of having insomnia (see the Dysfunctional Beliefs and Attitudes about Sleep–16 [DBAS-16] questions in Table 6.3 and Appendix B) |
| "What do you do to produce sleep?"<br><br>"What do you do to make up for lost sleep?" | Covert and overt examples of sleep effort (e.g., taking substances, increasing the amount of time spent in bed); avoidance behaviors (e.g., avoiding social activities in the evening) |
| "What do you do to cope with not getting enough sleep?" | Sleep-interpreting thoughts (e.g., belief that one cannot cope with sleep loss) |

*Note.* Text in brackets provides a specific example that is meant to illustrate a general point; this text can be replaced with other wording as appropriate to a particular patient.

late or early sleep schedule is sometimes dictated by current life circumstances, and therefore additional features should be probed. There are validated questionnaires (e.g., Horne & Ostberg, 1976; Smith, Reilly, & Midkiff, 1989) to assess morningness–eveningness. However, because patients' responses to these questionnaires may be skewed by social desirability, we recommend direct assessment of circadian tendencies during the insomnia intake interview, and we provide guidelines for this assessment below.

According to research discussed in Chapter 2, eveningness and morningness tendencies are correlated with delayed and advanced circadian clocks, respectively. Moreover, people with circadian rhythm sleep–wake disorder, delayed sleep phase type, have an eveningness tendency. Similarly, people with circadian rhythm sleep–wake disorder, advanced sleep phase type, have a morningness tendency. However, in either case, the reverse is not always true. When a patient describes features consistent with an eveningness or morningness chronotype, differential diagnosis between insomnia and circadian rhythm sleep–wake disorders, delayed or advanced sleep phase types, needs to be considered. As discussed in Chapter 4, these differential diagnoses hinge upon the following key distinguishing feature: Unlike persons with either of these two types of circadian rhythm sleep–wake disorder, persons with insomnia have disturbed sleep even when going to sleep at a time consistent with their chronotype (i.e., very late for a person with a delayed type, and very early for a person with an advanced type). To enhance the flow of the insomnia intake interview, we have included in the assessment of circadian tendency a question about a key factor that differentiates insomnia from circadian rhythm sleep–wake disorders. The interview flows well in this way, because the diagnoses of these two types of circadian rhythm sleep–wake disorders are applicable only for those with eveningness or morningness tendency.

## TABLE 6.3. Items from the Dysfunctional Beliefs and Attitudes about Sleep (DBAS–16) Scale

1. I need 8 hours of sleep to feel refreshed and function well during the day.

2. When I don't get the proper amount of sleep on a given night, I need to catch up on the next day by napping or on the next night by sleeping longer.

3. I am concerned that chronic insomnia may have serious consequences on my physical health.

4. I am worried that I may lose control over my abilities to sleep.

5. After a poor night's sleep, I know that it will interfere with my activities the next day.

6. In order to be alert and function well during the day, I believe I would be better off taking a sleeping pill rather than having a poor night's sleep.

7. When I feel irritable, depressed, or anxious during the day, it is mostly because I did not sleep well the night before.

8. When I sleep poorly on one night, I know it will disturb my sleep schedule for the whole week.

9. Without an adequate night's sleep, I can hardly function the next day

10. I can't ever predict whether I'll have a good or poor night's sleep.

11. I have little ability to manage the negative consequences of disturbed sleep.

12. When I feel tired, have no energy, or just seem not to function well during the day, it is generally because I did not sleep well the night before.

13. I believe insomnia is essentially the result of a chemical imbalance.

14. I feel insomnia is ruining my ability to enjoy life and prevents me from doing what I want.

15. Medication is probably the only solution to sleeplessness.

16. I avoid or cancel obligations (social, family) after a poor night's sleep.

*Note.* Adapted from Morin, Vallieres, and Ivers (2007). Copyright 2007 by Charles M. Morin. Adapted by permission.

### Assessing Evening Tendency

The assessment of an evening tendency is summarized in Table 6.4. It is best to start by focusing on the patient's experience of waking up in the morning, because a lifelong pattern of difficulties with morning waking is the most prominent aspect of having an eveningness chronotype. The assessment can begin thus: "How easy it is for you to wake up in the morning? Do you need to hit the snooze button several times in the morning? If so, how long has this been a problem?" In interpreting the responses, the therapist should keep in mind that some life circumstances, such as needing to attend to young children's needs every morning, can cause a physiological advance in the circadian clock and make it easier to wake up in the morning. However, difficulties in waking up usually resurface when such a patient stops maintaining an early and fixed rise time, as life circumstances change. Therefore, it is good to be particularly curious about preferred wake times

---

**TABLE 6.4. Assessment of Eveningness Tendency**

---

1. **Ease of waking up on the morning at a socially conventional time**

   *Lead-in questions*: "Is it difficult for you to wake up in the morning?"
   "When you wake up in the morning, are you usually fully awake within half an hour or so, or does it take you much longer than that?"

   *Follow-up questions, depending on response, to assess level of potential eveningness*: "How many times do you use the snooze button on your alarm clock?"
   "When you were in high school, how late did you sleep in on the weekends?"
   "What about college? Did you avoid morning classes?"

2. **Bedtime preference**

   *Lead-in questions*: "If you did not have to wake up early and there were no negative consequences if you woke up late, would you prefer go to bed very late? If so, when?"

   *Follow-up questions, depending on response, to assess level of potential eveningness*: "Do you find it difficult to stop what you are doing and go to bed?"

3. **Associated features**

   "Do you sleep better in the first or second part of the night?" (Patients with eveningness tendency report their best sleep is in the second part of the night.)

   Do the patient's sleep habits (explored earlier) evidence an irregular sleep–wake schedule?

4. **Self-identification**

   "Some people think of themselves as 'night owls.' Are you one of them?"

5. **Differential diagnosis of circadian rhythm sleep–wake disorder, delayed sleep phase type**

   "Do you have difficulty falling asleep when you go to bed at a conventional clock time?"

   "Do you still have problems falling asleep when you go to bed very late?"

---

during periods of life during which people tend to be relatively free to wake up when desired (e.g., on weekends and holidays, or during adolescence and the young adult years). For example, the therapist can ask, "When you were in high school, did you sleep in late on weekends? If so, how late?" (A response endorsing preference for waking up after 10 in the morning is consistent with an eveningness tendency; a preference for waking up after the noon hour reflects a very strong eveningness tendency.) If the patient went to college, it can help to ask, "Did you avoid morning classes when you were in college?" (People with a definite eveningness chronotype usually whole-heartedly say yes.) Another useful question is "How long does it take for you to feel fully awake after you first wake up in the morning?" People with an eveningness chronotype take a while to feel fully alert. Then the therapist can focus on the period around bedtime: "If you did not have to wake up early and there were no negative consequences if you did, would you prefer go to bed very late? If so, at what time? Is it difficult for you to disengage from what you do in the evening?" As discussed in Chapter 7, difficulty in disengaging from activities before bedtime may also make it difficult for a patient to follow some behavioral components of CBT-I.

When a therapist is assessing a person with an eveningness chronotype, it is also necessary to consider the possibility that circadian sleep–wake disorder, delayed sleep phase type (Chapter 4) may be present. For example, if the patient has difficulty falling asleep, the therapist can ask, "Would you still have difficulty falling asleep if you went to bed very late [or at the patient's stated preferred bedtime]?" (Recall that people with circadian sleep–wake disorder, delayed sleep phase type, have normal sleep if they go to bed very late.)

### Assessing Morning Tendency

The assessment of morning tendency is summarized in Table 6.5. Maintaining an early sleep schedule is not always an indication of morning tendency. Waking up early may be dictated by life circumstances (such as job start time or child care) or by having depression (see Chapter 5). The focus should be on a lifetime pattern. If the current sleep schedule is early relative to conventional time, the therapist can ask:

"Have you always gone to sleep earlier than most people you know?"
"Is it difficult for you to stay up until a conventional bedtime? For example, if you were attempting to stay up later, would you doze off unintentionally in the evening?"
"Have you always woken up early in the morning, even when you could sleep in as long as you wished?"
"Do you still wake up early even if you went to sleep late?"

When a therapist is assessing a person with a morningness chronotype, it is also necessary to consider the possibility that circadian rhythm sleep–wake disorder, advanced sleep phase type (Chapter 4), may be present..

## Common Comorbid Sleep Disorders

There is not enough time during an insomnia intake interview to conduct a comprehensive assessment of all existing sleep disorders. It is therefore most parsimonious to limit the focus

## TABLE 6.5. Assessment of Morningness Tendency

1. **Difficulty staying up until a desired (socially conventional) bedtime**

   *Lead-in questions:* "Is it difficult for you to stay up in the evening?"
   "Do you doze off in the evening when you are not engaged in stimulating activities?"
   "Have you always gone to sleep earlier than most people you know?"

   *Follow-up questions, depending on response, to assess level of potential morningness:*
   "Are you avoiding social activities in the evening because it is difficult to stay awake?"

2. **Lifelong tendency to wake up early to start the day**

   *Lead-in questions:* "Are you able to sleep in if you wish and if circumstances allow?"
   "Have you always awakened early in the morning, even when you could sleep in as long as you wish?"

   *Follow-up questions, depending on response, to assess level of potential morningness:*
   "When you were in high school, how late did you sleep in on the weekends?"
   "Did you still wake up early even if you went to sleep late?"

3. **Self-identification**

   "Some people think of themselves as 'morning people.' Are you one of them?"

4. **Differential diagnosis of circadian rhythm sleep–wake disorder, advanced sleep phase type**

   "Do you wake up much earlier than you wish at a time that is earlier than is conventional?"

   "Do you still wake up early even if you go to bed very late?"

---

to sleep disorders that are most likely to be experienced by patients with insomnia. These are circadian rhythm sleep–wake disorder (delayed and advanced sleep phase types), obstructive sleep apnea hypopnea (OSAH), restless legs syndrome (RLS), and nightmare disorder. The form Assessment of Other Sleep Disorders (see Appendix A) can be used as a guide for assessing these sleep disorders. Examples of this form as used in the assessment of the two cases introduced at the beginning of the book can be found in Chapters 11 and 12, respectively. The diagnostic and clinical features of each of these disorders have been discussed in Chapter 4; here we focus on their assessment. In Chapter 10, we discuss how to use the information gathered during the assessment when planning and implementing treatment.

### Circadian Rhythm Sleep–Wake Disorder, Delayed and Advanced Sleep Phase Types

Having just completed the assessment of circadian tendencies, including the extra questions distinguishing insomnia from circadian rhythm sleep–wake disorder, the therapist has most of the information needed for a diagnosis of either type of this disorder. Circadian rhythm sleep–wake disorder, delayed or advanced sleep phase type, will be diagnosed if there is a recurrent inability to fall asleep and wake up at desired conventional clock times, but there is no problem

with sleep when patients are allowed to use their preferred schedules. That is, there is no problem with sleep except for when sleep occurs early relative to the biological clock among patients
with the delayed sleep phase type, and later relative to the biological clock for those with the
advanced sleep phase type.

### Obstructive Sleep Apnea Hypopnea

As discussed in Chapter 4, a diagnosis of OSAH requires an overnight sleep study. However, clinical symptoms of OSAH can and should be assessed, both because it may be important for the
patient's health and therefore when suspected should be followed by referral for further assessment and treatment, and also because the presence of OSAH may require some modification to
the standard CBT-I protocol. (See Chapters 7 and 11.) The therapist should ask about the most
prominent features of OSAH, which are loud snoring, witnessed apnea, experiences of waking
up gasping for air or choking, and marked daytime sleepiness. The presence of any one of these
symptoms indicates that OSAH is likely; the greater the number of symptoms, the greater the
likelihood. A greater frequency or severity of symptoms also increases the likelihood of OSAH.
Suggested questions for these symptoms are as follows:

- *Loud snoring*: "Have you been told by others that you snore loudly? If so, is the snoring
  loud enough that it can be heard in a different room?"
- *Witnessed apnea*: "Has anyone told you that they saw you stop breathing while you sleep?"
- *Gasping/choking experience*: "Have you ever awakened gasping for air or choking?"
- *Marked sleepiness*: "Are you sleepy during the day? If so, do you fall asleep or doze off unintentionally during the day?" If yes, "Describe situations during which you are likely to fall
  asleep. How likely are you to doze off during the day in the following situations: sitting in
  a meeting, watching TV, reading, driving, performing your work?"

A note about sleepiness is in order: The greater the number of situations the patient endorses
as likely to be associated with dozing off, the greater the severity of daytime sleepiness. Similarly,
the more unusual and uncommon the situations the patient endorses as likely to be associated
with dozing off, the greater the severity of daytime sleepiness. For example, dozing off in situations that are dangerous (e.g., while driving) or in situations in which most people will not (e.g.,
while talking) suggests marked and excessive daytime sleepiness.

Mild OSAH may be present even if none of the four core symptoms are present. For example, snoring may be present, but may not be loud. In such cases, additional clinical features can
be assessed, particularly if the patient is at risk for OSAH (e.g., obese [body mass index* > 30],
older, or hypertensive). These include waking up in the morning feeling unrefreshed despite
adequate sleep duration, or with a headache, dry mouth, or drooling. The latter two may be
signs of mouth breathing, common when there is an obstruction in the nasal passages. Frequent
urination (more than twice per night; can also be a consequence of OSAH (Pressman, Figueroa,
Kendrick-Mohamed, Greenspon, & Peterson, 1996).

---

*Body mass index is computed by dividing weight in pounds (or kilograms) by height in inches (or centimeters) and,
if using the nonmetric system, multiplying the result by 703.

In the case of a patient previously diagnosed with OSAH, the therapist should inquire about treatment. If OSAH was previously diagnosed and successfully treated but the patient reports loss of some benefits, such as feeling less refreshed in the morning or more sleepy during the day compared to when first treated, the therapist should reassess OSAH. For example, some patients who have been treated surgically may experience recurrence of OSAH. As discussed in Chapter 4, continuous positive airway pressure (CPAP) is the standard treatment for OSAH, but adherence can be challenging. Some patients who were prescribed CPAP do not use it at all or use it "every once in a while." Others may begin the night with the mask on, but remove it knowingly or unknowingly in the middle of the night. The insomnia intake interview provides an opportunity to identify patients who were prescribed CPAP but do not use it at a therapeutic level. For minimal meaningful benefits, CPAP should be used at least 4 hours per night for at least five nights per week, but more frequent and longer nightly use is better. If CPAP was prescribed, the therapist should ask how many nights a week it is used and for how many hours per night. (Most contemporary CPAP units monitor adherence.) Sam had OSAH. He was prescribed CPAP and used it nightly, but his insomnia intake interview revealed that when he woke up, the mask was often no longer on his face. He did not remember having taken it off, and therefore it was not clear if he was using it for at least 4 hours. If adherence is suboptimal, as in Sam's case, the therapist should encourage a follow-up with a sleep specialist to explore obstacles to adherence and address them. In Sam's case, a simple instruction to replace the mask when he found it removed in the middle of the night was helpful in improving his overall CPAP use (see Chapter 12). As we discuss in Chapter 10, when OSAH is not or inadequately treated, the therapist should consult with the patient's sleep specialist to decide jointly on whether to proceed with CBT-I or postpone CBT-I until after the patient's OSAH has been adequately treated.

### Restless Legs Syndrome

The clinical features of RLS have been described in Chapter 4, where we have also indicated that a diagnosis of RLS does not require an overnight sleep study. A positive diagnosis of RLS requires the presence of an urge to move the legs. This urge is often associated with unpleasant, restless feelings in the legs. When asked to describe the feeling preceding the urge to move the legs, patients may struggle to find a good description. It is certainly unpleasant and felt deep in the leg, and it is associated with an urge to move the leg. Some words used by patients to describe the sensation include *tingling, pulling, burning, grabbing, itching,* and *electric.* In addition to the urges to move the legs, the diagnosis requires that the urge be worse during rest or inactivity, that it be temporarily relieved by moving, and that it begin or get worse in the evening or at night. The following single question has high specificity and sensitivity for diagnosis of RLS: "When you try to relax in the evening or sleep at night, do you ever have unpleasant, restless feelings in your legs that can be relieved by walking or movement?" (Ferri et al., 2007, p. 1016). Notice that this is a compound question that incorporates all four diagnostic symptoms of RLS. For a patient previously diagnosed with RLS, the therapist should inquire about treatment. If RLS is present but not treated, the patient should be referred for medical treatment. As discussed in Chapter 4, the majority of patients with RLS also have periodic limb movement disorder (PLMD), a disorder that is diagnosed mostly on the basis of PSG and is difficult to assess in its absence.

*Nightmare Disorder*

As discussed in Chapter 4, the most difficult aspect of assessing nightmare disorder is determining the presence of nightmares, because sometimes what patients refer to as *nightmares* may not meet the diagnostic criteria discussed in Chapter 4. The therapist may begin with an open-ended question: "Do you have nightmares?" Depending on the response, the therapist may need to clarify what a nightmare is (i.e., an elaborate dream that is remembered and associated with strong negative emotions, such as intense fear). Follow-up questions to ascertain that the experience reported by the patient is indeed a nightmare will probe the features of this definition. For example, because some patients report nightmares based on having been told by observers that they thrash or otherwise appear distressed in their sleep, the therapist can ask:

"Do you wake up when you have this kind of nightmare?"
"When you wake up, do you remember what you were dreaming about? Can you give me an
    example?"
"How do you feel when you wake up from a nightmare?"

Having ascertained that the phenomenon described is indeed a nightmare, the therapist can ascertain other clinical features:

"What time of night would you be likely to experience a nightmare?" (Nightmares are more
    common during the second than the first half of the night.)
"How does having a nightmare affect you?"
"Do you have trouble returning to sleep?"
"Does it cause problems during the day?"

## Comorbidities Other Than Sleep Disorders

Providing a full medical and psychiatric history intake section in the context of an insomnia assessment is beyond the scope of this book. Instead, we focus on identifying comorbid disease-specific sleep issues. For example, when assessing a patient with OCD, the CBT-I therapist does not need to know all aspects of the disorder, but does need to know about compulsive behaviors that interfere with sleep (such as repeatedly checking that the doors are locked at bedtime or in the middle of the night). In Chapter 5, we have discussed disease-specific sleep issues in these comorbid disorder categories: depression, bipolar disorders, anxiety disorders (including PTSD and OCD, although these now have their own categories in DSM-5), chronic pain, and feeding and eating disorders. Here we focus on their assessment. Given the limited time available for full medical and psychiatric history, the therapist will focus on current rather than lifetime conditions, except for bipolar disorders, which are diagnosed on the basis of historical information.

• *Presence of comorbidity*. Begin by asking the patient to list all current medical and mental disorders. If the clinical presentation suggests a condition that has not been previously diagnosed or reported by the patient, the therapist assesses it and either refers the patient for treatment or develops a treatment plan that includes treatment of the comorbid condition (see Chapter 10 for a discussion of sequencing CBT-I and treatments of comorbid conditions).

• *Treatment of comorbid condition(s)*. For each comorbid disorder, the therapist needs to gather information about its treatment and the potential impact of that treatment on sleep. An example would be whether there are sedating or alerting side effects of medications used to treat the comorbid condition. The focus should be on current medical conditions and treatments, as well as medical history relevant to the onset of or worsening of insomnia.

• *Temporal relation between insomnia and a comorbid condition*. For each comorbid disorder, the therapist also ascertains whether the patient perceives that the sleep problem and comorbid condition wax and wane with one another or if there is some independence.

• *Sleep-related clinical features of comorbid disorders*. Table 6.6 summarizes how to assess sleep-related clinical features of several comorbid conditions discussed in Chapter 5.

Sophie's insomnia intake interview revealed no significant comorbidities. Sam's interview assessed the impact of fibromyalgia pain on his sleep and evaluated the possibility that some of his sedentary lifestyle might be due to depression.

## Treatment Goals

At the end of the insomnia intake interview, the therapist should inquire about treatment goals and help the patient to set and operationalize such goals, so that progress can be tracked. For example, a patient whose goal is to "sleep like a normal person" will be asked to clarify what this means. When more than one goal is expressed, it is wise to rank-order them. In addition, the expressed goals should match the domains about which the patient expressed distress at the beginning of the interview. The goals also need to be realistic. One of Sam's goals was to be pain-free; this was certainly not a realistic goal, because CBT-I is not a treatment for fibromyalgia. However, his other goals were more realistic (to sleep more and feel less sleepy during the day so that he could spend more time with his grandchildren). Sophie's goal of falling asleep within 5–10 minutes and not waking up at all through the night were not consistent with norms for middle-aged adults and were revisited during CBT-I. Her goal of sleeping normally once again was a realistic goal, but one in which the definition of "sleeping normally" needed to be revised slightly to be more realistic.

THERAPIST: What is your goal for this treatment?

SOPHIE: I want to fall asleep when my head hits the pillow and never wake up until I have to in the morning.

THERAPIST: What do you mean when you say "my head hits the pillow"?

SOPHIE: I would like to fall asleep quickly like I used to, in 5 to 10 minutes. This is how it used to be.

THERAPIST: When you say "never wake up until I have to in the morning," how late in the morning would that be?

**TABLE 6.6.** Assessment of Common Sleep–Related Clinical Features among People with Comorbidities Other Than Sleep Disorders

| Clinical feature of a comorbidity | Assessment of impact on sleep |
|---|---|
| **Bed as an escape from suffering** (depressive episode and chronic pain) | How does the patient decide when to get into and out of bed? |
| | In someone with a depressive episode:<br>• Is increased time in bed an escape from emotional suffering, or is it a strategy for coping with sleeplessness (a reflection of sleep effort)?<br>• Does mood before bedtime or upon waking impact getting into/out of bed? |
| | In someone with chronic pain:<br>• Is increased time in bed an avoidance strategy to manage reinjury fears? |
| **Anhedonia** (depressive episode) | Is it difficult for the patient to get out of bed in the morning? What gets in the way? Is it related to anhedonia/low motivation? Does the patient spend time in bed during the day? If so, why? Is it related to anhedonia/low motivation? |
| **Diurnal mood variation** (depressive episode) | Does the patient experience worse mood in the morning [evening]? Does this have an impact on getting out of bed [getting into bed or falling asleep]? |
| **Hopelessness** (depressive episode and chronic pain) | Is the patient expressing hopelessness about resolving insomnia? Does the patient believe that insomnia will not improve unless he or she is pain-free [unless comorbid condition remits]? |
| **Waking up more than an hour earlier than desired** | Has this symptom emerged during an episode of depression or anxiety disorder? If this is not the first depression or anxiety episode, does this symptom improve when the depressive episode or anxiety disorder improves? If the patient stays in bed, is it due to anhedonia, a wish to escape from suffering, or just an effort to sleep more? |
| **Agitation** (hypomanic or manic episode) | Has the patient experienced a significant decrease in the need for sleep during a previous (hypo)manic episode? Has the patient previously experienced a (hypo)manic episode following a period of sleep deprivation? |
| **Sleep symptoms of a comorbid condition** Nightmares (PTSD) | Does the patient experience nightmares? If so, how long is the patient up? What does he or she do upon waking? How often do nightmares occur? Does the patient postpone bedtime fearing nightmare occurrence (sleep avoidance)? |

*(cont.)*

**TABLE 6.6** (*cont.*)

| Clinical feature of a comorbidity | Assessment of impact on sleep |
|---|---|
| Nocturnal panic (PD) | Does the patient wake up with a panic attack in the middle of the night? If so, how often does this occur? Does the patient postpone bedtime because he or she fears the occurrence of a panic attack (sleep avoidance)? |
| Pain | Does pain wake the patient up or make it difficult to return to sleep? If so, how often does this occur? Explore pain management strategy and ambivalence about taking pain relief medications at night. Refer to pain specialist as needed. |
| Nighttime OCD rituals | Does the patient engage in obsessive or compulsive behaviors that interfere with sleep? If so, what are they? Do they interfere with initial sleep onset? Do they interfere with returning to sleep after waking up in the middle of the night? How often do these behaviors occur? |

SOPHIE: Well, I have to be up at 7:30 on workdays, but I want to sleep until 9:00 on weekends.

THERAPIST: I see. Do you mean that you want to sleep longer when you do not need to go to work, or that you would prefer to also go to bed later?

SOPHIE: Both.

THERAPIST: I also hear that you want your sleep to be uninterrupted.

SOPHIE: Definitely; this is the most important part.

THERAPIST: It sounds like you have three goals. Let's list them in the order of their importance for you. You just said that the most important one is not to wake up in the middle of the night.

SOPHIE: Yes. I would say the next one is to fall asleep quickly.

THERAPISTS: You said this means within 5 or 10 minutes?

SOPHIE: Yes.

THERAPIST: Sounds like you want to (1) have your sleep uninterrupted; (2) fall asleep within 10 minutes; and (3) sleep a little longer (and later) on weekend nights.

SOPHIE: Yes. Do you think I am dreaming?

THERAPIST: I think these are good goals. It sounds like you want to sleep like you used to before you had insomnia.

SOPHIE: Yes. I used to sleep really well.

THERAPIST: Back then, you were not in bed as long as you are now. There may be a connection here. We will talk about it next time.

# THE SLEEP DIARY

The sleep diary (see filled-in examples in Chapters 11 and 12) is an essential tool for assessing sleep habits, nighttime symptoms of insomnia, and progress in treatment. The diary is completed daily, thus providing prospective data on current sleep. Specifically, the sleep diary provides information about the most salient aspects of sleep, such as bedtime, rise time, time to fall asleep, and time awake after sleep onset. It is also essential for the implementation of treatment, because certain aspects of CBT-I rely on its data and because it allows daily tracking of adherence and progress.

Reliance on retrospective estimates of sleep parameters to guide treatment is not advisable, because such reports can be inaccurate due to poor recall and may be biased by the patient's emotional state at the time of recall and/or by the most recent or worst night. Retrospective estimates of sleep parameters are poorly correlated with sleep diary estimates of the same parameters. Retrospective reports tend to depict problems as much worse problem than the daily charting does, and the latter is likely to be closer to reality (Babkoff, Weller, & Lavidor, 1996). Moreover, the correlation between retrospective estimates and objective estimates of sleep parameters, such as those obtained from PSG studies, are not as good as the correlations between daily sleep diaries and objective estimates of sleep (Carskadon et al., 1976). Because night-to-night variability in sleep behaviors and insomnia symptoms are common among people with insomnia (Suh et al., 2012), it is recommended that a minimum of 7 (and ideally 14) days of data collection be used in order to assess a patient's sleep reliably (Wohlgemuth, Edinger, Fins, & Sullivan, 1999). Copies of the sleep diary form can be sent to patients ahead of the initial assessment, along with written instructions. However, this may not always be practical.

## Enhancing Accuracy of Sleep Diary Information

Understanding what each diary item is asking, and recording information as soon as possible after waking up in the morning, can enhance the accuracy of the data recorded. An effective way of ensuring that each item is understood is to ask the patient to complete last night's data and answer questions as they arise. To illustrate that recollection of information about sleep becomes less accurate as time passes, the therapist can ask the patient to complete sleep diary data for last night, as well as two and three nights ago. Most people spontaneously say that they do not remember previous nights. If a patient does not spontaneously do so, the clinician can ask the patient to contrast how it was to complete the diary for last night and three nights ago. It has been our experience that a patient's completion of the sleep diary for the last few nights during the session, and a discussion of this experience, increase the likelihood that the patient will complete the diary every day (ideally, shortly after waking up).

Although accurate data are important, it is also important to prevent the very act of recording information about sleep from interfering with sleep. To that end, clock watching should be discouraged. Looking at the clock when unable to sleep creates performance anxiety that may prolong latency to sleep onset. Looking at the clock in the middle of the night could lead to anxiety and/or frustration about how little time remains for sleep or how long wakefulness has lasted. A therapist should discourage clock watching, and reassure a patient that the best time estimate will suffice: "I realize that it is impossible to be exact, and I do not expect precision."

The therapist can then explain that the way people estimate time at night tends to stay consistent over time. That is, if they underestimate time, they are likely to underestimate each night. Therefore, although the data recorded may not be exact, they will still allow tracking of changes in sleep over time.

## Enhancing Adherence with Sleep Diary Completion

To promote adherence, the clinician should take the time to identify and discuss obstacles to completing the sleep diary. The first question can be "How likely are you to remember to do this every morning?" If the patient is uncertain, the therapist can ask, "What may get in the way?" One barrier is anticipatory anxiety about getting it "right" (i.e., being 100% accurate), as just discussed. Some barriers are related to time management, such as being pressed for time in the morning and later forgetting to complete the diary, or being disorganized. In such cases, the therapist can work with the patient to think of ways that will support being disciplined about timely diary completion. For example, the patient can link diary completion to an existing morning routine, such as breakfast, getting out of the shower, or taking a train or bus to work.

Failure to understand the relevance of the sleep diary data to treatment is another common detriment to the diary's timely completion. It is therefore very important to explain the importance and relevance of the diary ahead of time. In doing so, it is also a good idea to convey the expectation that CBT-I is a collaborative effort. Patients who understand that sleep diary data are seriously considered during treatment will make diary completion a priority and be able to troubleshoot obstacles. If the importance of the diary data is not clear initially, it will become more so as treatment progresses, because each therapy session will begin with a review of sleep diary data and a discussion of missing or spotty data. If a person expresses concern that diary recording will result in less or worse sleep, it is best to acknowledge that this might be the case for the first few days, but that most people find that monitoring their sleep helps rather than hurts their sleep. Pitching diary completion as a time-limited experiment (e.g., "just until the next session") to test the idea that sleep will worsen may also be helpful. Patients may be less anxious if the diary recording is just for a short time. The experimental data they bring back will be seriously examined, thus underscoring the importance of the data, and their observations about the results of the experiment will inform the therapist about their beliefs regarding sleep. In the rare case when a patient reports that recording in the sleep diary has indeed led to worse sleep, the therapist can either modify the diary to obtain minimal information about sleep that the patient can provide without causing sleep worsening (e.g., time in bed and time asleep) or stop diary recording altogether.

## Reviewing Sleep Diary Data: Nocturnal Portion

The discussion below pertains to the use of the sleep diary as an assessment of sleep habits. In Chapters 7, 8, and 9, we discuss various ways in which diary data are used in treatment. During the assessment phase, the sleep diary data complement the clinical interview. The following aspects of sleep can be obtained from the daily sleep diary data. (Abbreviations commonly used in calculating sleep diary data are presented below and summarized in Table 6.7.)

1. *Night-to-night variability in sleep times.* Scanning the diary data can help the therapist assess variations from night to night in the time the patient gets into bed, the time lights are turned off, the time the patient wakes up, and the time the patient gets out of bed in the morning. Many people go to bed and wake up later on weekends. But this is not the only source of night-to-night variability. The therapist needs to explore the reasons for large variability. For instance, a patient may go to bed earlier than usual when the previous night was particularly "bad" or short. Sometimes wake time is determined by activities scheduled for the day. People with a mild eveningness chronotype may be particularly prone to waking up later if there is nothing scheduled.

2. *Night-to-night variability in sleep symptoms.* Scanning the diary data can also help the therapist assess night-to-night variability in the time it takes to fall asleep and, separately, the time awake in the middle of the night and number of awakenings. Most people with insomnia experience some variability in their sleep difficulties. The therapist can point to one or more nights that stand out as relatively good (or bad), and open up a discussion about why that might be.

3. *Lingering.* This is time elapsed between the time of final awakening and the time the patient gets out of the bed for the day. The therapist should find out what the patient does during this time. One patient may be lying in bed with eyes closed, trying to get more sleep; another may start the day in bed (e.g., by checking emails).

4. *Sleep quality.* The therapist should pay attention to self-rated sleep quality, as well as to what factors into the rating. Different aspects of sleep may influence ratings of sleep quality. For example, some patients assess their sleep quality based on its quantity; others base their assessment on how many times they woke up or how long they were awake at night.

5. *Time in bed (TIB).* This is the time elapsed from when the lights are turned out until the patient gets out of bed in the morning. TIB represents the period of sleep opportunity. It is

**TABLE 6.7. Abbreviations of Sleep Terms**

| Abbreviation | Term | Definition |
| --- | --- | --- |
| TIB | Time in bed | The time elapsed from when the lights are turned out until the patient gets out of bed in the morning |
| TWT | Total wake time | The total time awake during the period allotted for sleep (time to fall asleep initially + time awake in the middle of the night + time awake in bed lingering) |
| TST | Total sleep time | The total duration of sleep (TIB – TST) |
| SE | Sleep efficiency | The percentage of time in bed that is spent asleep (100*[TST/TIB]) |
| SOL | Sleep onset latency | The time it takes to fall asleep at the beginning of the night |
| WASO | Wakefulness after sleep onset | The time awake in the middle of the night (between initially falling asleep and waking up) |

referred to as the time in bed even when some of this time is actually spent out of bed (e.g., sitting in the living room watching TV in the middle of the night).

6. *Total wake time (TWT).* This refers to the total time the patient was awake during the period allotted for sleep—that is, time to fall asleep initially (sleep onset latency, or SOL) + time awake in the middle of the night (wakefulness after sleep onset, or WASO) + time awake in bed lingering.

7. *Total sleep time (TST).* This refers to the total duration of sleep. It can be calculated by subtracting TWT from TIB. We refer to this value as the *calculated TST*. The computed TST values may differ from the retrospective appraisal the patient has provided during the interview. When discrepancies are large (more than 1 hour), the therapist can point them out and discuss them. For example, it is possible that the retrospective value(s) the patient provided during the interview were based on a different time period than the diary (e.g., retrospective values may pertain to when the patient's sleep was at its worst—perhaps 2 months ago—and the diary to the last 2 weeks).

8. *Sleep efficiency (SE).* This provides an index of sleep quality that may or may not correlate with the patient's self-reported sleep quality. SE is defined as the percentage of time in bed that is spent asleep (100*[TST/TIB]). It is also used to guide certain aspects of treatment, as discussed in Chapter 7.

Therapists can also compute weekly averages of key sleep diary variables. For example, the average TIB is computed by adding the TIB for each night of the week for which a value is available, and dividing the result by the number of nights for which values were available that week. Most sleep specialists consider an average derived from fewer than five nights an unreliable estimate of the weekly TIB. We illustrate the computations by using data from Sophie's sleep diary.

## Example: Sophie's Sleep Diary Data

The interpretation and feedback from the review of Sophie's sleep diary are described in full in Chapter 11. Figure 11.4 in that chapter presents a week of sleep diary data completed by Sophie; below, we provide a discussion of how key variables derived from those data were computed. Here are the calculated values for Sunday:

- TIB was 11 hours and 55 minutes. This was derived by subtracting the time between when she started trying to sleep (diary item 2), which on Sunday was 9:15 P.M., and the time she got out of bed for the day, which for Sunday night was 9:10 A.M. on Monday morning (diary item 7).
- TWT was 4 hours and 35 minutes. This was computed by adding the following three times: the time it took her to fall asleep at the beginning of the night (SOL, diary item 3); the time she was awake between when she first fell asleep and her final awakening (WASO, diary item 7); and the time she was lingering in bed (the time spent in bed in the morning after her final awakening (diary item 6a) until she got out of bed to start the day (diary item 7).
- TST was 7 hours and 20 minutes. This was derived by subtracting TWT from TIB, mak-

ing sure that the TIB and TWT were first expressed in the same metric (i.e., both in minutes or both in hours).

- SE was 61%. As described above, SE was computed by using the formula 100*(TST/TIB). On Sunday night, Sophie's SE = 100*(440 minutes/715 minutes), or, equivalently, 100*(7.33 hours/11.92 hours).

The therapist computed TIB and TST for each day, and noted these values at the bottom of the corresponding column. The therapist also calculated SE for each day. Weekly averages of key sleep diary variables were as follows:

- *Average SOL:* The average time it took to fall asleep (diary item 3) was 1 hour and 55 minutes.
- *Average WASO:* The average time awake in the middle of the night (diary item 5) for the first week was 52 minutes.
- *Average TIB:* Average TIB was 10 hours and 30 minutes.
- *Average TST:* Average TST was 6 hours and 15 minutes.
- *Average SE:* Average SE was 40%.

Diary-based computations may appear daunting, but become less so with experience. The therapist can explain how to compute variables that will be relevant later in treatment (Chapter 7). With repeated exposure and involvement, patients can learn how to compute sleep variables. This will prepare them to self-administer CBT-I later, if the insomnia should ever return. (See Chapter 10 for discussion of relapse prevention.)

There are many variants of a sleep diary. We have included in this book a version of a validated sleep diary called the Consensus Sleep Diary (Carney et al., 2012), so called because it was created by a consensus of 20 sleep experts. In addition to the sleep variables, the diary includes items about napping, as well as use of common substances that have an impact on sleep (such as caffeine, alcohol, and sleep medications). A blank diary form adapted for this book, the Consensus Sleep Diary–M, can be found in Appendix B.

## THE INSOMNIA SEVERITY INDEX

The Insomnia Severity Index (ISI), also provided in Appendix B, is a validated 7-item self-report questionnaire that measures patients' perceptions of their sleep symptoms, their perceived consequences, and the level of concern or distress caused by these sleep symptoms (Bastien, Vallieres, & Morin, 2001; Morin et al., 2011). Specifically, items assess the severity of sleep onset and maintenance difficulties (including middle-of-the-night and early-morning awakenings), satisfaction with current sleep, interference with daily functioning, how noticeable the impairment attributed to the sleep problem is, and distress caused by poor sleep. Each item is rated on a 0–4 Likert scale, with the total representing overall severity level (a higher score indicates more severe insomnia). It is easy to administer in the waiting room (it takes less than 5 minutes to complete) and easy to interpret (it can be scored in less than 1 minute). The validation study divided the range of ISI scores into four categories (Bastien et al., 2001):

0–7: No clinically significant insomnia
8–14: Subthreshold insomnia
15–21: Clinical insomnia, moderate
22–28: Clinical insomnia, severe

More recently, a score of 10 was validated as a cutoff for distinguishing between insomnia disorder cases and noncases in the community (Morin et al., 2011).

### KEY PRACTICE IDEAS

- The insomnia intake interview is an important first step in ascertaining the problem and planning treatment. Components of the interview include the following:

  - Nature of the presenting sleep problems and their history, including identification of the most distressing aspects of these problems.
  - Sleep–wake patterns, with careful attention to factors that can weaken the sleep drive.
  - Circadian tendency and circadian factors relevant to the presenting problems.
  - Evidence of sleep effort.
  - Evidence of hyperarousal (including likelihood of conditioned arousal).
  - Contribution of comorbidities and their treatment to insomnia (including psychiatric, medical, and other sleep disorders).
  - Other relevant factors, including the sleep environment, use of substances, and timing of eating and exercising.
  - Identification of treatment goals that can be operationalized and (if more than one) prioritized.

- A sleep diary provides prospective data on sleep habits and sleep difficulties that complement to the interview. At least 7 days (and preferably 14 days) of sleep diary data are needed for meaningful interpretation.

# CHAPTER 7

# Behavioral Components of CBT-I
## *Part I*

In this chapter, we describe the two core behavioral components of CBT-I: *stimulus control* (Bootzin, 1972) and *sleep restriction therapy* (Spielman, Saskin, & Thorpy, 1987). Other behavioral components, including strategies to reduce hyperarousal in bed and sleep hygiene recommendations (e.g., optimizing the sleep environment and timing the consumption of food, caffeine, alcohol, and nicotine, as well as exercise), are described in Chapter 8. Stimulus control and sleep restriction therapy are effective when applied separately or combined (Morin, Bootzin, et al., 2006; Morin, Hauri, et al., 1999). We describe these two core components separately, including rationales, standard instructions, anticipated obstacles to adherence, and variants of the standard instructions. We then present a protocol for combining them.

## STIMULUS CONTROL

In Chapter 3, we have discussed conditioned arousal and its role in the etiology of insomnia. Briefly, through repeated pairing of the bed with frustration, fear, agitation, and anxiety (i.e., states of hyperarousal), the bed and sometimes the bedroom become conditioned or learned cues for arousal and wakefulness rather than sleep (Bootzin, 1972; Bootzin & Epstein, 2000). In other words, whereas for good sleepers the bed is a cue for sleep, for people with insomnia the bed has become a cue for arousal, which is incompatible with sleep.

Stimulus control instructions reverse conditioned arousal by strengthening the bed as a cue for sleep. This is done primarily through being in bed only when asleep or sleepy and eliminating from the sleep environment behaviors that are incompatible with sleep. The most important behaviors to eliminate from the sleep environment are those associated with anxious or otherwise unpleasant emotional states. Patients are encouraged to recognize when they are sleepy (as distinct from tired), to use sleepiness as a cue for getting into bed at night (Instruction 1 below), and to use its absence (e.g., when it becomes clear that sleep is not imminent) as a cue for getting out of bed after waking up in the middle of the night (Instruction 2 below). They are told to use the bed and bedroom only for sleep and sex (Instruction 3 below), and to wake up at the same time every morning, regardless of the amount or quality of sleep (Instruction 4 below). It is also recommended that they avoid napping (Instruction 5).

We elaborate below on each of the five instructions (summarized in Table 7.1), explaining its rationale, and discussing ideas to help with common adherence issues. As will become clear from the discussion below, together the five instructions address the three aspects of the sleep regulatory system that we have discussed in the first part of the book: the sleep drive (Chapter 2), the circadian clock (Chapter 2), and the arousal system (Chapter 3). In Chapter 9, we discuss how to use cognitive therapy techniques to work through some of the adherence issues, including some of those discussed in this chapter. Before introducing this set of instructions, the clinician should explain the idea of conditioned arousal, using examples pertinent to the patient. The main points to convey are these:

• Through repeated pairing of the bed with negative experiences such as being upset, frustrated, or tense, the bed becomes a cue for the body to be tense. In other words, the body has learned to become alert when getting into bed, and when seeing and even thinking about the bed. To remove self-blame, it helps to add that this learning occurs without awareness. The explanation can be enhanced by using personalized examples relevant to each patient, as well as examples of other conditioning experiences. For instance, if patients report struggling to stay awake on the sofa in the living room at night, yet becoming wide awake upon getting into bed, the therapist can explain the experience as a sign that being in bed has become a cue for alertness rather than sleepiness. The classic Pavlov conditioning experiment can be used to explain the idea of learned behaviors. Most people have some familiarity with this example, so the experiment can be summarized briefly by explaining that dogs in that experiment learned to drool at the sound of the bell because food (which naturally induces salivation) and the bell were repeatedly paired together. Over time, the dogs began to salivate when the bell rang, even in the absence of food. Just as food naturally leads to salivation, frustration and tension naturally produce alertness. Similarly, just as pairing the dogs' food with a bell made the bell a cue for salivation, pairing the bed with tension and frustration makes the bed a cue for alertness. (See Figure 7.1.)

• *What is learned can be unlearned.* This is an important point to convey, because it promotes hope. The plan for unlearning involves breaking this association through consistently avoiding the bed when a patient is not sleepy or asleep. Again, the therapist can refer to the example used

## TABLE 7.1. Summary of Stimulus Control Instructions

1. Go to bed only when sleepy (not just fatigued or tired).

2. If unable to sleep, get out of bed and return to bed only when sleepy.

3. Use the bed and bedroom only for sleep (and sex).

4. Wake up at the same time every day, regardless of how much you slept, and get out of bed within 10–15 minutes.

5. Do not nap.

| Pavlov's Classical Conditioning | | | | | Unintended Conditioned Arousal in Insomnia | | | | |
|---|---|---|---|---|---|---|---|---|---|
| FOOD<br>something<br>that makes<br>dogs drool | + | BELL | = | DROOL | TENSION<br>something<br>that makes<br>you alert | + | BED | = | ALERT |
| FOOD | + | BELL | = | DROOL | TENSION | + | BED | = | ALERT |
| FOOD | + | BELL | = | DROOL | TENSION | + | BED | = | ALERT |
| FOOD | + | BELL | = | DROOL | TENSION | + | BED | = | ALERT |
| FOOD | + | BELL | = | DROOL | TENSION | + | BED | = | ALERT |
| FOOD | + | BELL | = | DROOL | TENSION | + | BED | = | ALERT |
| FOOD | + | BELL | = | DROOL | TENSION | + | BED | = | ALERT |
| FOOD | + | BELL | = | DROOL | TENSION | + | BED | = | ALERT |
| | | BELL | = | DROOL | | | BED | = | ALERT |

**FIGURE 7.1.** Understanding and explaining conditioned arousal.

for explaining the learning process through pairing. In the Pavlovian experiment, for instance, the dogs eventually learned to stop salivating at the sound of the bell after the experimenter consistently rang the bell in the absence of food. Over time, the bell stopped being a cue for salivation. In the same way, if a patient repeatedly avoids being in bed when in a state of frustration/ alertness/tension/nondrowsy wakefulness, the bed will eventually stop being a cue for alertness.

In the excerpt below, the therapist explains to the patient the idea of conditioned arousal.

THERAPIST: Do you remember how it felt when you went to bed 5 years ago, when you did not have insomnia?

PATIENT: Not much. It wasn't an issue. I went to bed, and before I knew it, I was asleep.

THERAPIST: It sounds like your bed back then was like a signal for your body to sleep.

PATIENT: My husband is still like that. His head hits the pillow, and 5 minutes later he is snoring.

THERAPIST: Exactly. So for him the bed is a cue for sleep, and for you it stopped being a cue for sleep.

PATIENT: (*Laughing*) For me, the couch is a signal to sleep. I fall asleep on the couch while I watch TV around 10 P.M., but when I go to bed, it now takes me at least an hour to fall asleep. I wonder, why does this happen?

THERAPIST: It happens through a process of learned association. Do you know what that is?

PATIENT: Not really.

THERAPIST: You told me you have a dog. Have you ever noticed your dog anticipating your next move?

PATIENT: Yes. My dog wags his tail and runs to the place where I keep his leash whenever I put my shoes with laces on.

THERAPIST: Your dog seemed to have learned to automatically associate your walking shoes with going on a walk, probably because historically whenever you put this kind of shoes on, you took him on a walk. Does it sound right?

PATIENT: Yes.

THERAPIST: In your case, when you had a problem in your relationship with your husband 5 years ago and you started having problems sleeping, you were in bed, and your mind would be flooded with thoughts that kept you awake. So your body learned to associate your bed with being alert. Now, even though your relationship is in a good place, your bed is still a signal to your body to be alert. Does this make sense?

PATIENT: Yes, but how can I reverse this?

THERAPIST: There are ways to unlearn associations. We will use a procedure called *stimulus control* to help us come up with a plan to unlearn poor bed–sleep associations.

## Instruction 1: Go to Bed Only When Sleepy (Not Just Fatigued or Tired)

Relying on materials presented in Chapters 2 and 3, the therapist can explain that sleepiness signals are present when the sleep drive is high and the person is calm enough to experience these two signals as sleepiness. Going to bed when sleepy increases the probability that the latency to sleep onset will be short, because it means that the net balance between sleep and wake factors is in favor of sleep. Instruction 1 contributes to the unlearning of bed–wakefulness associations, because less time awake means fewer opportunities for a continued association between the bed and wakefulness. Below we discuss several issues related to the implementation of this instruction.

### Sleepiness versus Fatigue

Recall from Chapter 2 that *sleepiness* refers to the propensity to fall asleep when given the opportunity, and *tiredness* refers to a low energy level that does not necessarily reflect the propensity to fall asleep. Thus, whereas tiredness signals the need for rest, sleepiness signals the need to seek sleep. The therapist should make sure that the patient understands this distinction. For instance, the therapist can say that sleepiness is being on the verge of dozing off and almost having to struggle to stay awake, whereas fatigue is having low energy and low motivation to stay awake. The following is a script that demonstrates explaining the distinction between being sleepy and being tired or fatigued.

THERAPIST: Let's discuss the difference between being sleepy and being tired. You may think of the word *sleepy* differently than I do. What comes to mind when I ask how it feels to you when you are sleepy?

PATIENT: Totally exhausted. I feel like this all of the time.

THERAPIST: It sounds like you experience quite a lot of fatigue. Being *fatigued* or *tired* means having low physical or mental energy. When you are fatigued or really tired, you need to rest. Does this sound like what you're experiencing?

PATIENT: Yes, exactly.

THERAPIST: OK, thanks for clarifying. I think of feeling sleepy a little differently than feeling fatigued or tired. For me and sleep specialists in general, being *sleepy* means having to put effort into staying awake. When you are sleepy and you are given the chance to sleep, you would fall asleep relatively quickly. If you feel wired, even when tired, you are not feeling sleepy. In that case, even though you may wish to sleep, you would have a hard time falling asleep if you are given the opportunity.

PATIENT: Sometimes I feel this way on the couch around 10 P.M., but if I go to bed, I don't feel sleepy any more.

THERAPISTS: It sounds to me that when you watch TV you are indeed sleepy, but then you become wired and no longer sleepy. You probably still feel tired.

PATIENT: Yes. I am very tired, but also wide awake. I see your point about the difference between sleepy and tired. It is interesting. I never thought about it this way.

## Masked Sleepiness

High arousal levels may override the homeostatic sleep drive and prevent the emergence of the sleepy sensation that is normally experienced when the homeostatic drive is very strong. This overriding is called *masking*. High arousal and/or hypervigilance masks sleepiness, just as caffeine does. For example, when a sleep-deprived person is anxious about having to appear before a traffic judge, this person generally does not feel sleepy at the hearing, despite getting insufficient sleep the night before. When the threat of the court appearance is over and this individual is relaxed, he or she may nod off while reading a magazine article, because the underlying sleepiness generated by sleep deprivation the night before rises to the surface and is unopposed by the hyperarousal that was caused by the thought of appearing in court.

When a person with insomnia reports never feeling sleepy, even when sleep-deprived, it is probably because the balance between the homeostatic sleep drive and the arousal level is tipped in the direction of arousal. This arousal may result from anxious thoughts about life stresses or about having sleep difficulties, or it may be present without clear preceding thoughts and may be experienced as body tension or an endless parade of thoughts. Regardless, the arousal masks sleepiness and is therefore an important target for treatment. Techniques to reduce arousal (e.g., relaxation and unwinding before bedtime) are integral to CBT-I and are discussed in Chapter 8. Even after a therapist has explained the difference and the idea of masking, some patients continue to have a difficult time judging when they are sleepy. Other patients may actually be avoiding going to bed out of fear of sleep, as is sometimes the case in patients with PTSD (see Chapter 5). In attempting to adhere to the recommendation to go to bed only when sleepy, these patients may wind up delaying the time they go to bed and escalating their arousal. In such cases, it may be necessary to instruct the patients to go to bed at a set time, regardless of how sleepy they feel—with the reminder that if they then do not fall asleep quickly, they should get out of bed and wait for sleepiness (Instruction 2 below). The hope is that over time, the bed will become a stimulus for sleep, and the patients will eventually feel sleepy when getting into bed at bedtime.

### Bed-Partner-Related Obstacles to the Implementation of Instruction 1

A patient who is used to going to bed at the same time as a bed partner may discover that he or she is not sleepy at the couple's habitual bedtime. This may raise concerns about loss of intimacy and, depending on who goes to sleep earlier, about waking or being awakened by the bed partner. When loss of intimacy is a concern, it may help to distinguish between spending time in bed together and going to sleep at the same time. For instance, the partners can go to bed at the same time and spend some time together, but if the bed partner is ready for sleep before the patient feels sleepy, the patient can leave the bed and return to bed only when feeling sleepy. Concerns about waking up the bed partner may or may not be valid. A partner without insomnia who goes to sleep before the patient does may not be awakened when the patient comes to bed, and even if awakened, is unlikely to have a problem falling back asleep. It is always a good idea to encourage a patient to explain the rationale behind the change in bedtime behaviors, and to discuss problems and solutions with the partner. Sometimes it is helpful to invite the bed partner to a session to discuss the issue and come up with a joint solution.

### Issues Related to Comorbid Depression and/or Chronic Pain

As discussed in Chapter 5, some people with depression go to bed not because they feel sleepy, but because they want to escape from emotional suffering or because not much else feels good to do. To explore whether this is the case, the therapist can ask, "How do you decide when to go to bed?" The answer can reveal whether and, if so, how anhedonia affects the decision to go to bed. For example, if a man who is depressed says that he goes to bed because he does not feel like doing anything else, the therapist can ask him to reflect how he decided when to go to bed when he did not have insomnia. The answer usually reveals that bedtime was later and followed a routine that usually involved engagement in activities outside of bed. The therapist can also ask whether the patient was sleepy at bedtime back then. The answer usually reveals that he was sleepy at bedtime or shortly after getting into bed. The therapist can then work collaboratively with the patient to identify activities that he may be willing to engage in as part an early evening routine. Such behavioral activation in the evening can prevent early retirement to bed and help the patient go to bed only when sleepy. This approach is also relevant to patients with chronic pain who go to bed early as a pain management strategy. In this case, the discussion will also include exploration of alternative pain management techniques.

## Instruction 2: If Unable to Sleep, Get Out of Bed and Return to Bed Only When Sleepy

Following Instruction 2 means that there will be fewer opportunities for pairing the bed with wakefulness, which will promote the unlearning process. Getting out of bed when unable to sleep also reduces sleep effort; that is, it interrupts the process of "trying to sleep." The instruction to leave the bed when unable to sleep, however, may not be easy to follow. Lying in bed can feel comfortable, and getting out of bed is counterintuitive. Therefore, it is particularly important that patients fully understand the concept of conditioned arousal. It is also important for them to understand that it takes time (usually more than a week) before consistently following this recommendation will translate into improved sleep. Continuing to be in bed when unable to sleep leads to frustration and worry about not sleeping, which are not compatible with sleep because they are associated with physiological and cognitive arousal (Chapter 3). Therefore, failing to follow Instruction 2 may further strengthen conditioned arousal. Trying to force sleep is ineffective and counterproductive. Below we discuss several issues related to the implementation of this instruction.

### Helping Patients Decide When to Get Out of Bed If Unable to Sleep

It is best to advise patients to use the sensation of alertness as a guide for when to get out of bed. For example, a therapist can use phrases such as " . . . when you start feeling that sleep is not about to happen" or " . . . when you start to feel frustrated." It is important not to dwell on this decision, because dwelling may promote wakefulness. It is also not a good idea to use a clock to decide when it is time to get out of bed, because it may promote performance anxiety and prolong sleep onset (Tang, Schmidt, & Harvey, 2007). An elegant study by Tang et al. (2007) supports the notion that clock watching prolongs sleep onset. In that study, people with insomnia who were instructed to watch a digital clock as they were going to sleep took longer to fall asleep than people with insomnia who were instructed to watch a digital display of four random digits. A clock can stay in a patient's bedroom and can be used as an alarm in the morning, but it is best to turn it away and/or avoid the temptation to turn on an electronic device to check the time. Ideally, patients learn to calmly observe their state of sleepiness–alertness and use it to guide them when they should stop trying harder to sleep and instead get out of bed.

### Things to Do When Out of Bed

The best activities to engage in when out of bed are pleasant and engaging, but not too activating. If the activity is boring, the risk is that the patient will be thinking about sleep or its absence. If the activity is too engaging or activating, it will mask sleepiness. The therapist and patient can work together to identify and list suitable activities ahead of time. Examples of engaging but nonactivating activities are reading nonsuspenseful, non-work-related materials; listening to an audiobook or a podcast (again, the topic and duration should be carefully selected); watching a light program on TV; or knitting or embroidering—to name just a few. We emphasize carefully selecting contents for reading or listening, because materials that are calming to one patient may be activating to another. A list from which a patient could select such activities is provided in the handout titled Buffer Zone Activities in Appendix C. Below we also discuss how to help patients who are afraid that getting out of bed may mean staying up the rest of the night.

### Difficulty Getting Out of Bed When Unable to Sleep

Leaving a warm bed in the middle of the night is not very appealing, particularly in the winter. It may help to prepare a comfortable sitting place, with a throw blanket and a space heater readily available, and to identify activities to engage in when out of bed in the middle of the night. Modifications to this instruction for patients who cannot or will not get out of bed in the middle of the night are discussed below.

### Concern That Getting Out of Bed in the Middle of the Night May Disturb a Bed Partner

Concern about a bed partner may be another reason a patient does not want to get out of bed; a similar concern has been discussed under Instruction 1 above. The therapist can discuss the validity of this concern, highlighting the following points:

- The bed partner may not be awakened by the patient's leaving and returning to bed.
- Even if awakened, the bed partner may well be able to fall back asleep easily.
- Getting out of bed is less likely to disrupt a bed partner's sleep than tossing and turning.

### Concern That Getting Out of Bed May Mean Staying Up for the Rest of the Night

When discussing the concern that getting up in the middle of the night may mean staying up till morning, the therapist needs to convey that this is part of a long-term strategy. Getting out of bed when unable to sleep is not meant to help the patient sleep better that same night; rather, it is meant to help in the long run. The bed–arousal association cannot be unlearned in one night. It is OK if getting out of bed keeps the patient awake that night, because being awake more in the short run means that the patient is building sleep drive, and getting out of bed consistently means that eventually the bed will be repeatedly paired with sleepiness and with falling asleep quickly. Whereas it is a good idea to engage in nonstimulating activities when out of bed, it is even more important to unlearn bed–wakefulness associations and avoid trying to sleep as part of a long-term strategy for resolving insomnia.

### Returning to Sleep in the Same Bed

Sometimes, when implementing stimulus control, patients get out of bed in the middle of the night and fall asleep on the sofa or in another bedroom. However, when a patient's goal is to sleep well in his or her own bedroom and bed, it is better to return to that bed in the middle of the night, because that way the association between the bedroom bed and sleep will be strengthened. The short excerpt below demonstrates how this idea can be explained to a patient. This conversation took place during the session in which the rationale for stimulus control had already been explained, and the therapist had ascertained that the patient understood that the aim was to strengthen the bed as a cue for sleep.

PATIENT: I get it. I will get out of bed and go to the living room and read.

THERAPIST: Do you think you will know when it is time to go back to bed?

PATIENT: Yes, but I'd rather sleep on the sofa the rest of the night. I am afraid that getting back to bed will make me more alert, and then I will again have problems falling back asleep.

THERAPIST: It looks like you understand why it is important to get out of bed when you are unable to fall back asleep in the middle of the night, and that you are on board with that idea.

PATIENT: Yes, I am. Tossing and turning in bed makes my brain associate the bed with being upset.

THERAPIST: Correct. Let's think about this idea from a different angle. You want to associate your bed with falling asleep.

PATIENT: Definitely.

THERAPIST: Getting out of bed when you cannot sleep is an important step in this direction. It will help break the association of your bed with being upset. The next step is to create a positive association between the bed and sleep. This means you should actually go back to sleep there.

PATIENT: I get the idea, and, ideally, I want to be able to sleep in my own room. But, as I said, if I go back to my bed it will be harder to fall back asleep, and I will end up with less sleep. I have to wake up to work. I cannot sleep in.

THERAPIST: You predict that it will be easier for you to fall asleep on the couch?

PATIENT: Yes. At least I will be sleeping.

THERAPIST: It sound like we are dealing with the same idea we discussed earlier today—the difference between short-term and long-term gains. I can see the short-term benefit of staying asleep on the sofa. But will that bring you closer to your long-term goal of sleeping well in your bedroom bed?

PATIENT: I see your point. I need to learn to sleep in my own bed.

THERAPIST: Yes. This means that although you find it easier to fall asleep on the couch, you should go back to bed. Assuming that your predictions are correct, there will be a few nights on which you will sleep less than if you stayed on the sofa—but eventually you will create a good automatic connection between your bed and sleeping.

PATIENT: It sounds hard. But I would like to sleep in my own bed. And besides, sleeping on the couch is not good for my back. But what if I get tense again? Just go back out to the couch?

THERAPIST: Yes. I think you know why.

PATIENT: I get it. If I want my body to get the idea that the bed is where I sleep, I need to bite the bullet and do it.

## Instruction 3: Use the Bed and Bedroom Only for Sleep (and Sex)

Engaging in waking activities while in bed—such as eating, studying, surfing the Internet, or talking on the phone—creates associations between the bed and wakefulness, and therefore weakens the association between bed and sleep. The most important activities to eliminate from the bed are those associated with arousal (e.g., worrying, "trying to sleep"). Avoiding arousing activities in bed will strengthen the bed as a stimulus or cue for sleep. The following are a few fine points regarding this instruction.

### *Reading in Bed*

Some people find that a short period of light reading in bed helps them to fall asleep. This is probably because reading eliminates sleep effort, and also because it has become a cue for sleep.

In this way, a brief period of reading helps unmask sleepiness. In such cases, reading suspenseful or otherwise arousal-producing content (e.g., work-related material), should be avoided, because doing so could strengthen the bed as a cue for arousal rather than sleep.

### Watching Television

As in the case of reading, a brief period of watching nonupsetting TV programs in bed can help unmask sleepiness. However, some people watch upsetting content or spend a long time watching TV in bed, thus associating the bed with wakefulness. Some even keep the television on all night, usually because they experience silence as aversive. As discussed in Chapter 8, noise can be detrimental to sleep. A better substitute for those aversive to silence is to use white noise.

### Modifications for Some Sleep Environments

Dorm rooms, studio apartments, and other types of cramped or crowded living quarters present a challenge for the implementation of Instruction 3, because the bedroom environment is inevitably associated with waking activities. In such cases, it may be possible to keep the spirit of Instruction 3 by separating the space used for sleep (i.e., the bed) from other spaces.

### Resting

To strengthen the bed as a cue for sleep, resting (as distinct from intentional napping) should not be done in the sleeping bed. This is relevant to patients with chronic pain and other medical conditions necessitating rest. If dozing is a problem, resting, even when not in the sleeping bed, should not occur while a patient is lying down or reclining. In the case of Sam, he suffered from fibromyalgia and spent considerable time on the couch dozing. (For more on Sam's treatment plan, read Chapter 12.)

### Safety

A modification called *countercontrol* is discussed below to address the problem of people for whom getting out of bed in the middle of the night is unsafe (e.g., because of physical frailty) or too painful.

## Instruction 4: Wake Up at the Same Time Every Day, Regardless of How Much You Slept, and Get Out of Bed within 10–15 Minutes

Anchoring wake time is the foundation of good sleep. Keeping a fixed wake time strengthens the signal from the circadian pacemaker (clock). The idea that one should get out of bed at the same time, regardless of how well or how much one sleeps at night, is counterintuitive to people with insomnia. On a morning that follows a night of poor sleep, it is very tempting to sleep in if the opportunity is available. Clear understanding of the importance of fixed wake and out-of-bed times for the regulation of sleep will promote adherence to this counterintuitive instruction. The rationale involves educating patients about the circadian sleep–wake clock; its role in sleep regulation; and factors that stabilize the clock, such as exposure to light and being vertical (see Chapter 2). The explanation does not need to be extensive and should be tailored to each patient. The therapist can explain that variability in wake-up times creates a "behavioral jet lag" and burdens the body with frequent adjustments to time shifts. The therapist should also emphasize that consistency in following this instruction is important, because occasionally giving in to the temptation to sleep in could weaken the circadian clock signal and offset the benefits of having been adherent on previous nights.

Many young individuals wake up an hour or two later on weekends to make up for having to wake up early during the week. This behavior could somewhat destabilize their circadian clock. On balance, for people without insomnia or insomnia disorder, the benefits of reducing sleep deprivation probably outweigh the detrimental effects on the circadian clock. In contrast, among patients with insomnia, irregular wake and out-of-bed times are often motivated by sleep effort. Many patients with insomnia base their decisions about waking and getting out of bed on how well they slept at night. For them, getting out of bed shortly after waking up, regardless of sleep quality or quantity on the preceding night, can also reduce sleep effort. Sometimes patients wake up at the same time even when their schedules permit a later wake time, and then stay in bed trying (and often failing) to sleep more. These attempts to sleep more create opportunities for pairing the bed with wakefulness. For these patients, the therapist can provide an alternative or additional rationale for Instruction 4 that is anchored in conditioned arousal. That is, getting out of bed shortly after the final awakening eliminates time awake in bed and can therefore help reduce conditioned arousal. Below we discuss common reasons for nonadherence to getting out of bed at the same time every morning.

### Strong Beliefs about Catching Up on Lost Sleep

When patients (e.g., Sophie) believe they must make up for lost sleep, it can be helpful to present Instruction 4 as a time-limited behavioral experiment, to test whether getting up at a set time for 1 week produces better results than lying awake in bed. The therapist and the patient can decide together what "better results" mean (i.e., the desired outcomes). The list of possible outcomes may include better-quality sleep, less time awake in bed, feeling more alert during the day, and/or feeling alert more quickly upon awakening. In general, inviting patients like Sophie to test a recommendation can be a useful way to increase their adherence to many behavioral changes. Additional discussion and examples of using behavioral experiments in CBT-I, and other cognitive techniques to address concerns about negative consequences of poor sleep, are discussed in Chapter 9.

### Eveningness Tendencies

Getting out of bed in the morning is particularly difficult for patients with eveningness tendencies. For them, waking up at a conventional time may mean waking up when their circadian clocks' alerting signals are still low, which is physiologically difficult. Even when they wake up later (at a time when their clocks' alerting signals are increasing), patients with eveningness tendencies find it harder than others to get going in the morning, because they have greater sleep inertia (Chapter 2) and therefore need more time to be fully awake after waking up. Two additional recommendations can help in these cases. The first is morning light exposure. Because morning light has a strong influence on the circadian clock and helps synchronized the internal clock with earth's clock (see Chapter 2), exposure to bright light at the same time each morning helps set and stabilize the clock. The therapist can recommend that these patients be consistent with their wake time and expose themselves to bright light (ideally outdoors) shortly (within 5–10 minutes) after waking up, and set the expectation that after a week or so it will become easier to wake up and start the day.

A second recommendation to help patients with eveningness tendencies wake up at the same time every day is for them to schedule activities that will provide motivation to get going shortly after the scheduled wake time. What motivates one person may not motivate another. Our combined clinical experience indicates that activities that involve commitments to others work best. It is also important to choose activities that a patient is likely to adhere to. For example, if a patient has always wanted to go to the gym in the morning but has never actually done so, it will not be wise to choose morning exercise at the gym as the motivating morning activity. In contrast, if a patient used to exercise in the morning but has fallen out of the habit lately, then morning exercise may be a good choice. Together these two strategies, if used consistently, may help such patients to shift their clocks to an earlier time so that waking up becomes easier over time.

### Depression-Related Anhedonia

People whose insomnia is comorbid with depression also report greater difficulty adhering to out-of-bed or rise times (Manber et al., 2011), but, unlike those with eveningness tendencies, they usually do not find it difficult to wake up in the morning. In fact, as discussed in Chapter 5, some may wake up earlier than when in a euthymic state. In depression, difficulty getting out of bed is often related to anhedonia. Here again, the therapist can help these patients schedule activities that will provide motivation to get going shortly after they wake up, following the same principles as those mentioned in our discussion above of eveningness-related morning difficulties. In general, it is easier to get out of bed for an activity that one is motivated to do. Activities that involve commitments to others may be particularly helpful for those with depression, because in addition to helping them get out of bed in the morning at the same time, these activities can reduce the social isolation that some patients with depression experience. The principles and strategies described in the book *Behavioral Activation for Depression* (Martell, Dimidjian, & Herman-Dunn, 2010) can be helpful for promoting adherence with the instruction to get out of bed at the same time every day (shortly after the fixed wake-up time). Martell and colleagues present ways to help patients to follow a behavioral plan rather than a feeling.

### A Fixed Wake Time May Lead to a Regular Bedtime

Finally, it should be noted that going to bed at the same time every night is *not* a stimulus control instruction and is not what Instruction 1 is about. Instead, Instruction 1 is to use sleepiness as a guide for when to go to bed. By strengthening the circadian clock, Instruction 4 (sticking to a fixed wake-up time) eventually leads to feeling sleepy at roughly the same time most evenings and hence to a regular bedtime. Sharing this expectation with patients can be helpful.

As discussed in regard to Instruction 1 above, going to bed at the same time every night is recommended in some cases, when fear of sleep and hypervigilance interfere with recognition of sleepiness.

## Instruction 5: Do Not Nap

As discussed in Chapter 2, napping (as distinct from resting) decreases the homeostatic sleep drive. In general, people with insomnia are not able to nap even when provided with opportunities (Chapter 2). However, people whose insomnia is comorbid with disorders that are associated with marked daytime sleepiness, such as sleep apnea, are usually able to nap and may need to nap to ensure that they do not fall asleep while driving or performing other activities that are dangerous when a person is not optimally alert. Drowsy driving is a safety issue that patients should be reminded of when Instruction 5 is discussed. Safety naps can be taken at any time, because safety supersedes all other sleep guidelines.

In rare cases that are unrelated to safety, a therapist may choose to relax this instruction somewhat, even though ideally it is best to avoid napping altogether. These cases usually involve extremely high sleep anxiety that interferes with a patient's engagement in other important aspects of treatment. When making this alteration, the therapist should try to minimize the detrimental effects of naps to the healthy regulation of sleep. Naps are least disruptive to the regulation of sleep when they are short (e.g., 20 minutes) and occur early in the day, preferably no later than early afternoon. Napping (or even dozing) that occurs close to bedtime may not leave enough time for the homeostatic sleep drive to rebuild sufficiently to support sleep at night. That said, patients should be advised that before they engage in activities for which high sleepiness levels pose a safety risk, preemptive naps are encouraged. Safety should always receive the highest priority. When a patient is taking a nap, an alarm can be used to ensure that the nap is short. The therapist should weigh the pros and cons of relaxing the nap instruction, keeping in mind that failed nap attempts provide additional opportunities for pairing the bed with sleeplessness and hence strengthen conditioned arousal.

## Countercontrol: An Alternative Form of Stimulus Control Therapy

*Countercontrol* is an alternative form of stimulus control therapy, in which the recommendation to get out of bed when unable to sleep is replaced by a recommendation to sit up in bed and engage in a calming activity, such as reading, watching TV, or listening to music or an audiobook (Davies, Lacks, Storandt, & Bertelson, 1986; Zwart & Lisman, 1979). Countercontrol is based on the premise that the most crucial element of stimulus control may be the dissociation of the bed from "trying to sleep" and/or suffering the frustration of not sleeping. Countercontrol has been found to be superior to a delayed-treatment control and nearly equivalent to stimulus control (Davies et al., 1986; Zwart & Lisman, 1979). The following are clinical situations in which the therapist may want to consider countercontrol as an alternative for stimulus control.

- *Safety concerns and medical necessity.* Getting out of bed in the middle of the night when unable to sleep can be dangerous for frail patients, such as those with restricted mobility and those with medical conditions involving an increased risk of falls (e.g., orthostatic hypotension). Getting out of bed is also not feasible for immobile or nonambulatory patients. Countercontrol is safer and more feasible in such situations.

- *High sleep-related anxiety.* Some patients react to the idea of getting out of bed when unable to sleep with very high levels of anxiety or resistance. They may understand the theory, but their anxious response creates high levels of arousal that could offset the potential benefits of following the stimulus control instructions. Countercontrol is a useful alternative to consider in such cases, as are motivational enhancement and other cognitive therapy techniques (see Chapter 9).
- *Patients who are overzealous.* Some patients are overzealous about getting out of bed in the middle of the night. They get out of bed immediately after waking, depriving themselves of any opportunity to fall back to sleep. Countercontrol is an option they may be willing to consider.

## A Word about Implementing Stimulus Control in PTSD

As discussed in Chapter 5, previous exposure to trauma that occurred in a sleep-related context (e.g., exposure to disaster, combat, brutality, or rape that started when the person was asleep) may lead to later experience of high levels of hypervigilance in bed and fear of going to bed. In such cases, the instruction to go (or return) to bed only when sleepy may not be feasible, because the fear and vigilance mask sleepiness. Although using the sensation of sleepiness as a guide for when to go (or return) to bed should be the rule, the therapist can consider modifications to Instructions 1 and 3 when poor recognition of sleepiness states related to PTSD hypervigilance is present.

- *Modified Instruction 1:* Go to bed at a set time.
- *Modified Instruction 3:* If unable to sleep, get out of bed and return to sleep after 20 minutes.

At the same time, it is also important to pay attention to presleep and middle-of-the-night activities when such a patient is out of bed, and to ensure that these activities are likely to reduce arousal.

# SLEEP RESTRICTION THERAPY

Sleep restriction therapy was first introduced in 1987 by Arthur Spielman and colleagues (Spielman, Saskin, & Thorpy, 1987). It is an iterative (i.e., gradual, multistep) process that starts with a focus on improving sleep quality (by reducing unwanted wakefulness) and then gradually on increasing sleep quantity. This is done by first reducing the TIB to be equal to the average amount of time the patient reports currently sleeping based on sleep diary data (but never below what will be safe) and avoiding daytime naps. Patients who adhere to the TIB restriction usually experience a marked decrease in unwanted wakefulness within a week or two. Their sleep becomes consolidated, and they report improved sleep quality. When the desired sleep consolidation is attained, the next step in the sleep restriction therapy process is to increase TIB by small increments (15–30 minutes per week), as described below. Subsequent increases in TIB are considered after at least a week on a new schedule and commence only if sleep remains consolidated and more sleep is needed (i.e., daytime alertness is not yet optimal). Because patients with insomnia tend to underestimate how much time they are asleep (Chapter 1), prescribing a TIB that equals their reported time asleep may lead to an actual reduction in their total sleep time (TST) and an associated increase in the drive for sleep (Chapter 2). For that reason, the first step of sleep restriction is in essence "harnessing the sleep drive" to reduce wakefulness and improve sleep quality. Sleep restriction therapy is particularly helpful for consolidating fragmented sleep (middle insomnia), but the increase in sleep drive can also reduce the time needed to fall asleep at the beginning of the sleep period. Sleep restriction therapy is now used for treating all aspects of insomnia in all age groups. Below we elaborate on the instructions and highlight clinically relevant implementation issues.

## Step 1: The Initial TIB Restriction

The first step is to determine the recommended TIB and its specific placement (starting with collaboratively determining morning wake time).

### The Initial TIB

The original sleep restriction therapy protocol recommended using the current average TST as the initial TIB. Ideally, this is based on data from 2 weeks of daily sleep diaries (discounting atypical nights such as those involving illness or travel). When 2 weeks of data are not available, then 1 week of data can be used. There is a large night-to-night variability in sleep among people with insomnia (Wohlgemuth et al., 1999). The greater the variability in a patient's sleep pattern, the longer the duration of the baseline sleep diary should be in order to enhance the accuracy of the estimated average TST. In some cases, 3 weeks of baseline diary collection may be necessary. The initial TIB is determined by using the following formula, but it should *never* be below 5 hours, even if the average TST is less than that:

TIB = Average of TST in the past week (based on sleep diary, rounded to the nearest quarter hour)

### Placement of the TIB Window of Opportunity for Sleep

After determining the patient's duration of time in bed, the therapist and patient select a wake-up time that fits the patient's life circumstances and circadian tendency or chronotype (examples are given below). Once TIB and wake time have been determined, bedtime is determined by counting back from wake time. For example, if TIB is 6 hours, and wake time is 6:30 A.M., then bedtime will be 6 hours before wake time (i.e., 12:30 A.M.). As in stimulus control, the wake time has to be the same every day even on nonwork days, and getting out of bed should occur 5–15 minutes after wake time. The rationale is the same as discussed above in the section on stimulus control.

The following two examples demonstrate the importance of paying attention to a patient's chronotype in making decisions about the initial TIB recommendation. If the patient has a morningness tendency and wakes up earlier than desired, it is best to choose a wake time that is as close to the patient's personal target wake time as the patient will tolerate, given that the chosen wake time and TIB usually imply that the patient will need to delay bedtime. For example, a 12:30 A.M. to 6:30 A.M. TIB may not be feasible for a patient with a morningness tendency, a 9:30 P.M. habitual bedtime, fast sleep onset, and an expressed desire to set wake time at 6:30 A.M., because the patient may have significant difficulty staying up until 12:30 A.M. In this case, the therapist and patient will need to identify the latest feasible bedtime, keeping in mind that it is best for it to be as late as possible.

Here is another example, concerning a person with an eveningness tendency, a variable habitual wake time between 10:30 A.M. and 12:30 P.M., a variable habitual bedtime between 12:30 A.M. and 3:00 A.M., sleep initiation difficulty, and an expressed desire to set the wake time at 7:30 A.M. A 12:30 A.M. to 7:30 A.M. initial TIB recommendation may not be a good fit for this person, for two reasons: (1) This TIB does not match the patient's chronotype and is therefore not likely to help the patient fall asleep faster, and (2) with variable habitual schedule, the patient may not be able to wake up consistently to an alarm at 7:30 A.M.

## Clinical Issues Relevant to Step 1 of Sleep Restriction Therapy

### PRESENTING THE RATIONALE FOR INITIAL TIB RESTRICTION

Before introducing this procedure, the clinician should explain the rationale, anticipating the potential for an anxiety response and trying to preempt it. It is best to avoid the professional term *sleep restriction*, because it may produce anxiety in some patients. Alternative terms, less likely to produce anxiety, are *time-in-bed restriction*, *sleep quality enhancement*, and *sleep efficiency training*. These terms also better describe the initial step, which in fact restricts TIB and increases sleep quality. Examples of presenting the rationale for sleep restriction therapy can be found in Chapters 11 and 12. Key ideas to convey can be selected from the following list:

- The plan is to improve sleep quality first by consolidating it before increasing its quantity. Within limits, longer, uninterrupted sleep bouts are more important for feeling refreshed in the morning than TST per se (see Chapter 2).
- The initial curtailment of TIB is only the first step in a gradual, multistep process. The sleep opportunity window will be expanded slowly as sleep becomes more consolidated. Knowledge of the overall plan and how it works may reduce anxiety in response to the idea of limiting TIB.
- The new sleep schedule could create mild sleep deprivation, which will strengthen the sleep drive. The sleep drive is a sleep-promoting factor.
- There is no single universally ideal amount of sleep. The slow expansion of the sleep opportunity window helps the patient discover his or her true sleep need (i.e., the amount of sleep needed for optimal alertness).
- The new sleep schedule is not likely to reduce TST much below what the patient is currently sleeping (unless the patient's anxiety about the process is so high that it overrides the stronger sleep drive).

## COLLABORATION

The best way to present sleep restriction therapy is to explain the process and its rationale, and then ask the patient to determine TIB and the optimal times to get out of and into bed. This is a two-way process, in which the clinician helps shape the discussion to ensure that the end result is feasible, especially in regard to the patient's chronotype. For example, Chapter 11 describes the process of deriving Sophie's TIB window. The therapist reviewed her sleep diary data before the session and computed her average TST, which was 6 hours and 15 minutes. Sophie first chose a 7:00 A.M. wake time, which was the time for which she was setting an alarm on work days; when she counted back to determine the earliest bedtime, however, Sophie realized that this meant she would have to go to bed at 12:45, which she considered too late. Sophie then volunteered an earlier alarm time, to make sure that she could adhere to both the "earliest bedtime" and the "latest rise time" rules. Such a collaborative process of determining TIB placement provides an opportunity to identify potential obstacles to adherence and therefore should not be rushed. Flexibility and sensitivity to what the patient can tolerate will promote adherence.

## SAFETY ISSUES

Concerns about safety are the reason for never restricting TIB to less than 5 hours. In the original sleep restriction protocol, the minimum TIB was 4.5 hours (Spielman, Saskin, & Thorpy, 1987) but a 5-hour minimum has been used in several subsequent implementations (e.g., Morin, Colecchi, et al., 1999). These concerns include emergence of daytime sleepiness as a side effect and the potential for exacerbating comorbid conditions, both of which are further discussed below. In either case, patients should be alerted. When safety is a concern, the therapist needs to consider alternative, more liberal versions of sleep restriction therapy (discussed below), or to avoid it altogether and rely on other CBT-I techniques as clinically indicated.

*Daytime Sleepiness.* Daytime sleepiness may emerge during the initial stages of sleep restriction therapy (Perlis et al., 2004). Concerns about sleepiness-related safety are particularly relevant to patients with sleep apnea and other medical illnesses associated with daytime sleepiness, as well as to patients taking medications that produce daytime sedation. Chapter 12 describes how Sam's sleep apnea was not adequately treated because Sam was not fully adhering to the use of his CPAP device. The therapist consulted with a sleep specialist to determine whether CBT-I should commence and whether any adaptations to CBT-I would be necessary for Sam. The sleep specialist suggested encouraging Sam to use CPAP as directed and to proceed cautiously with CBT-I.

Regardless of the cause of sleepiness, patients should be alerted and advised to avoid driving or conducting other potentially dangerous activities (such as using power tools) while sleepy, and to take safety naps as needed. In Sam's case, cautious implementation of CBT-I included encouraging him to nap at times when there were possible safety concerns. Although it is best to avoid naps (because sleep decreases the sleep drive), safety concerns preempt this rule, as noted earlier. In some implementations (e.g., Morin, Colecchi, et al., 1999), daytime napping was made optional but limited to less than 1 hour taken before 3:00 P.M. When daytime sleepiness (as distinct from tiredness and fatigue) is severe, it is best to avoid sleep restriction therapy altogether and instead utilize other CBT-I components.

*Exacerbation of Comorbid Conditions.* Restricting TIB may aggravate some comorbidities. In addition to its impact on illnesses that are associated with excessive daytime sleepiness, restricting TIB may cause sleep loss, which in turn could lower seizure thresholds in epileptic patients (Fountain, Kim, & Lee, 1998), lower the panic threshold in those with PD (Roy-Byrne, Mellman, & Uhde, 1988), exacerbate sleep walking and night terrors (Pressman, 2007), and precipitate mania (or hypomania) in patients with bipolar disorder (Colombo, Benedetti, Barbini, Campori, & Smeraldi, 1999). (Some research suggests that the risk of a switch into (hypo)mania following sleep deprivation is not more pronounced than the risk associated with typical pharmacological antidepressant treatment; Riemann et al., 2002.)

## THE IMPORTANCE OF THE SLEEP DIARY

The sleep diary is essential for proper administration of sleep restriction therapy. As discussed in Chapter 6, retrospective information about sleep habits is subject to reporting biases, and therefore its use may result in a less accurate estimation of TST than that based on prospective data. In addition, the sleep diary provides a better method for accurate and detailed monitoring of changes in sleep over time than does the patient's global reflection.

However, despite multiple reminders and despite emphasis on the importance of diary data, some patients do not complete a sleep diary. When a patient reports that completing the sleep diary "makes me too anxious," the therapist needs to decide whether or not completion of the sleep diary may be contraindicated for the case. Sometimes the expressed concern is based on a belief rather than on data. Therefore, before relaxing the request for daily sleep diary data, it may be helpful to ask the patient to test whether monitoring sleep in the diary will actually lead to worsening of sleep. In our collective clinical experience, many but not all previously reluctant patients come to the conclusion that this is not the case. If completion of the daily sleep diary does lead to worsening of sleep, or if the patient is not willing to engage in the experiment, the clinician can consider proceeding with sleep restriction therapy in the absence of sleep diary data. In such a case, the initial TIB will be based on self-reported sleep schedule. The clinical decision about whether to proceed without sleep diary data is based on balancing all the clinically relevant aspects of the case. Factors to consider include the possibility that a recommended TIB based on retrospective report may not be accurate and may result in unsafe levels of daytime sleepiness; the patient's level of anxiety about keeping a sleep diary; and other clinically relevant factors, such as the possibility that the patient is not making diary recording a priority.

## DEALING WITH OBSTACLES TO ADHERENCE

*Difficulties with Adhering to the TIB Window.* Difficulties (anticipated or actual) in waiting until the designated bedtime and wake time may have different causes. Some of the adherence issues relevant to sleep restriction therapy are similar to those already discussed in the section on stimulus control. For instance, we have already discussed planning activities that will assist patients in adhering to fixed wake times and out-of-bed times, and in dealing with some partner-related issues. We now discuss additional issues.

- *Difficulty delaying bedtime.* Implementation of sleep restriction therapy may involve delaying bedtime relative to baseline. This may be difficult for people with morningness tendencies, because they may doze off before the recommended bedtime. To help these patients, the therapist can recommend that they engage in stimulating rather than calming activities in the evening, in order to avoid dozing off too early.

- *Partner-related adherence obstacles to implementing sleep restriction therapy.* Again, in the section on stimulus control, we have discussed several partner-related issues. In regard to stimulus control Instruction 1, we have suggested encouraging patients to work on solutions with their partners collaboratively. For example, we have recommended that a patient who is not sleepy at a couple's habitual bedtime negotiate visiting with the bed partner at the couple's current bedtime and then leaving the bed until sleepy. A similar strategy may apply to a patient whose designated sleep restriction bedtime is later than the couple's habitual bedtime. This strategy may work well for a patient with an evening chronotype, but may not be feasible for a morning person, because it may be difficult to stay awake while visiting with the bed partner. In such cases, the couple will need to come up with alternative solutions. For instance, the couple may decide to have different bedtimes during the early stage of sleep restriction therapy, or the bed partner may agree to go to sleep later and help the patient stay awake until the designated bedtime. In either case, it helps to know that these alterations in the couple's habits are likely to be needed only for a relatively short time, until the patient's bedtime becomes earlier.

*Heightened Anxiety in Response to Sleep Restriction Therapy.* Sometimes the idea of restricting TIB leads to very high anxiety; as discussed in Chapter 3, this can compete with and override the increase in sleep drive that typically accompanies the restricted TIB. Under such circumstances, alternative versions of sleep restriction therapy (discussed below) may be considered. In extreme cases, other components of CBT-I (cognitive therapy and anxiety reduction skills) may need to be implemented before sleep restriction therapy is introduced.

## Step 2: Instructions for TIB Alterations

Alterations to TIB are considered at each session after the initiation of TIB restriction. These sessions are typically scheduled 1–2 weeks apart. In the original sleep restriction protocol, study participants called in daily to report their sleep diary data, and alterations to TIB were considered every 5 days (Spielman, Saskin, & Thorpy, 1987). Each session begins with a review of the sleep diary and assessments of adherence to the previously recommended TIB, improvement in sleep quality (defined by sleep efficiency or SE; see Chapter 6 and below), and a clinical assessment of the need for more sleep (see below).

### Sleep Quality

In sleep restriction therapy, sleep quality is operationalized as SE—that is, the percentage of TIB that was spent asleep (TST). The reader has already encountered this term in Chapter 6, where we have discussed variables that can be derived from the diary data. As a reminder, SE is computed by using the formula (TST/TIB)*100. Table 7.2 is an example summary of 7 days of sleep

**TABLE 7.2. Sample Sleep Efficiency (SE) Calculations over 7 Days**

| Day | Time in bed (TIB) | Total sleep time (TST) | Sleep efficiency (SE) |
|-----|-------------------|------------------------|------------------------|
| 1 | 12.9 | 7.2 | 55.8% |
| 2 | 12.7 | 8.9 | 70.1% |
| 3 | 13.6 | 7.9 | 58.1% |
| 4 | 13.3 | 8.3 | 62.4% |
| 5 | 13.2 | 9.1 | 68.9% |
| 6 | 10.9 | 7.9 | 72.5% |
| 7 | 13.6 | 10.5 | 77.2% |
| Mean | 12.9 | 8.5 | 66.4% |

diary data. The columns include the TIB and TST values for each of the 7 nights. The last row gives the averages (means) of TIB (12.9 hours), TST (8.5 hours), and SE (66.4%). Each average is computed as the sum of the seven daily values divided by 7. (When data are missing, the sum should be divided by the number of days for which data are available. As discussed in Chapter 6, averages based on less than 5 days of data should be considered unstable.) The sleep restriction protocol uses the average SE as an index of a patient's sleep quality. Two cutoff values for SE, 85% (Edinger, Hoelscher, Marsh, Lipper, & Ionescu-Pioggia, 1992) and 90% (Spielman, Saskin, & Thorpy, 1987), have been used to define "good sleep quality" when sleep restriction therapy is implemented. In this book, we use the 85% cutoff.

## Sleep Need

In sleep restriction therapy, sleep need is determined by the subjective perception of alertness during the day. Higher alertness during the day means lower need for sleep. Although people may have other reasons for wanting to sleep more than they do, sleep restriction therapy is focused on optimizing daytime alertness. In other words, sleep need is distinct from sleep want. How refreshing sleep was judged to be may be less pertinent, particularly for people with evening chronotypes; because they experience sleep inertia, they tend to judge their sleep as nonrefreshing and infer that they need more.

## The Rules for Changing TIB

- *If SE in the prior week was at least 85%,* then the TIB is increased by 15 minutes. The focus is on last week's SE, even when 2 or more weeks of data may be available. This is because SE increases over time, when adherence is high, and also because initial daytime sleepiness is transient. Therefore, data from the week just before the appointment provide more clinically relevant information on what to do next than the grand mean of all available data does. For example, if the first week of sleep restriction resulted in 81% SE, but in the most recent week the SE was

87%, the mean of the 2 weeks is less than 85%. Using the grand mean will result in a different course of action than using the most recent week. The fact that SE is now quite high (87%) suggests that the patient is improving and could benefit from a longer TIB. If the patient experiences daytime sleepiness (distinct from fatigue and tiredness), the TIB is increased by 30 minutes (or more, if daytime sleepiness is very high), and other safety measures are taken as indicated. (See Step 1 above.)

• *If SE is less than 80%,* then a new TIB is calculated, based on the current sleep diary data and Step 1 guidelines. We refer to this strategy as *recalibrating* TIB. As in Step 1 of sleep restriction therapy, obstacles to adherence need to be identified and worked through to facilitate adherence to the new TIB. Another tested implementation is to further curtail the TIB by 15–30 minutes (Morin, Colecchi, et al., 1999) instead of recalculating TST based on last week's data. The disadvantage of this approach is that TIB reduction can be experienced as punitive.

• *If SE is between 80 and 84%,* then the therapist can consider one of the following options:

  • Leave TIB unaltered, as indicated in the original sleep restriction therapy algorithm (Spielman, Saskin, & Thorpy, 1987).
  • Recalibrate TIB. That is, assign TIB based on the current sleep diary data and Step 1 rules.

In either case, the therapist chooses a TIB that should facilitate adherence, promotes safety, and focuses on identifying and working through obstacles to adherence (see Figure 7.2).

### Clinical Issues Relevant to Step 2 of Sleep Restriction Therapy

Clinical issues relevant to Step 2 include those already discussed for Step 1 above, as well as the following:

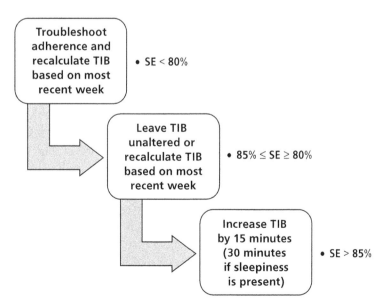

**FIGURE 7.2.** Decision tree for altering time in bed (TIB).

- Poor or inconsistent adherence is a common reason for failure to improve sufficiently, but by no means the only reason to consider.
- There may be changes in the patient's life circumstances, such as increased stress, illness, or travel. In such cases, the therapist can restart the sleep restriction therapy protocol afresh (recalibrate).
- The TIB window may have not been ideal for the patient's chronotype, possibly because it has been hard to identify the patient's morningness–eveningness tendency. In such cases the therapist shifts the TIB window for a better match to the patient's estimated chronotype as needed and feasible, based on schedule contraints.
- There was an unforeseen increase in sleep-related anxiety. This may indicate that one of the alternatives to sleep restriction therapy may need to be considered (see below), or that the patient is not yet ready for sleep restriction therapy.

## Alternative Sleep Restriction Protocols

We present below a few proposed and studied variants of sleep restriction therapy. Deciding which variant to use requires consideration of the costs and benefits. The standard protocol given above is ideal for patients who can tolerate and are likely to adhere to it, and for whom there are no safety concerns. It produces fast improvement in sleep quality (i.e., higher SE). More liberal alternatives may work better for patients with high sleep-related anxiety, those with high levels of daytime sleepiness, those who routinely nap, and those with certain comorbidities (e.g., bipolar and seizure disorders).

### More Liberal Initial TIB Prescription in Step 1

More liberal initial TIB prescriptions have been tested in the literature. For example, focused on improving adherence, Friedman, Bliwise, Yesavage, and Salom (1991) modified Spielman and colleagues' protocol and negotiated with each participant an acceptable TIB window that was as close an approximation of the average current TST as the patient could tolerate. Edinger and colleagues reasoned that the SE of people with no sleep complaints is not 100%, because even the best of sleepers take a few minutes to fall asleep and have some brief awakenings from sleep. They first proposed to add to the average current TST age-appropriate times to fall asleep and middle-of-the-night wakefulness (Edinger et al., 1992; Hoelscher & Edinger, 1988), and a decade later they used TST + 30 minutes as the initial TIB recommendation (Edinger et al., 2001). In addition to being tested in older adults (Edinger et al., 2001), this variant was proven effective when used as a component of CBT-I for people with comorbid MDD (Manber et al., 2008), patients with mixed psychiatric disorders (Edinger et al., 2009), and patients with fibromyalgia (Edinger et al., 2005). We should note, however, that strict versions have also been used and shown to be effective when implemented as part of CBT for patients whose insomnia is comorbid with cancer (Savard, Simard, Ivers, & Morin, 2005), chronic pain (Vitiello, Rybarczyk, Von Korff, & Stepanski, 2009) or with mixed medical and psychiatric conditions (Perlis, Sharpe, Smith, Greenblatt, & Giles, 2001), as well as for older adults (Morin, Kowatch, et al., 1993). We therefore recommend that clinicians use clinical judgment to decide which version will best suit a given case, and consider a liberal TIB recommendation for patients who manifest daytime sleepiness.

Another liberal variant of sleep restriction therapy is to base TIB on the total amount of sleep per 24 hours, rather than just at night. This version may be particularly relevant to patients who nap regularly. We illustrate this strategy in Chapter 12 with Sam. Sam, a 60-year-old man with insomnia, fibromyalgia, and sleep apnea, spent 8 hours and 15 minutes in bed each night and slept an average of 4 hours and 5 minutes (his average SE was 51%). He also spent considerable time during the day resting, dozing, and napping, averaging 2 hours per day. If only his nighttime sleep were considered, his TIB prescription would have been 5 hours—the minimum we recommend (because his TST was less than the minimum recommended). However, Sam had comorbid sleep apnea and some sleepiness, raising safety concerns. Moreover, his sleeping for an average of 2 hours during the day suggested that his current sleep need might be more than 5 hours. Therefore, the therapist considered the total sleep time in the 24-hour period and recommended that Sam's initial TIB should be 6.5 hours (6 hours of sleep over 24 hours, plus a 30-minute safety margin). Sam was also reminded to take safety precautions. At his next appointment, Sam's SE increased to 80%, and his prescription remained unchanged. At a subsequent appointment, his SE further increased to 93%, which would typically trigger a 30-minute increase. However, Sam was nervous that any further increase would result in worsened sleep. The therapist was concerned that this might not be optimal for Sam, and encouraged Sam to test this belief by increasing the TIB modestly (15 minutes) and then evaluating the evidence on whether his sleep worsened significantly.

Another example where a more liberal TIB should be considered is in work with parents of infants, who are up in the middle of the night to feed or otherwise care for the infants. Most are able to fall back asleep right away, but those with insomnia may have difficulty. In such a case, we recommend that sleep restriction therapy make allowance for the time spent tending to the infant. That is, the TIB recommendation should be TST plus the time spent tending to the infant. This recommendation is based on our clinical experience, and at this writing one of us (Rachel Manber) is testing it in a study of CBT-I for perinatal insomnia.

### Different Criteria for TIB Alterations in Step 2

The protocol outlined above uses an 85% SE threshold for increasing TIB and an 80% threshold for decreasing TIB. The original sleep restriction protocol used 90% and 85% cutoffs, respectively. In practice, clinicians use thresholds that are based on their clinical judgment and experience. Based on our collective experience, we recommend basing the decision cutoffs on a patient's baseline SE, adherence, and progress. For example, if a patient's baseline SE is at or above 80%, then it would be reasonable to increase TIB only when SE increases to 90% or more, particularly if in addition the level of adherence is low. Regardless, in cases with low levels of adherence where the initial TIB is low, clinical judgment regarding alteration of TIB should be based on what is most likely to improve adherence.

### Sleep Compression

*Sleep compression therapy* (Lichstein et al., 2001; Riedel, Lichstein, & Dwyer, 1995) is a variant of sleep restriction therapy that consists of a gradual, rather than abrupt, restriction of TIB. It is a form of shaping that may be very useful for patients with extreme anxiety about restricting TIB, for people with high levels of daytime sleepiness, and for older adults. The idea is to reduce excess TIB (the difference between the average TIB and the average TST at baseline) gradually. The gradual decrease can be designed in a flexible manner. Lichstein and colleagues recommend that in a six-session treatment, the initial reduction should be one-sixth of the baseline TIB excess per therapy session. For example, for a patient who at baseline spends an average of 8 hours in bed but sleeps an average of 6 hours, TIB will be reduced each week by 20 minutes (Lichstein, Thomas, & McCurry, 2011). At each subsequent session, an additional 20-minute reduction can be implemented. Alternatively, the next reduction can be based on the current TIB excess and the number of remaining sessions. The process stops when there is no longer clinical justification for further compression. See Table 7.3 for an example of a sleep compression protocol.

### A Word about Implementing Sleep Restriction in PTSD

Some patients with PTSD, particularly those with trauma related to nighttime combat experiences, do not allocate enough time for sleep at night. This may be due to discomfort with silence, fear of having a nightmare, or the need to monitor for safety (hypervigilance). Because their time in bed is already restricted, sleep restriction therapy will not be useful. In fact, these patients will need to learn to tolerate spending more time in bed through the use of stimulus control, cognitive therapy, and carefully selected counterarousal measures. Some of these patients make up for curtailed sleep at night by sleeping more during the day. In such cases, the aim is to increase TIB gradually, while reducing and eventually eliminating daytime napping.

## COMBINING SLEEP RESTRICTION THERAPY AND STIMULUS CONTROL

Stimulus control and sleep restriction therapy are often combined. The combined instructions are essentially the five stimulus control instructions, modified by specifying times for going into and out of bed. These are summarized in Table 7.4 and in Combined Sleep Guidelines (Appendix C), a handout for patients. Clinical examples of using the combined instructions can be found in Chapters 11 and 12.

**TABLE 7.3. Example of a Sleep Compression Protocol**

| Pretreatment values | Week | TIB prescription |
|---|---|---|
| TIB = 8 hours<br>TST = 6 hours | 1 | 7 hours, 40 minutes |
| | 2 | 7 hours, 20 minutes |
| | 3 | 7 hours |
| | 4 | 6 hours, 40 minutes |
| | 5 | 6 hours, 20 minutes |
| | 6 | 6 hours |

**TABLE 7.4. Combining Stimulus Control and Sleep Restriction Therapy: Combined Sleep Rules**

1. Wake up at _____ every day (set an alarm), regardless of how much sleep you actually get, and get out of bed within a few minutes after your alarm rings.

2. Go to bed when you are sleepy (remember that being sleepy is different from being tired), *but not before* _____. (If you do not feel sleepy at this time, wait until you *do* feel sleepy.)

3. If you can't sleep, *stop trying.* Get up and do something calming, and return to bed only when you are sleepy again. When you lie in bed awake trying to sleep, wanting and hoping to go back to sleep, you are training yourself to be awake in bed.

4. Use the bed only for sleeping. Do not read, eat, watch TV, etc., in bed. Sex is an exception. The most important activity to eliminate from the bed is the activity of "trying to sleep," because it inevitably interferes with the natural sleep process.

5. Avoid daytime napping—but if you believe that sleepiness compromises your safety, do take a nap.

## SUMMARY OF PRINCIPLES FOR SUCCESSFUL DELIVERY OF STIMULUS CONTROL AND SLEEP RESTRICTION

1. The therapist should provide a rationale anchored in a solid understanding of sleep regulation (Chapters 2 and 3) and tailored to each patient's clinical presentation.

   a. This rationale should include only information relevant to the patient. For instance, a patient with a normal circadian chronotype does not necessarily need to be provided education about the circadian process.
   b. The therapist should consider the patient's sleep-related anxiety, and provide information that will help preempt an anxious response to the recommended behavioral changes.
   c. The therapist needs to avoid overwhelming the patient.
   d. The therapist should elicit feedback to track the patient's understanding.

2. Collaboration with the patient is vital! The therapist should explain the principle(s), and ask patients to state how these apply to them.

3. Although flexibility is important, the therapist should use the strictest guidelines that a patient can tolerate and adhere to. Understanding and following the spirit of the law, rather than getting caught up in the letter of the law, should be the aim.

4. Nonadherence may be an indication of problems with the delivery of these behavioral components, and hence may call for reappraisal and appropriate adjustment of the therapist's behaviors.

   a. The therapist may have failed to obtain sufficient feedback to ascertain that the patient understood the rationale. (The patient's understanding should be checked now.)
   b. The rationale provided may have not been optimal for this patient. If so, the therapist should try again.

c. The therapist may have failed to identify potential obstacles to adherence. If so, reasons for nonadherence should be explored, and the guidelines should be adjusted accordingly.

5. Consistent adherence must be emphasized and promoted. The therapist and patient should collaboratively create a list of activities to promote adherence to the prescribed into- and out-of-bed times.

## KEY PRACTICE IDEAS

- Together, stimulus control and sleep restriction therapy work to normalize the three sleep regulatory systems discussed in earlier chapters: the sleep drive (Chapter 2), the circadian rhythm (Chapter 2), and the arousal system (Chapter 3).

- The sleep drive is stabilized by limiting naps (both stimulus control and sleep restriction) and TIB (sleep restriction).

- To some extent, stimulus control also limits TIB, because it instructs patients to get out of bed when unable to sleep and always to wake up at the same time, regardless of how much sleep was obtained.

- A fixed wake time, common to both interventions, also strengthens the circadian clock signals, because it means that two factors that help entrain the circadian clock are consistently present (see Chapter 2).

- Conditioned arousal is decreased by eliminating sleep-incompatible behaviors (the most important of which is sleep effort) from the bed and bedroom (see Instructions 1, 2, and 3 for stimulus control).

# CHAPTER 8

# Behavioral Components of CBT-I

## *Part II*

In this chapter, we describe additional behavioral components of CBT-I that are helpful adjuncts to stimulus control and sleep restriction therapy. These include (1) techniques to reduce arousal in bed, and (2) sleep hygiene therapy (i.e., timing the use of food, caffeine, alcohol, nicotine, and exercise, and optimizing the sleep environment). Whereas stimulus control and sleep restriction therapy, as described in Chapter 7, are effective when applied separately or combined (Morin, Bootzin, et al., 2006; Morin, Hauri, et al., 1999), arousal reduction methods and sleep hygiene instructions are not effective as stand-alone therapies (Morin, Bootzin, et al., 2006; Morin, Hauri, et al., 1999) but are often included in the CBT-I package as adjunctive to the two core behavioral interventions. Relatedly, properly timed light exposure is recommended for the treatment of circadian rhythm sleep–wake disorders (Chesson et al., 1999), and it is also sometimes used to help facilitate the treatment of insomnia in patients with morningness or eveningness tendencies. We therefore include a brief discussion of this vast and evolving topic.

## ADDRESSING HIGH AROUSAL/ACTIVATION

Most mental health clinicians are familiar with relaxation and other behavioral techniques for reducing arousal levels. In this section, we highlight a few techniques that are relevant or unique to insomnia.

### Creating a Time to Unwind before Bedtime

As discussed in Chapter 3, hyperarousal and hypervigilance are detrimental to sleep even when the sleep period is at a time of high homeostatic sleep drive and low alerting circadian signals. It is therefore important to take measures to promote a quiescent presleep state of mind. One such measure is to set aside time to unwind before bedtime. This creates a buffer between being active and engaged in striving activities, and being quiet and calm (i.e., in a state of low arousal that facilitates surrender to sleep). We call this quiet and calm time a *buffer zone*. This should be a time spent in a nonstriving state of being—doing pleasant activities that are not activating and are not done as means to an end, but rather for their own enjoyment. These activities do not hasten sleep directly. Instead, buffer zone activities are designed to facilitate sleep by reducing sleep-interfering arousal. In the language of sleep regulation that has been introduced in Chapters 2, 3, and 7, arousal counteracts the homeostatic drive and masks sleepiness. A buffer zone activity then serves two functions: by reducing arousal it facilitates sleep onset and by unmasking sleepiness it allows patients to use sleepiness as a guide for when to go to sleep (stimulus control instruction 1). People who state that they do not have time for a buffer zone are likely to need it the most and usually come to recognize that they can benefit from it. A therapist and patient collaboratively decide when the unwinding period should begin and what activities will be undertaken during the buffer zone time.

The specific presleep activities will vary among patients. Most people choose to read or watch TV as their primary buffer zone activities. It is important to ensure that the materials a patient is reading or watching are not upsetting or overstimulating—and, in the case of reading, not so suspenseful that they cannot be easily put down. Moreover, reading and TV/movie watching are by no means the only possible buffer zone activities. Other examples include listening to music, knitting, embroidering, stretching, and taking a warm bath. We emphasize the importance of carefully selecting the activities, because activities that are calming to one patient may be activating to another. Any activities that facilitate winding down can be buffer zone activities. The handout Buffer Zone Activities (see Appendix C) is a sample list of activities. Ideally, patients will generate lists of their own.

## Addressing Intrusive Presleep Cognitions

Thinking at bedtime or in the middle of the night about issues that have not been adequately addressed or resolved during the day, and worrying about future things not in one's control, are experienced by almost everyone as intrusive. In an attempt to eliminate the intrusive thoughts, people may try to clear their minds and to "not think," particularly upsetting thoughts. However, ironically, suppressing presleep thoughts is not an effective method for quieting the mind. Research has shown that continued attempts to suppress thoughts may lead to more intense worries and hence may interfere with sleep. This is because thought suppression requires mental effort, which may lead to mental fatigue and subsequently to rebound of the suppressed thoughts when the mental effort decreases (Ansfield et al., 1996).

CBT-I includes strategies for helping patients reduce their worries and intrusive thoughts when in bed, because these are incompatible with sleep. Worries and other unpleasant thoughts that are experienced in bed also exacerbate insomnia, because they weaken the bed as a cue for sleep. The latter (conditioned arousal) is addressed with stimulus control (Chapter 7). The former (intrusive thoughts) can be addressed with one of the following strategies, as further discussed below: (1) *scheduled worry*, an effective method to reduce intrusive worries in people with GAD (Borkovec, Wilkinson, Folensbee, & Lerman, 1983); (2) *constructive worry*, a technique tested for reducing presleep worries (Carney & Waters, 2006); (3) writing about presleep thoughts and concerns, another technique tested in people with difficulties getting to sleep because of such thoughts and worries (Harvey & Farrell, 2003); and (4) creating a "to-do" list, a common-sense approach to reducing mental load at night.

## Scheduled Worry

The instructions to patients for scheduled worry are as follows:

1. Learn to identify worrisome thoughts and other thoughts that are unnecessary or unpleasant. Distinguish these from necessary or pleasant thoughts related to the present moment. In the context of sleep, all worries are intrusive.
2. Establish a worry period to take place at the same time and in the same location each day.
3. When you catch yourself worrying, postpone the worry to the worry period, and replace it with attending to present-moment experience.
4. Make use of the worry period to worry about your concerns and to engage in problem solving to eliminate those concerns.

Scheduling worry time may sound counterintuitive and even foolish, but it is rooted in the idea that thought suppression is not an effective strategy to deal with unwanted intrusive thoughts. Instead, facing these intrusive thoughts diffuses their intensity and reduces their frequency. In the context of insomnia, it is best to schedule the time to worry not too close to bedtime. The original recommendation was to dedicate half an hour to worry daily (Borkovec et al., 1983). Our clinical experience indicates that a shorter duration is more feasible and is quite effective. In the context of insomnia, postponing worries may help break existing associations between worry and bed. As such, scheduled worry can be theoretically and practically integrated into stimulus control.

## Constructive Worry

The instructions to patients for constructive worry—first described by Espie and Lindsay (1987) as "worry control," and later by Carney and Waters (2006)—are as follows:

1. In the early evening, record three or more problems/worries that you think have the greatest likelihood of keeping you awake at bedtime.
2. For each problem listed, write down what will be the next step that could contribute to the resolution of the problem.
3. Place a worry worksheet on the nightstand next to your bed.
4. If you experience worry before bed, tell yourself that you have already dealt with your problems when you were at your problem-solving best, and there is nothing better you can do now that you are so tired.

This procedure is based on the idea that intrusive worries reflect ineffective problem solving (Wicklow & Espie, 2000), thwarted by anxiety (Davey, Hampton, Farrell, & Davidson, 1992); hence more effective problem solving should reduce intrusive worries.

*Presleep Writing*

The instructions for the presleep writing task are based on Pennebaker's (1997) work on therapeutic effects of writing as an emotional processing task. The protocols tested for addressing sleep-interfering thoughts in two studies were to write for 20 minutes before bedtime (Harvey & Farrell, 2003) or early in the evening (Mooney, Espie, & Broomfield, 2009) about "thoughts, concerns, or things on your mind," and to "be honest and explore the very deepest emotions and thoughts" (Harvey & Farrell, 2003, p. 118). These studies tested the effects of using this strategy for 3 or 4 days; they found a small or no reduction in the time to fall asleep compared to no writing, but not compared to neutral writing tasks (i.e., writing about hobbies or completing worry questionnaires). These findings suggest that presleep writing may reduce sleep effort and other sleep-incompatible behaviors. It is possible that writing about things on one's mind in the evening is too arousing and such writing earlier in the day or for more than a few days could be beneficial; but this possibility needs further testing.

*"To-Do" List for Tomorrow*

In today's busy life, multitasking is common, and many tasks remain unfinished at the end of the day. People with insomnia report thinking in bed about what needs to be done the next day, and they experience these thoughts as intrusive. Taking time at the end of the day (but before the buffer zone time) to list what needs to be done the next day can help a patient put these worries aside, so that they will not intrude when the patient is trying to sleep at the beginning or middle of the night. Having a written plan for the next day is likely to reduce intrusive thoughts about tomorrow's tasks. Critically examining the feasibility of the list can be additionally helpful for people who tend to hold unrealistic expectations about what they should be able to accomplish in a day.

## Relaxation

There is no single relaxation method that is best for everyone. Progressive muscle relaxation, meditation, and diaphragmatic breathing can all help calm an active mind. Together, a therapist and patient should select a relaxation method that best fits the patient, and the therapist should recommend practice during the before-bedtime wind-down period. Regardless of the relaxation method used, it is a good idea to tell the patient that relaxation is a skill that, like many other skills, requires training and practice. The key to relaxation around bedtime is letting go of sleep effort. Relaxing in order to sleep may become sleep effort in disguise. It is as if the person is in part relaxing and in part anxiously vigilant about whether they are falling asleep. One metaphor to explain this idea of co-existence of relaxation and arousal comes from the animal kingdom—specifically, from whales. Whales sleep one brain hemisphere at a time, allowing them to continue monitoring their environment while they are asleep (Lyamin et al., 2002). In Chapter 9, we discuss cognitive therapy techniques to address sleep effort.

Some people have difficulty learning relaxation procedures, and some become even more anxious when they try to relax (relaxation-induced anxiety). The anxiety is often about relinquishing control or hypervigilance, as is often the case in patients with PTSD. Relaxation-induced anxiety can be dealt with by providing further guidance or recommending methods that may be less likely to be perceived as relinquishing control or letting go of hypervigilance. Examples include using methods that emphasize attention to, rather than control of, breath (e.g., mindfulness breath-based meditation) and recommending indirect relaxation (i.e., engaging in activities that produce relaxation indirectly as a side effect, such as stretching and listening to certain music).

## Other Arousal Reduction Issues

Certain behaviors of people with insomnia stem from and perpetuate sleep effort and preoccupation with sleep, and therefore should be identified and discouraged. Examples of such behaviors include the following:

- Following rigid sleep rules (e.g., avoiding evening activities that are perceived as threats to sleep, such as occasionally staying up late for a show or other social activity).
- "Praying for sleep": Whereas praying can be a good meditative activity before bedtime, praying for sleep specifically may reflect anxious concerns, which are likely to interfere with sleep. As prayer is a very personal issue, this subject needs to be addressed respectfully, sensitively, and delicately.
- Complaining about sleep to others.
- Monitoring the clock.

Again, in Chapter 9 we discuss cognitive therapy techniques to address sleep effort—including avoidance behaviors and monitoring, as well as other sources of arousal in bed—and demonstrate how the idea of sleep effort can be explained to patients.

## SLEEP HYGIENE

*Sleep hygiene* refers to a set of behaviors that influence sleep. Poor sleep hygiene includes the use of sleep-disturbing substances (e.g., caffeine, alcohol, nicotine); improper timing of exercise and eating relative to the desired sleep period (see Chapter 6); and environmental factors (e.g., light, temperature, noise). *Sleep hygiene therapy* refers to a set of recommendations aimed at correcting sleep-interfering behaviors. Sometimes *sleep hygiene* is more broadly defined to include engaging in calming activities close to bedtime and sleep–wake scheduling. The narrowly defined sleep hygiene factors may be less relevant to patients with insomnia than to good sleepers: Among good sleepers, almost all domains of sleep hygiene correlate significantly with sleep ratings, whereas among patients with insomnia, only the arousal-related behaviors correlate with sleep ratings (Yang, Lin, Hsu, & Cheng, 2010). Similarly, Gellis and Lichstein (2009) found that the narrowly defined sleep hygiene factors did not distinguish well between poor and good sleepers; the most robust differentiating factor was that of engaging in arousal activities while in bed (worry, planning, and thinking about important matters). Moreover, sleep hygiene therapy does not have empirical support for use as a monotherapy (Morin, Bootzin, et al., 2006; Morin, Hauri, et al., 1999). It is thus probably best regarded as a sometimes necessary, but rarely sufficient, treatment strategy.

## Sleep-Disturbing Substances

### Alcohol

It is common for patients with insomnia to self-medicate with alcohol (Ancoli-Israel & Roth, 1999). In individuals with no alcohol abuse or dependence (as defined by DSM-IV), alcohol use has mixed effects on sleep. Shortly after consumption, alcohol leads to relaxation, which facilitates sleep onset. However, later in the night, elimination of alcohol from the bloodstream induces sleep fragmentation (Landolt et al., 1996; Roehrs et al., 1993). Sophie reported that she had experimented with drinking a glass of wine just before going to bed to help her fall asleep (see Chapter 11). She stopped the practice because, although drinking wine helped her fall asleep, she became aware that it increased her wakefulness in the middle of the night. Alcohol before bedtime suppresses REM sleep in the first half of the night, resulting in a rebound of REM episodes in the second half (i.e., REM episodes are longer and involve a greater number of rapid eye movements, a correlate of dreaming). Alcohol also increases sleep apnea severity (Taasan et al., 1981). For most people with no history of alcoholism, one glass of wine or beer with dinner scheduled 3–4 hours before bedtime is not likely to have a negative impact on sleep, because it is likely to be metabolized before bedtime. For some very sensitive individuals, elimination of alcohol in the evening altogether may be advisable.

Insomnia is prevalent among those with DSM-IV-defined alcohol dependence in early recovery (Cohn, Foster, & Peters, 2003). Sleep difficulties often persist for months despite continued abstinence, and their presence has been associated with higher rates of relapse (Brower, Aldrich, Robinson, Zucker, & Greden, 2001; Drummond, Gillin, Smith, & DeModena, 1998). Initial indications suggest that CBT-I is effective for insomnia in those recovering from alcohol dependence (Arnedt et al., 2007).

### Caffeine

As discussed in Chapter 6, caffeine, which is a stimulant, has negative effects on sleep (longer sleep onset and more fragmented sleep); the severity of these effects depends on the amount consumed and the timing of consumption. Caffeine is a relatively long-lasting stimulant: Its half-life is on average 4.5 hours, and even longer when consumed in conjunction with some substances (such as oral contraceptives, hormone replacement therapy, and SSRIs). Therefore, caffeine consumption should be limited to the equivalent of no more than three 8-ounce cups daily, and consumption after lunch should be avoided.

### Nicotine

As discussed in Chapter 6, nicotine is another stimulant that causes sleep fragmentation and sleep initiation difficulties. Although nicotine has a short half-life (approximately 2 hours), smokers tend to consume it close to bedtime and sometimes even in the middle of the night.

There are many health reasons to avoid nicotine altogether. Smokers with insomnia who do not wish to stop nicotine consumption are advised to avoid smoking in the evening (for at least 2 hours before bedtime) and in the middle of the night.

## Exercise and Diet

Depending on the timing of exercise relative to an individual's circadian rhythm, as well as its duration and intensity, exercise can cause shifts in the circadian rhythm (Buxton et al., 2003). Much less is known about the impact of late-night exercise on sleep quality. However, because of its potential phase-shifting effects, avoiding rigorous exercise 3–4 hours before bedtime is generally recommended. Gentle stretching exercises before bedtime are all right; they may, in fact, be relaxing and therefore supportive of sleep.

A heavy meal close to bedtime may lead to indigestion and gastrointestinal reflux during the night, both of which may cause wakefulness. Going to bed before food is fully digested is therefore a poor sleep practice. Eating in the middle of the night is also not a good idea, because it sends alerting signals to the brain and may prolong the time awake. Because feeling hungry may also disrupt sleep, eating a light, easily digestible snack at bedtime to alleviate hunger may sometimes be advisable.

## Sleep Environment

The ideal sleep environment is safe, quiet, dark, and comfortable. The following are a few relevant facts.

### Sound

Acoustic stimuli are processed during sleep, with intermittent noise having greater negative effects on sleep quality than continuous noise (Öhrström & Rylander, 1982). This is one reason why sleeping with the television, radio, and other sound entertainment devices is not a good idea: Abrupt changes in volume can cause arousals. Although listening to a TV or radio program may facilitate sleep by taking one's mind off unwanted thoughts, changes in sound level can cause wakefulness after sleep is attained.

White noise can be used for masking abrupt environmental noises (by reducing the difference between background noise and intermittent peak noise), thus making a noisy sleep environment less disruptive of sleep. For example, white noise has been used to improve sleep in noisy intensive care units (Stanchina, Abu-Hijleh, Chaudhry, Carlisle, & Millman, 2005). White noise can be generated without cost by setting a television on a station with no reception, by running a fan, or by using a smartphone application. White noise machines can also be purchased inexpensively.

### Light

Light is greatly attenuated by the eyelids. However, because light exposure has significant influence on the circadian clock, either waking up in the middle of the night in a lit room or using a bright-screen electronic device when awakened has the potential to cause circadian rhythm disruptions, depending on the timing and duration of the exposure to the light. It is generally recommended to keep the bedroom environment dark and to avoid prolonged use of bright-screen devices. If light is needed for safety, particularly during the execution of stimulus control, dim light should be used. Emerging research on the potential detrimental effects of light emanating from electronic devices, such as tablets, telephones, and computers, suggest a measurable but small impact on the circadian clock of 1–2 hours of exposure to light equivalent to that emitted from such devices (Figueiro, Wood, Plitnick, & Rea, 2011; Heath et al., 2014). At present, the available data cannot be translated into specific guidelines about when the use of bright-light emission from electronic devices is detrimental to the circadian clock. (However, an important aspect of using electronic devices in bed at night that should be considered is the potential of content to be alerting, as is the case with thrilling games.)

## Comfort

### MATTRESS

Among people free of chronic pain, studies linking the type of sleeping mattress with sleep quality have not yielded consistent results. However, for people with chronic musculoskeletal pain, using a mattress of medium firmness has been shown to decrease pain and disability (Kovacs et al., 2003).

### TEMPERATURE

In Chapter 2, we have discussed the links between core body temperature and sleep, in terms of both the circadian rhythm and thermoregulation. In general, falling asleep is associated with a drop in core body temperature (Barrett, Lack, & Morris, 1993). The temperature to which the body is exposed during sleep, which we refer to as *environmental temperature*, depends on the net effect of room temperature, sleep attire, and bedding. Excessively high and low environmental temperatures can both have a negative impact on sleep. In the naturalistic environment, sleep is more likely to be disturbed by exposure to heat than exposure to cold (Okamoto-Mizuno & Mizuno, 2012). The key is to maintain a room temperature that is personally comfortable, which is usually between 65° and 72°F; however, individual comfort rather than absolute values should be the guide, because people differ in what temperature range they perceive as comfortable.

## Aversion to Silence

Some patients may be averse to silence and therefore may keep the television on all night. However, as previously mentioned, the television's changes in sound volume and light may be perceived during sleep and thus may disrupt it. A better substitute for silence is white noise. White noise may not be a good strategy for patients who are simultaneously receiving exposure therapy for PTSD, because its use constitutes a safety behavior, which is discouraged in such therapy. As stated in Chapter 5, we do not recommend using CBT-I with patients concurrently undergoing exposure therapy for PTSD. However, white noise may also be contraindicated for patients with

PTSD who have recently completed exposure therapy. For these patients, an alternative strategy is to modify stimulus control instructions by allowing the patients to stay in bed for 20 minutes before getting out of bed. In other words, although clock watching is generally discouraged, it will be allowed in these cases. Experiencing the anxiety-provoking silence in bed may initially increase arousal in bed and exacerbate insomnia. In the long term, however, the patients will learn to reassociate bed and silence with sleep. This modification to stimulus control is useful whenever hypervigilance interferes with a patient's ability to recognize signs of sleepiness—an important ability for implementation of standard stimulus control instructions.

## Use of Light for Patients with Eveningness and Morningness Chronotypes

Our clinical experience and some research (Lack, Wright, & Paynter, 2007) indicate that patients with insomnia who have an eveningness chronotype can benefit from exposure to light shortly after waking up. After a few days, they report an easier time waking up in the morning; with continued exposure, many report that they also start feeling sleepy earlier in the evening than they used to. These benefits probably reflect a shift in their core body temperature curve (which is an indicator of the circadian sleep–wake clock). In Chapter 2, we have mentioned that, depending on the time and brightness of exposure, light can shift the phase of the circadian clock. Circadian researchers have determined that light exposure shortly after the minimum core body temperature is reached shifts the whole circadian rhythm curve to an earlier time (for a summary, see Chesson et al., 1999). Exposure to light immediately after waking up also helps shift the clock to an earlier time, but it may take longer for the shift to occur. In general, the better the timing relative to the core body temperature minimum (the formula is complex), and the more intense the light, the faster the shift will occur.

The American Academy of Sleep Medicine has published practice parameters for the use of light therapy in the treatment of circadian rhythm sleep disorders (Chesson et al., 1999), which in the DSM-5 are called circadian rhythm sleep–wake disorders in the middle of the night. The guidelines include recommendation for delayed sleep phase syndrome (which in the DSM-5 is call delayed sleep phase type) but do not include recommendations about the use of light exposure for patients with insomnia and an eveningness chronotype who do not meet full diagnostic criteria. Nonetheless, many sleep specialists use morning light exposure to help patients with insomnia and mild evening tendencies improve their sleep. When outdoor light is feasible, the recommendation is simply to be outside for an hour. It is not necessary to be out in the sun, and it is not recommended to look at the sun. Light at dawn may be sufficiently intense. If an hour is not feasible, shorter durations will help too, though to a lesser degree. Commercially available artificial light sources may help if natural light is unavailable (Chesson et al., 1999). This approach is relatively easy to implement in patients whose eveningness tendencies are mild (i.e., their sleep–wake schedules are no more than 3 hours later than they desire). Those with larger discrepancies between their desired and current sleep schedules, and those with circadian rhythm sleep–wake disorders, should be referred to a sleep specialist with experience in treating these disorders. This is because wrong timing of light exposure can result in a shift of the circadian clock in the opposite of the desired direction, and also because additional interventions may be required.

Evening light exposure can sometimes be used to help patients with insomnia and a morningness chronotype maintain a later sleep schedule when they desire to do so. This recommendation is based on findings from circadian research that a morningness chronotype is associated with an advance in the circadian clock, and that evening light exposure can shift the whole circadian rhythm curve to a later time (Czeisler et al., 1989). In a small study, participants with insomnia who felt sleepy in the evening and woke up at least 2 hours earlier than they wished benefited from 4 hours of bright-light exposure (8:00 P.M. to midnight) in the laboratory (Lack & Wright, 1993). This intense experimental manipulation is not feasible in clinical settings. Our clinical experience indicates that some patients with insomnia and a morningness chronotype benefit from exposure to light in the evening, particularly in the summer, when days are long. To the best of our knowledge, there are no published guidelines for the use of bright-light exposure for patients with insomnia with a morningness chronotype. It is not yet known when to begin the light, how long each light exposure session should be, or how many days a week it should take place.

## KEY PRACTICE IDEAS

- Counterarousal techniques are used to manage hyperarousal and therefore can be helpful adjuncts to the core behavioral strategies. Counterarousal strategies include the following:
  - Implementing a buffer zone or wind-down period an hour before bed.
  - Scheduling worry, problem solving, or "to-do" list making in the early evening for those who are prone to worrying about how they will solve a particular problem.
  - Presleep writing for those who have difficulties with establishing closure to their days.
  - Relaxation techniques, which can include muscle relaxation, imagery, or meditation, for those with presleep tension or anxiety.

- Sleep hygiene therapy is rarely sufficient but sometimes necessary to address sleep-disruptive behaviors. Such therapy includes the following:
  - Limits on alcohol, caffeine, and tobacco, as well as advice on the timing of the last consumption of these substances.
  - Keeping the bedroom safe, comfortable, quiet, and dark.
  - Avoiding heavy meals before bed, but consuming a light snack if patients are prone to waking up in the night hungry.
  - Exercising, but stopping any activating exercise 3–4 hours before bedtime.

- Properly timed light exposure may help patients with insomnia and eveningness or morningness chronotypes.

# CHAPTER 9

# Addressing Sleep-Related Cognitions

Cognitive therapy teaches patients to notice, identify, evaluate, and respond in constructive ways to thoughts and beliefs that contribute to their presenting problems. It has been used effectively across multiple problems and disorders; as discussed below, although it has been tested as part of a multi-component treatment (CBT-I), tests of its utility as a single-modality treatment for insomnia are limited. This chapter is not a primer on cognitive therapy. The reader is referred elsewhere for general resources for cognitive therapy techniques (e.g., Beck, 2011; Greenberger & Padesky, 1995). Instead, assuming readers' familiarity with cognitive therapy theory and practice, we provide guidelines and examples of how cognitive therapy techniques can be applied to reduce psychological arousal and promote adherence with the behavioral components of CBT-I.

As discussed in Chapter 3, psychological arousal may be present when a person's bedtime is approaching, when the person initially tries to fall asleep or wakes up in the middle of the night or too early, and even during the day. We have also discussed in Chapter 3 different sources/types of psychological arousal. Briefly, psychological arousal in insomnia is related to sleep-specific cognitions (e.g., worries about sleep) or to thoughts and emotions that are not related to sleep, such as fear, anxiety, and excitement. Examples of worries about poor sleep are predicting sleep difficulty (e.g., anticipatory anxiety); predicting negative, and sometimes catastrophic, consequences of poor or insufficient sleep; and misattributing poor daytime functioning exclusively to poor sleep. In turn, these worries increase the sense of urgency or pressure for sleep (i.e., sleep effort). These same sleep-related worries can also compromise adherence to behavioral guidelines, such as getting out of bed when unable to sleep (i.e., stimulus control) and waking up at the same time each morning regardless of the amount or quality of sleep obtained on the preceding night (i.e., stimulus control and sleep restriction therapy).

## COGNITIVE THERAPY IN CBT-I

In CBT-I, cognitive therapy is typically applied fluidly throughout treatment, along with the behavioral components. At this writing, only one randomized controlled study has evaluated the efficacy of cognitive therapy as a monotherapy for insomnia disorder. This study (Harvey et al.,

2014), which compared cognitive therapy alone, behavioral therapy alone, and their combination (CBT-I), concluded that CBT-I is superior and should be the treatment of choice. The study found that immediately after treatment, cognitive therapy led to lower rates of response (42.4%), defined by clinically significant reduction in insomnia severity, than CBT-I and behavioral therapy (67.3% and 67.4%, respectively). However, at a 6-month follow-up, participants who received cognitive therapy alone made significant additional gains (response rates increased to 62.3%); those who received behavioral therapy alone showed a significant loss (response rates dropped to 44.4%); and those who received CBT-I maintained their gains (67.6%). Together, the results from the important Harvey et al. (2014) study suggest that although cognitive therapy may have a delayed action, it is likely that it contributes to the documented long-lasting therapeutic effects of CBT-I.

The cognitive therapy component of CBT-I is employed in order to help patients understand how some of their thoughts and beliefs about sleep contribute to their insomnia and to come up with alternative, more helpful, and often more accurate thoughts. The modified thoughts and beliefs lead to reduced arousal and facilitate changes in behaviors that are incongruent with sleep. Addressing maladaptive cognitions in insomnia affects the sleep regulation system directly by reducing arousal, and indirectly, by promoting behavioral changes congruent with strengthening the sleep drive and/or the circadian clock. The cognitive therapy component of CBT-I involves (1) providing scientific information pertinent to correcting inaccurate thoughts and beliefs about sleep; (2) collaboratively evaluating the validity, relevance, and/or usefulness of thoughts and beliefs through Socratic questioning, behavioral experiments, and cost–benefit analysis; (3) helping patients replace inaccurate/unhelpful thoughts and beliefs with alternative, more accurate/relevant ones; and (4) helping patients apply the insights they have gained to help them behave in ways that promote sleep and cope better with less than ideal sleep when it does occur. Cognitive therapy can help reduce sleep-related arousal and increase the likelihood of adherence with treatment recommendations. We discuss below some of the most common thoughts and beliefs that interfere with sleep, as well as specific cognitive therapy techniques that can be used with each.

## ADDRESSING THOUGHTS AND BELIEFS THAT INTERFERE WITH SLEEP

### Worries about the Negative Impact of Poor Sleep on Daytime Performance

In addressing a patient's worries that poor or insufficient sleep will impair daytime performance, an important first step is to understand the meanings and implications of the consequences that the patient fears. The *downward arrow technique* is a cognitive therapy technique that consists of a series of successive related questions used for exploring unexpressed anticipated consequences that underlie the anxiety response to the expressed worry. For example, the therapist can ask, "What would happen if X [the stated feared consequences] were true?", and then ask the same question with regard to the response: "And what would happen if [the feared answer to the previous question] were true? What implications would that have?" When the true nature of the worry becomes clear, the therapist can explore evidence that does and does not support the anticipated negative consequences and their likelihood, using Socratic questioning and behavioral experiments. In doing so, the therapist can also provide scientific information that can help the patient adapt a realistic perspective about the subject of worry. We illustrate this with the following example about fears of work-related consequences.

THERAPIST: You said that at night when you are having difficulty falling asleep, you keep worrying that you won't be able to function during the day. Let's take a closer look at your concern. Can you tell me what you mean when you say that you will not be able to function?

PATIENT: I mean I will make mistakes at work.

THERAPIST: I can understand that this is a real concern. What will happen if you make a mistake at work?

PATIENT: I usually catch my own mistakes, but then I have to start over and then I fall behind. I am just less efficient.

THERAPIST: What are the ramifications of being less efficient?

PATIENT: I hate being inefficient. I am also concerned I will get bad reviews. I will probably not get promoted.

THERAPIST: It sounds like you are concerned that a lot is at stake. I hear you say that you believe that if you do not sleep well, then you will be less efficient at work and you will eventually get bad reviews.

PATIENT: Yes.

THERAPIST: Let's think for a moment about the effect of your worries about not sleeping and therefore getting unfavorable performance evaluations. Imagine that just before you went to bed, you got upsetting, worrisome news. How would this affect your ability to fall asleep?

PATIENT: Well, I know it would take me much longer to fall asleep.

THERAPIST: Do you think that worrying about how efficient you could be at work tomorrow at work could have a similar effect on your ability to sleep?

PATIENT: Definitely! I can't fall asleep fast when I am worried. But I can't stop worrying.

THERAPIST: I am wondering if we can look at the relationship between your sleep and your level of efficiency and errors at work. Have there been times when you did not sleep well, and then the next day you made mistakes at work?

PATIENT: I can remember a time when I slept very little, because we picked up our daughter from the airport and her flight was delayed. So I ended up sleeping only 4 hours that night. I remember it well, because the next day I deleted an important file that was not backed up. This was a costly mistake. This file was important for a deadline we had a day later. I ended up staying at work until 11 that night to recover it.

THERAPIST: This does not sound very pleasant, particularly for someone who likes to be efficient. Is this the only time you remember making mistakes at work after not sleeping well the night before?

PATIENT: Nothing stands out as much, but I know there have been other times when I made programming errors and had to spend time recovering from them.

THERAPIST: Would you say that every time you had a poor night's sleep, you made programming errors the next day?

PATIENT: Well, not every time. I am sleeping pretty lousy every night nowadays, but I don't make errors every day.

THERAPIST: It sounds like there are times when you are able to function fairly well during the day, despite having slept poorly the preceding night. You have told me that even now some nights are better than others.

PATIENT: Yes.

THERAPIST: Have there been times when you made programming errors after nights when you slept relatively better?

PATIENT: (*Thinking*) Yes, that has happened several times as well.

THERAPIST: So it sounds like your errors and inefficiency at work are not entirely dependent on how well you sleep. Would you agree?

PATIENT: Yes, I do now.

THERAPIST: Can you think of other things that have a negative impact on your work performance and efficiency?

PATIENT: Well, when I am distracted, I don't do as well.

THERAPIST: This is quite a common reason for making errors. Would you say that being worried about something tends to distract you?

PATIENT: Of course.

THERAPIST: Given our discussion, can you revisit your statement, "If I don't sleep well at night, I don't function well the next day," and make it a bit more accurate?

PATIENT: I guess I can say, "Even if I do not sleep well at night, I can sometimes function just fine."

THERAPIST: Right now worrying seems pretty automatic, but do you think that you could catch yourself worrying about what will happen if you do not fall asleep soon, and then remind yourself of this more accurate fact?

PATIENT: Maybe. I can try. I am not sure.

THERAPIST: OK. I understand. Perhaps it will help to know what science has to say about the relationship between how well we sleep and how well we perform on certain tasks.

PATIENT: OK.

THERAPIST: Scientists have found that moderate sleep loss has little negative impact on tasks that involve logical thinking, which is what your work seems to entail. So, realistically, your routine work is not likely to suffer as much as you fear.

PATIENT: I didn't know that. This makes me feel a bit less worried.

THERAPIST: Good. Would you be interested in collecting your own data to find out how closely your performance is tied to your sleep quality and whether your work is negatively affected by your sleep quality?

PATIENT: I like this idea. I am already tracking my sleep in the diary you gave me. I can keep track of my performance every day on the back of the diary.

THERAPIST: Tracking both sleep and work sounds like a good idea. I recommend that you track your work performance on a different sheet of paper, and that you not compare it to your sleep diary until your next session.

PATIENT: It makes sense. I can do that.

In this example, the therapist started the conversation by using the downward arrow technique to explore the patient's concerns, and then used Socratic questioning to explore how tight the relationship between the patient's sleep quality and work performance was. In some cases, it may be necessary to continue using the downward arrow technique until the patient's most extreme feared consequences are reached. For instance, in the example above, at the point at which the patient was concerned about a bad review, the therapist could have followed up with "And what would happen if you got a bad review?" In response, it is not uncommon for a person with insomnia to express fear that the sleep problem will end not only in joblessness, but in disability, homelessness, or death. In such a case, it is helpful for the patient to see that lurking under a seemingly harmless worry about job performance is a highly unlikely catastrophic outcome. In the example above, the therapist periodically provided relevant scientific information and checked to make sure that the patient understood the explanations. The therapist concluded with a plan to track daily performance in order to examine the validity of the feared association (a behavioral experiment).

When patients are concerned about next-day performance following a night of poor sleep, they often respond well to what science has to say about the issue. Below we provide information about the relationship between insufficient or poor sleep and performance, which a clinician may find helpful when addressing expressed feared consequences of poor sleep:

• Routine performance is usually not compromised, and even if it is compromised, it is usually to a much lesser degree than a patient predicts. Although it is true that people with insomnia experience impaired functioning on some tasks (e.g., slower reaction time to complex vigilance tasks that require multitasking; Altena, Van Der Werf, Strijers, & Van Someren, 2008; Edinger, Means, Carney, & Krystal, 2008; Schneider, Fulda, & Schulz, 2004), other neuropsychological functions, such as logical thinking, are not impaired (Fulda & Schulz, 2001). Importantly, observed deficits in performance improve following CBT-I (Altena et al., 2008).

• Among good sleepers, moderate sleep loss has little negative impact on novel logic-based tasks, such as rule-based deduction and identifying whether a logical conditional statement is true or false (Blagrove, Alexander, & Horne, 1995). In contrast, divergent-thinking tasks, such as tasks that involve innovation, risk assessment, insight, and multitasking, are particularly vulnerable to sleep loss (Durmer & Dinges, 2005). It should be noted, however, that results from sleep deprivation research conducted with good sleepers may not apply to people with insomnia. As discussed in Chapter 3, those with insomnia have high cortical arousal, which could protect them from some of the performance deficits following sleep deprivation that are observed in good sleepers; therefore, results from sleep deprivation studies may not apply to them equally.

• Research on the negative consequences of insufficient sleep on memory and cognitive performance has received much attention in the mass media. Such media reports often increase patients' concerns and fuel worries about negative consequences of poor sleep. Again, however, most of this research has been conducted with healthy adults who were experimentally sleep-deprived, and the results from these sleep deprivation experiments do not always generalize to patients with insomnia. For example, as discussed in Chapter 3, individuals with insomnia are less able to nap during the day than individuals without insomnia whose sleep is experimentally manipulated to simulate insomnia.

• Although research is mixed with regard to cognitive performance in insomnia, one consistent finding is that poor sleep usually compromises one's resources for dealing with extra burden. People with insomnia feel that they need to put more effort into activities that they can perform effortlessly after good sleep.

## Unrealistic Expectations about Sleep

Examples of beliefs that reflect unrealistic expectations about sleep include the belief that one must sleep well (or a minimum set number of hours) every night, or that one must wake up rested every morning. Below is an example of an unrealistic expectation expressed by a retired man with insomnia, who believed that now that he was retired, he should finally be able to sleep 8 hours per night.

PATIENT: I've always thought that it will be nice to sleep 8 hours. Now that I am retired, I should be able to finally get that.

THERAPIST: How long did you sleep before you retired?

PATIENT: About 6½ to 7 hours.

THERAPIST: And do you think you functioned well during the day on 6½ to 7 hours of sleep?

PATIENT: Yes, I did well. I just hated to have to get up in the morning.

THERAPIST: I am wondering. If you do well with 6½ to 7 hours of sleep, why do you want to sleep more now?

PATIENT: It is nice to be able to sleep in, like I used to do on vacations when I was younger. I always wanted to not have to wake up at a set time. Now I can do it. I can afford to sleep as much as I want.

THERAPIST: There is a difference between how much sleep you need and how much you want. Although many people say they sleep 7 or 8 hours a night, some, like you used to, do well with less than that.

PATIENT: I see. I heard that older people need less sleep.

THERAPIST: Although there are some changes in sleep as we age, it is not at all clear that how much sleep we need really changes. For example, when people get older, they tend to wake up more in the middle of the night. They do not necessarily sleep less overall, but their sleep tends to be more broken and shallower than it used to be when they were younger.

PATIENT: I suppose it is because they have prostate problems, like me.

THERAPIST: That may be the reason for some men. I also wanted to tell you an interesting scientific fact: When good sleepers are asked to try to sleep more than they normally do, they start having problems sleeping. What do you make of that?

PATIENT: Interesting. But how do I know how much sleep I need? I heard that if you sleep more, your memory is better—and as I as I get older, I am very concerned about that.

THERAPIST: You are asking two interesting questions. You are asking how you can tell how much sleep you need, and I am also hearing you ask me if what you heard about sleep and memory is correct. Let's start with the first question.

PATIENT: OK.

THERAPIST: The best way to find out how much sleep you need is to experiment with different sleep durations and see how you feel during the day. What would be important information for you to collect to decide if you sleep enough?

PATIENT: I would like to have energy during the day to do all the things I like to do.

THERAPIST: OK. So what would be a good scale to keep track of your energy during the day?

PATIENT: I suppose we can say that 10 is very good energy and 1 is very low energy.

THERAPIST: So you can use the "Comments" row in your sleep diary form every day to record your energy level that day. What time of day would be a good time to do that?

PATIENT: I will do it before I start getting ready for sleep. This way I will have a perspective on the whole day.

THERAPIST: OK. Now we need to decide on the different durations of sleep you will try, and how many nights you should try each duration.

PATIENT: I would like to try 6½, 7, 7½, and 8 hours.

THERAPIST: Let's look at your sleep diary forms and see the range of sleep you are getting now. There is no point in designing an experiment that cannot be followed.

PATIENT: (*Looking at his sleep diary forms*) I sleep between 6 and 7 hours; one night I only slept 5 hours.

THERAPIST: What do you think about experimenting with durations that fall in the range of 5 to 7 hours)?

PATIENT: I do not really want to experiment with 5 hours. It sounds like a punishment.

THERAPIST: Fair enough. What would you propose?

PATIENT: How about a few nights 6, a few 6½, and a few 7?

THERAPIST: This is a good start. Our next appointment is in 2 weeks. How about we mark on this blank sleep diary form that the first 5 days you will only be in bed 6 hours; the next 5 days, 6½ hours; and the remaining 4 days, 7 hours?

PATIENT: I can do that. And then I will note my energy level in the diary.

THERAPIST: On second thought, it may be better if you don't look at the results of this little experiment before you complete it. It might be best to record your energy level on a different piece of paper, and then you can look at it on the last day and we can discuss what you find out.

PATIENT: OK.

THERAPIST: You were also curious about the relationship between sleep and memory. Would you like to add a rating of your memory to this experiment?

PATIENT: Good idea. I will do that.

In this example, the therapist used Socratic questioning to examine the validity and helpfulness of the patient's expectation, discussed the difference between needing and wanting sleep, provided relevant information about the impact of aging on sleep, mentioned a scientific study demonstrating that trying to extend sleep leads to worsening of sleep, and helped the patient design a behavioral experiment to discover what his personal sleep need really was. The therapist encouraged the patient to be involved in the design of the experiment and its implementation details. This was intended to increase the patient's investment in and adherence to the experiment.

When therapists are treating older adults, and particularly when they are using cognitive therapy with older patients, it helps to know a few facts about sleep that are relevant to this population. This knowledge can help clinicians be effective in answering the questions about sleep that older patients frequently pose or express. Below are a few relevant points.

- More than half of older adults have symptoms insomnia, but fewer than a quarter experience sleep difficulties frequently (Schubert et al., 2002). (This fact can be used to reduce the hopelessness associated with certain beliefs, such as the belief that there is nothing to do about insomnia because it is one of the inevitable features of aging.)
- Even older adults without insomnia experience some changes in their sleep and daytime energy as they age. (This and the following facts can be used to provide a realistic perspective and help promote realistic expectations about sleep with advancing age.)
- Sleep architecture changes with aging.

  - Aging is associated with more awakenings (i.e., sleep becomes more fragmented).
  - Deep sleep (stage N3) gradually decreases, and lighter sleep (stage N1) increases.

- Sleep loss is less detrimental to older than to younger adults. Older adults sustain alertness and performance better, and report being less sleepy, than their younger counterparts do. This has been interpreted by some as an indication of reduced sleep need (Duffy, Willson, Wang, & Czeisler, 2009). These findings can be used to help alleviate worries about negative consequences of poor sleep.
- Some older adults are more distressed about the possibility that sleep loss will cause memory impairment and other impairments in cognitive functions than they are about their poor sleep at night per se. Even when this worry is not explicitly expressed, it may be clinically useful to explore, because, such a concern may increase sleep effort and objections to implementing sleep restriction therapy.
- Fatigue in older adults can be due to low physical activity and/or poor health. These factors may contribute more to the experience of fatigue than sleep quantity or quality may. Moreover, levels of physical activity and health both generally decrease with age. These facts can be used in working with older adults' beliefs about the relationship between sleep and fatigue.

## Beliefs Related to Sleep Effort

As discussed in Chapter 3, sleep effort—that is, an insomnia sufferer's attempt to control sleep—is often at the core of the insomnia experience. In accordance with Wegner's research on ironic processes (Ansfield et al., 1996), efforts directed at the elimination of specific thoughts, emotions, and sensations are likely to have the paradoxical effect of increasing their frequency. Letting go of the agenda to control sleep can help restore the automaticity that is essential for healthy sleep. A Chinese finger cuff (see Chapter 3) can provide a useful experiential metaphor to help patients see that the effort they are exerting to sleep is counterproductive, and that letting go of effort to sleep may be a viable solution. The patients are then left with the challenge of translating this knowledge into the practice of ceasing to "try to sleep." Techniques used in acceptance-based therapies can help the patients in this translation.

Acceptance-based approaches to insomnia, such as mindfulness meditation and acceptance and commitment therapy (ACT; Hayes, Strosahl, & Wilson, 2012), focus on patients' relationships to their thoughts about sleep rather than on the accuracy or utility of these thoughts. For example, in an acceptance-based approach, a patient reporting the thought "I have to sleep well tonight, because tomorrow is an important day" will be encouraged to observe the thought as a present-moment mental event ("I am having this thought"), rather than to engage in the process of examining the validity or utility of the underlying belief. The shift to observing, rather than engaging with, one's thoughts can give rise to recognition that such a thought about sleep is just that—a thought about sleep, and nothing more. This can allow a patient to observe the worrisome thought as it is, without trying to fix it or not think it. The shift from engaging with to observing one's thoughts creates an objective (decentered) space that facilitates letting go of an expectation of meeting certain sleep needs, and permits the emergence of willingness to accept sleeplessness and its assumed consequences. The accepting stance can reduce arousal, which in turn can facilitate sleep at night and coping the next day.

Adapting an accepting stance also promotes flexibility in the approach to sleep, thus expanding the range of response options and making more room for sleep-compatible behaviors. For example, when unable to fall back to sleep after a middle-of-the-night awakening, patients with insomnia typically react by "trying to sleep"; this often feels as if it is the only option. If instead they accept that at this moment they are not in a state of mind that is conducive to sleep, they can then consider other options. For example, they can choose to engage in a pleasant waking activity until a state of mind more conducive to sleep emerges. In that way, the stimulus control instruction to get out of bed when unable to sleep can emerge organically when an acceptance stance is adopted. In his book *Full Catastrophe Living*, Jon Kabat-Zinn (1990) relates a personal story of how adopting an accepting stance helped him during a long bout of insomnia: It led him to stop struggling with sleeplessness, get out of bed when unable to sleep, and return to bed when sleepiness reemerged. This approach eventually alleviated his insomnia.

As they begin to adopt an accepting stance in their approach to sleeplessness and fatigue, some patients realize that sleep has become overvalued—a "centerpiece" of their lives—and has been overshadowing other values they consider important. People with insomnia may get to this point by making concessions to their other values in an effort to manage their insomnia symptoms. For example, an individual who places high value on health promotion may forgo adherence to a previous morning exercise regimen, and instead "sleep in" to compensate for lost sleep on the previous night. The saying "Sleep to live, rather than live to sleep" can be a helpful mantra for some of these patients. Borrowing from ACT, a therapist can help such patients to recognize how excessive focus on sleep compromises their pursuit of other important values, and then help them recommit to acting in accordance with these other values even after a night of poor sleep. This in turn reduces the personal cost of poor sleep, which helps reduce sleep effort.

Adopting an observing and accepting stance can also allow an individual to view sleeplessness as an occurrence or an event, rather than as a personal, immutable characteristic. Whereas perceiving insomnia as an immutable trait leads to helplessness, the observer stance, by contrast, opens the door to the possibility of engaging in behavioral changes that will lead to improved sleep. For additional discussion of mindfulness and acceptance-based approaches to the treatment of insomnia, see Ong et al. (2012).

Below we provide a sample discussion of "living a valued life," a construct central to ACT. This principle is also illustrated in the treatment of Sam (Chapter 12), in which the therapist asked Sam to examine his decisions and goals regarding sleeping separately from his wife in relation to his values.

THERAPIST: You told me that because you are such a light sleeper, you started sleeping in the guest bedroom. How is this working for you?

PATIENT: It's OK. My husband is very understanding. He knows I am a light sleeper, and he wants me to sleep well.

THERAPIST: It sounds like the two of you have a very good relationship.

PATIENT: Yes, we do.

THERAPIST: How do you like this sleeping arrangement?

PATIENT: It's OK. I still have insomnia, but it was even worse when I slept in our bedroom. My husband wakes up early. This wakes me up, and I have a hard time falling back asleep.

THERAPIST: I see. So the upside is that your insomnia was worse when you slept in the same room than it is now that you sleep apart. But are there any downsides to the current arrangement?

PATIENT: Well, I do not think this is a long-term solution. My husband said he would like to have me back in our bedroom.

THERAPIST: And what about you? Do you also want to be back in your bedroom?

PATIENT: Yes. Of course! But I am not ready. But I also would not like to sleep alone forever. I do miss our cuddle time before we went to sleep.

THERAPIST: It sounds like you really value your relationship with your husband.

PATIENT: I do.

THERAPIST: Do you think your relationship has been affected by your sleeping in separate rooms?

PATIENT: A little. We have a little less touch. He is patient and understanding, but I do think it is not perfect for us.

THERAPIST: And you value your sleep.

PATIENT: I do.

THERAPIST: You are trying to do everything you can think of to sleep well.

PATIENT: Yes. I do not know what else to do.

THERAPIST: I am wondering if you are doing too much. I am wondering if you are trying so hard that you've lost touch with something that may be more important than sleep.

PATIENT: I always knew that this was not a long-term solution. I can already see that our relationship is affected by our not sleeping together.

THERAPIST: Are there other things that you value, but have been ignoring because of your insomnia?

PATIENT: Yes. My exercise routine has always been important to me. I used to wake up early and get to the gym before work. Now I am too tired in the morning. I go to the gym only on the weekend.

THERAPIST: And you also told me that this year you decided to cancel your planned trip to Australia to see your son, because you are afraid that you will not be able to cope with the jet lag.

PATIENT: That too. I see what you are saying. I am letting this insomnia affect my life too much. I wish I could stop.

THERAPIST: I noticed you used the words "I am *letting* this insomnia affect my life." Can you think of a way you can let it affect your life less?

PATIENT: I think I will start sleeping in our bedroom again. I can wake up early when my husband wakes up and go to the gym. This is what I used to do before I had insomnia.

THERAPIST: You sound happy about this decision.

PATIENT: I am.

THERAPIST: This will also help you sleep better. Let me tell you why I say that . .

In this example, the therapist used a technique called *cost–benefit analysis* to help the patient realize that she was compromising the ACT principle of living a valued life. Cost–benefit analysis is a type of Socratic questioning that helps make patients explicitly aware of hidden costs that are associated with certain beliefs and behaviors. This technique is also helpful for addressing beliefs related to safety behaviors, which we discuss next.

## Beliefs Related to Safety Behaviors

Safety behaviors, as discussed in Chapter 3, are behaviors aimed at avoiding a feared outcome. In the context of insomnia, the feared outcomes are difficulties in sleeping and the expected consequences of poor sleep. In the example just given, the patient exhibited safety behaviors such as changing her sleep environment and trying to sleep past her premorbid wake-up time. Many people with chronic insomnia engage in these and other safety behaviors, such as canceling social engagements or avoiding certain work tasks following a night of poor sleep, and avoiding social events in the evening for fear that they might interfere with their sleep. These behaviors are counterproductive. They reflect excessive cognitive preoccupation with sleep, are often associated with strong negative emotions that increase arousal levels, and reinforce the patients' belief that they cannot cope (e.g., helplessness). Safety behaviors may produce short-term gains, in part because they reduce the intensity of the associated negative emotions; in the long run, however, they prolong the insomnia problem.

Persons engaged in safety behaviors are focused on what they fear and tend to be unaware of or to ignore the costs of engaging in these behaviors. Examining the accuracy of thoughts that precede and lead to the safety behaviors is often not effective, because even if the patients recognize that what they fear has low probability, they are not likely to stop engaging in the safety behaviors because the high negative emotions associated with the fear overpower their logical reasoning. This overpowering is sometimes referred to as *emotional reasoning*. In such cases, examining the utility of holding onto a belief is more likely to lead to behavior change than is focusing on its accuracy. Cost–benefit analysis, introduced in the preceding section, is a cognitive-behavioral technique that is helpful for discussing the utility of a belief; it is particularly powerful for unraveling the hidden costs of safety behaviors that involve a loss of living in accordance with one's values. Realizing such a loss is usually associated with an emotional reaction, which can offset the negative emotion that has led to the safety behavior in the first place. In the example above, becoming aware of the costs helped the patient to abandon two safety behaviors: sleeping in the guest room and trying to sleep in. Another strategy for addressing safety behaviors is carefully designing behavioral experiments. Behavioral experiments are helpful for testing the validity of a belief that motivates engagement in a safety behavior, as well as the utility of the safety behavior. This is illustrated in the following example of a behavioral experiment for testing how helpful it really was to forgo exercising after a night of poor sleep.

THERAPIST: You told me that you used to exercise every morning, but you stopped because you are trying instead to use the time to get more sleep.

PATIENT: Yes. I have always enjoyed a workout before going to work. I used to wake up at 5:30 and be at the gym at 6:00; then I'd go directly to work.

THERAPIST: When do you get out of bed now?

PATIENT: At 6:45. The way I sleep now, I cannot imagine working out at 6:00.

THERAPIST: What do you mean when you say you cannot imagine exercising?

PATIENT: I don't think I would have the energy, and it is hard to get going. I just stay in bed and rest.

THERAPIST: What would you imagine would happen if you pushed yourself to go to the gym, even though you do not sleep well?

PATIENT: It would be hard. And then I would not have energy the rest of the day.

THERAPIST: Are you speaking from experience?

PATIENT: Well, I tried one morning to go to the gym. My wife was going, and she said I should join her, since I am not falling back asleep most mornings anyway.

THERAPIST: And what happened?

PATIENT: I headed to the gym, but then I decided I might as well head straight to work to catch up on some stuff I had to do. This way I could return home early and try to catch a nap.

THERAPIST: I am wondering if we can think of an experiment to find out if when you go to the gym before work, you have less energy at work.

PATIENT: You mean just do it for a few days and see what happens?

THERAPIST: Yes. But we want to be scientific about it so we can draw meaningful conclusions. For example, what do you mean by "see what happens"? What would be important to observe?

PATIENT: I suppose I can see how much energy I have.

THERAPIST: That sounds good. When will you do the rating?

PATIENT: I think it would be best to do it at the end of my workday, on the train home.

THERAPIST: Good. How about using a scale from 1 to 10, where 1 means low energy and 10 means very energetic?

PATIENT: I can do that.

THERAPIST: And what will you compare it to?

PATIENT: I suppose I can compare it to my energy at work now.

THERAPIST: What is your energy level now on this scale?

PATIENT: It's a 5. But I am sure it will be lower at the end of the day.

THERAPIST: You have a point. It will be important to know your energy level at the same time every day. How about collecting some data before changing anything, and then start going to the gym and see if there is a difference?

PATIENT: I got it.

THERAPIST: Our next appointment is in 10 days. You will have 8 workdays. How about the first 4 of these days, you will not go to the gym and rate your energy level at the end of work, and the next 4 days, you will go to the gym and do the same rating at roughly the same time?

PATIENT: I can do that.

THERAPIST: Do you see any problems with this? Will you be able to go to the gym?

PATIENT: I think I can try the gym for a few days.

THERAPIST: Do you think you might change your mind, like you told me you did that one time before?

PATIENT: That is a danger. But I think that if I go to the gym with my friend from work, I will stick to it.

THERAPIST: I think it is a great idea. If you promise your friend to meet him at the gym at 6, it will be easier to keep your word. Do you think there is anything else that might be a problem for this experiment?

PATIENT: Not really.

THERAPIST: Do you think you can make the rating each day without looking at your previous ratings?

PATIENT: Yes. I see why I should do it this way, to be fair. I can tell the rating to my wife, so she keeps the record.

# ADDRESSING OBSTACLES TO ADHERENCE WITH BEHAVIORAL COMPONENTS

Cognitive therapy can be used to address obstacles to adherence with the behavioral components of CBT-I preemptively (i.e., to remove anticipated obstacles in advance), as well as to address nonadherence when it emerges in subsequent sessions. Here we discuss using cognitive therapy to address common obstacles to adherence with two instructions: the stimulus control instruction to get out of bed when unable to sleep, and the instruction to wake up at the same time every morning (which is part of both stimulus control and sleep restriction therapy). The principles and techniques we discuss below can also be used to address obstacles to adherence with other behavioral aspects of CBT-I. Cost–benefit analyses may be particularly effective for addressing beliefs that interfere with adherence, particularly beliefs that are associated with strong emotions. In such cases, examining the cost and utility of holding onto the beliefs is more likely to lead to adherence than is focusing on the beliefs' accuracy.

## Concern about Getting Out of Bed When Unable to Sleep

In Chapter 7, we have discussed how to address concerns about disturbing a bed partner when a patient is following the stimulus control instruction to get out of bed if unable to sleep. Here we discuss how to use cognitive therapy to address another common concern that patients express in response to this stimulus control instruction—the concern that getting out of bed will result in staying up for the rest of the night. There is some reason for this concern. Getting out of bed may indeed prolong time awake in the middle of the night, and sometimes (e.g., when the awakening is close to the time a patient needs to be up in the morning) the patient *will* not fall back to sleep for the rest of the night. Focusing on examining the validity of this concern (through a behavioral experiment and/or Socratic questioning) may not be an effective way of addressing this concern—particularly when the patient is engaged in strong emotional reasoning, or when an initial examination reveals that in the past, getting out of bed in the middle of the night *has* resulted in being awake the rest of the night.

We discuss here two alternative cognitive therapy approaches. One approach, anchored in acceptance theory, is to invite the patient to accept that there is merit in sleeping less for a few nights (i.e., by getting out of bed and possibly prolonging wakefulness), because this strategy might eventually improve insomnia. The use of analogies is an acceptance-based technique to promote acceptance in general (see Hayes et al., 2012) and can be used in this example. For instance, chess players routinely sacrifice a few chess pieces in order to win the game; that is, they focus on long-term goals rather than short-term goals. Or a war analogy, sacrificing a battle to win the war, may resonate with some people. Such analogies were important in addressing Sophie's concerns about reduced time in bed (see Chapter 11).

A second approach is to use cost–benefit analysis: A therapist can ask a patient to identify the benefits and costs of the concern that getting out of bed when unable to sleep will result in more time awake. Figure 9.1 is a sample list of such costs and benefits. An additional cost of staying in bed (besides the ones listed in Figure 9.1) is that it results in continued association of the bed with not sleeping; this is counterproductive for the patient's goal of resolving insomnia. Weighing the costs and benefits can thus help reinforce the idea that it may be necessary to sleep less on some nights as a strategy for improving sleep in the long run. A patient who decides that the costs outweigh the benefits may be at a lower stage of readiness for change at this point, and this is all right. Placing the reasons for and against making the change is often an effective motivational enhancement strategy, and even if it doesn't lead to change right away, it may facilitate change later. That is, at a future time at which the benefits are seen to outweigh the costs, the patient may be readier to implement this strategy. (See below for a fuller discussion of motivational enhancement.) In the Figure 9.1 example of cost–benefit analysis, the patient concluded after reviewing the costs and benefits that the costs of staying in bed when awake in the middle of the night outweighed the benefits: Most of the time, staying in bed did not result in the patient's getting more sleep or feeling more rested. The patient decided to try the stimulus control recommendation for a week to see what would happen.

## Concern about Getting Out of Bed at the Same Time Every Morning

In Chapter 7, we have discussed behavioral strategies to improve adherence to getting out of bed at the same time every day, regardless of the amount of sleep obtained the night before; such strategies include scheduling morning activities and increasing morning light exposure. Here we

| *If I get out of bed in the middle of the night, I will never be able to fall back asleep.* | |
|---|---|
| **Benefits** | **Costs** |
| Staying in bed is easier and more comfortable than getting out of bed. | If I stay in bed, I worry more. |
| If I rest in bed, I may fall back to sleep. | This has not really worked for me. If I keep doing this, I may not get better. |
| If I stay in bed, I may feel more rested tomorrow. | I don't usually feel more rested when I stay in bed. Sometimes I feel worse. |
| | My wife always tells me I should do it, and she is frustrated that I don't. |

**FIGURE 9.1.** A cost–benefit analysis of getting out of bed at night.

focus on cognitive therapy techniques. The choice of strategies should be based on the reasons why individual patients have difficulty adhering to this recommendation. For example, when sleeping past the designated wake time is a safety behavior (e.g., trying to sleep more as a strategy to avoid feared consequences of insufficient sleep), then the strategies discussed above in the section on safety behaviors can be used. When sleeping past the designated wake time is related to anhedonia, then morning-focused behavioral activation is called for. When the patient has an eveningness chronotype, it will also be important to include morning light exposure, because over time this will facilitate getting up at the same time every morning. In all of these instances, *motivational enhancement* may further help with adherence.

Motivational enhancement is a CBT technique that is based on a transtheoretical model, first described by Prochaska and DiClemente (1994), to explain how people change addictive behaviors. The technique has since been applied to prepare people to engage in behaviors needed for other desired changes and can be used to enhance adherence to behavioral changes in CBT-I, such as getting out of bed at the same time every morning. Motivational enhancement is designed to mobilize a patient's own change resources and to support intrinsic motivation for change. Motivation for change occurs when people perceive a discrepancy between where they are and where they want to be. In CBT-I, a therapist seeks to raise a patient's awareness of the personal adverse consequences of poor sleep, and to focus the patient's attention on the discrepancy between current and desired sleep.

Patients are more likely to engage in this type of discussion when they are in a psychologically safe, empathic environment, and when the patient, and not the therapist, voices the arguments for change. Practically, this essential principle translates into the following five basic therapeutic guidelines (Miller & Rollnick, 2013):

- Express empathy.
- Develop discrepancy (i.e., help patients consider how they sleep vs. how they want to sleep).
- Avoid direct argumentation.
- Roll with resistance.
- Support self-efficacy.

Following these principles, the therapist gently helps the patient realize that changes in current sleep-related behaviors (e.g., getting out of, rather than staying in, bed when unable to sleep, or curtailing the time allotted for sleep) are possible. For additional reading on motivational enhancement, please see Miller and Rollnick (2013). We demonstrate this technique with another example.

THERAPIST: . . . This is why it is important that you get out of bed at the same time every morning.

PATIENT: I don't want to get up at the same time every day, because I fall asleep at a different time every night.

THERAPIST: It is hard to get out of bed if you fell asleep late and have not slept much. I expect that the first few days of doing this may be hard. It will get easier if you persist, because, as we discussed before, getting up at the same time every morning will strengthen your biological clock. Eventually your clock's alerting signals will start to decrease earlier at night, and you will be able to fall asleep earlier.

PATIENT: I see your point, but I don't think I can do it. I don't think I've ever gotten up at the same time every morning. Even in high school, sometimes I missed classes because I slept in.

THERAPIST: It sounds like there are good reasons why you cannot imagine you will be able to get up at the same time every day. You have never done it consistently before. Can you think of other reasons why getting up at the same time would be a bad idea for you?

PATIENT: I will feel worse in the morning.

THERAPIST: I imagine you may.

PATIENT: I will lose my freedom. I hate to be on a schedule.

THERAPIST: I understand.

PATIENT: How will I ever get over my insomnia problem?

THERAPIST: Well, let's see. I have written on this side of the page all that you said about why getting up at the same time is not very attractive to you. Let's see if we can think of what might make getting out of bed a good idea.

PATIENT: I will be at work on time every day.

THERAPIST: Have you been reprimanded for coming late to work?

PATIENT: My schedule is flexible, but there are some important morning meetings that I have not been able to make.

THERAPIST: Anything else?

PATIENT: I will be able to plan my weekends and do things with my friends.

THERAPIST: And how important is this for you?

PATIENT: Very important. I have been meaning to do it for a long time. It will help get my friends off my back. They have been teasing me about always saying I will do things and then not keeping my promises.

THERAPIST: I have been writing down what you said in favor of getting out of bed reliably at the same time every day. Now that you look at both sides, which side do you think pulls you more?

PATIENT: I think I can give it a try.

THERAPIST: So what time will you get out of bed?

The therapist continued to work with the patient to support the patient's self-efficacy by devising a plan to make sure he kept his commitment, asking what might get in the way, and helping to troubleshoot. The therapist suggested writing on an index card the recommended new behavioral strategy and the reasons that led to the decision to try it.

# ADDRESSING COGNITIONS UNIQUE TO NIGHTMARE DISORDER AND PTSD

## Cognitions Related to Awakenings from Nightmares

Chapter 4 has discussed nightmare disorder and its treatments; Chapter 5 has discussed PTSD. Here our discussion is limited to helping patients with nightmare disorder or PTSD deal with their reactions to nightmares. Upon waking up from a nightmare, a sleeper may replay the nightmare or memories it has triggered, or try to figure out what it might mean or its significance. Barry Krakow has suggested that these common reactions should be avoided, because they may create a habitual nightmare response and perpetuate the nightmare experience (Krakow & Zadra, 2006). Cognitive therapy can be used to help a patient accept a nightmare without trying to figure out its meaning, and to promote getting out of bed and engaging in activities that can help to quiet the mind. Grounding (i.e., reconnecting with the present moment/place) is helpful if a nightmare awakening is associated with confusion. The use of stimulus control in patients with insomnia and nightmares is underscored by Krakow's conceptualization of the nightmare experience as a learned behavior.

## Beliefs Related to Sleep Avoidance and Hypervigilance

Cost–benefit analysis is also useful in addressing some unique features of insomnia that are experienced by patients with PTSD: fear of loss of vigilance (or hypervigilance) and sleep avoidance, both of which can lead to sleep deprivation (see Chapter 5). To help such patients see the costs of hypervigilance and sleep avoidance, the therapist may want to provide relevant scientific information. For example, whereas under normal conditions people can detect meaningful stimuli while asleep and wake up to respond to the stimuli, this ability is compromised when people are sleep-deprived. As discussed in Chapter 2, sleep deprivation leads to increased arousal thresholds (i.e., the strength of the stimulus needed to wake someone up increases) during a subsequent sleep episode. This is because sleep deprivation increases sleep drive. Ironically, by increasing the arousal threshold, sleep deprivation compromises the ability to wake up in the case of a true emergency; when awakened from sleep, the sleeper is likely to experience confusion and to have poor judgment and suboptimal responses. This can be disastrous if, for example, a patient has a loaded gun in the bedroom, as some combat veterans do. This information about the impact of sleep deprivation on arousal threshold and normal sleep vigilance can make patients aware that by engaging in hypervigilant behaviors (e.g., sleeping with the lights on and/or repeatedly checking the locks and/or perimeter), they are less likely to detect real threats when they finally succumb to sleep, and their response when awakened will be compromised. In other words, their hypervigilant behaviors backfire.

The same costs apply to sleep avoidance when the fear of sleep stems from viewing sleep as a dangerous "off-guard" state, as well as to avoidance of sleep for other reasons. For example, some patients with PTSD do not like going to sleep because they are afraid they will have nightmares. Here too, information about the effects of sleep deprivation on REM sleep and the likelihood of experiencing dreams may be important to convey. As discussed in Chapter 2, sleep deprivation leads to increased REM sleep and dreams during subsequent sleep. Periods of REM sleep may occur earlier in the night, last longer, and include more rapid eye movements, which can mean more and/or higher-intensity dreams and nightmares than usual. In other words, sleep avoidance for fear of nightmares actually increases the likelihood of experiencing nightmares and is thus counterproductive. It should also be noted that refraining from safety checking may initially increase anxiety and sleep loss, but over time, as anxiety attenuates and the checking behavior is reduced/eliminated, sleep will improve.

## COGNITIVE THERAPY TECHNIQUES RELEVANT TO INSOMNIA

We have demonstrated above the application of cognitive therapy techniques in CBT-I. In general, cognitive therapy techniques include a wide range of interventions, including eliciting predictions; imagining the worst-case scenario (and evaluating why it's unlikely); examining the costs and benefits of holding certain beliefs; asking, "What advice would you give a friend?"; and other techniques (Leahy, 2003). Here we summarize and discuss other applications of cognitive therapy techniques as applied to insomnia.

### Socratic Questioning

Socratic questioning consists of a series of questions designed to draw the patient's attention to information that is relevant to the issue discussed but is outside the patient's attention or awareness, so that the patient can reevaluate previous notions or come up with new ideas (Beck, 2011; Padesky & Greenberger, 2012). During the first part of this process, the aim is to gather information to help both the patient and therapist get insight into, and concrete understanding of, the patient's statement that is being examined. Important questions are "What do you mean by [part of the patient's statement]?" and "What is the implication of [the answer]?" Once the therapist and patient have reached a better understanding of what specifically the patient is concerned about, they can continue exploring the cognition and gathering information to arrive at a more helpful perspective. When relevant, at key points in the process, the therapist can add information that the patient does not have (e.g., scientific facts about sleep regulation or the impact of insufficient sleep on next-day performance or mood). In the second example given in this chapter, for instance, the therapist provided information about how sleep changes with aging. The patient can then be guided to examine the implications of the new information for his or her situation.

### Thought Records

*Thought records* are used for helping patients learn to self-administer a series of questions to examine the validity of sleep-related thoughts and the impact of these thoughts on their sleep. Thought records are integral to general cognitive therapy (e.g., Padesky & Greenberger, 2012; Beck, 2011). They provide a structured format prompting patients to examine the association between what they think and how they feel (see the second and third columns in Figure 9.2, which is a filled-in version of the Thought Record form provided in Appendix C), explore evidence consistent and inconsistent with the thought (the fourth and fifth columns in Figure 9.2), and come up with revised (e.g., more accurate and/or relevant thoughts) alternatives (the sixth

| Situation | Mood (intensity 0–100%) | Thoughts (underline the most emotionally charged thought) | Evidence for the underlined thought | Evidence against this thought | Adaptive/coping thoughts | Do you feel any differently? |
|---|---|---|---|---|---|---|
| I was parking my car at the mall and started to cry. | Anxious (80%)<br><br>Tired (95%)<br><br>Sad (60%) | I need to get a solid 8 hours of sleep tonight.<br><br>I had no sleep last night.<br><br>I'm going to crash my car again.<br><br>I have to get all my shopping done, but I can't focus or concentrate.<br><br>This is NEVER going away.<br><br>I will go nuts if this sleep problem continues. | I had an accident once when I was super tired.<br><br>Fifteen years ago, I could have gotten all the things on my list done before noon.<br><br>I forgot which store I was supposed to go to first. | When I fell asleep at the wheel, I had an undiagnosed sleep apnea—now that my apnea is treated, it is not as likely to happen.<br><br>Fifteen years ago, I was 15 years younger and could do many things better!<br><br>The afternoon is my sluggish time. I can do these errands in the morning.<br><br>I sometimes feel tired even when I have a good night's sleep. | I always feel this way in the afternoon, even when I sleep well—it will pass (80%).<br><br>Just because I feel crappy, this doesn't mean there is going to be a disaster (75%).<br><br>I could have tea and go over my to-do list—this would be better than freaking out (100%). | Anxious (40%)<br><br>Tired (50%)<br><br>Sad (0%) |

FIGURE 9.2. Filled-in Thought Record example.

136

column in Figure 9.2). By observing, reporting, and evaluating thoughts related to sleep, patients can gain some distance from their thoughts and recognize that thoughts can be unreliable. This then facilitates an open-minded approach to the task of testing the validity of thoughts. In the example shown in Figure 9.2, the patient uses the seven-column Thought Record form in Appendix C to examine the thought "I will go nuts if this sleep problem continues." By examining the evidence, the patient realizes that the thought is probably untrue and certainly unhelpful, and arrives at some alternative thoughts that are associated with better mood.

## Behavioral Experiments

Behavioral experiments are used to test sleep-interfering beliefs between sessions. The therapist and the patient collaboratively decide how, when, and where a belief will be tested. During the session, the therapist discusses possible outcomes. For instance, the therapist can ask the patient to think what will be the implications if the experiment confirms, disconfirms, or partially confirms the belief that is being tested. The use of behavioral experiments in insomnia has been promoted by Ree and Harvey (2004). In some of the examples earlier in this chapter, we have demonstrated the use of behavioral experiments to test various beliefs: about the negative impact of poor sleep on daytime performance; about personal sleep need; about the helpfulness of skipping morning exercise routine after a night of poor sleep; and about the costs of getting out of bed at the same time every morning. Figure 9.3 provides a few additional examples of behavioral experiments relevant to insomnia.

## Cost–Benefit Analysis

Cost–benefit analysis is a type of Socratic questioning that helps make patients aware of the costs of certain beliefs and behaviors that they may be ignoring. In some of the earlier examples, we

| Aim | Experiment |
| --- | --- |
| Test this belief: "If I am tired, I should conserve energy (e.g., cancel plans)." | Expend energy (do not cancel plans) when tired for a few days, and compare level of fatigue to a few days of conserving energy (canceling plans) (Ree & Harvey, 2004). |
| Test this belief: "People notice when I am sleeping poorly, because I look bad." | Take a series of photos, and test people's ratings (Ree & Harvey, 2004). |
| Test this belief: "If I go to bed later, I will disturb my bed partner." | Try it for a few nights (alternatively, ask the partner). |
| Test the impact of clock watching at night. | Keep the clock in the bedroom, and check the time as often as you like for a few nights. Then take all time-keeping devices from the bedroom for a few nights. |

**FIGURE 9.3.** Examples of behavioral experiments.

have demonstrated the usefulness of this technique for addressing beliefs related to sleep safety behaviors, and thoughts and beliefs that interfere with adherence to changes in sleep behaviors. We have also provided an example of using cost–benefit analysis in the context of PTSD-related sleep avoidance. Whereas most other cognitive therapy strategies are useful for examining the validity of a belief, cost–benefit analysis is helpful for discussing the utility of a sleep-related belief.

## Acceptance–Based Techniques

As we have discussed in the section on sleep effort above, the principles of acceptance-based therapies, such as ACT and mindfulness, can help patients abandon their efforts to control sleep—which, as observed in Chapter 3, almost always backfire. Acceptance-based techniques include the use of metaphors, such as the experiential Chinese finger cuff exercise described in Chapters 3 and 8. They also include promoting a shift from engaging with to observing one's thoughts through mindfulness meditation, which enhances willingness to accept sleeplessness and its assumed consequences, as well as to recognize how an excessive focus on sleep compromises pursuing other important personal values.

## Motivational Enhancement

Motivational enhancement is particularly relevant for increasing adherence to the behavioral components of CBT-I. It is intended to mobilize a patient's own resources for change. The therapist gently yet emphatically assists the patient to develop personal responsibility for change, and shapes progress toward commitment to behavior change by supporting self-efficacy (Miller & Rollnick, 2013).

### KEY PRACTICE IDEAS

- Cognitive therapy techniques are useful for addressing the following:
    - Worries about the negative impact of insufficient or poor sleep on daytime performance.
    - Unrealistic expectations about sleep.
    - Beliefs related to sleep effort.
    - Beliefs related to safety behaviors.
- Cognitive therapy techniques are also useful for addressing adherence to the behavioral components of CBT-I.
- Cognitive therapy techniques commonly used in CBT-I include the following:
    - Behavioral experiments, to allow patients to directly experience the advantages and disadvantages of an unhelpful belief.
    - Cost–benefit analysis, to help make patients aware of the costs of certain behaviors (e.g., safety behaviors) that often have a short-term benefit but long-term detrimental effects of which the patients may not be aware.

- Acceptance-based techniques, to help patients abandon their efforts to control sleep and fatigue, and to help patients see how their excessive focus on sleep has interfered with their other personal values.
- Motivational enhancement, to highlight the competing motivations for change versus the status quo. This awareness can be helpful in moving patients from a less action-ready stage to a stage in which they are motivated to adhere to the behavioral components of CBT-I.
- Socratic questioning, to help a patient discover information that is currently outside the patient's awareness, so that the patient can reevaluate the utility or validity of the thought or behavior.
- Thought records, to interrupt emotionally charged thought chains and allow patients to take a look at whether their thoughts are unhelpful and/or distorted. By selecting a more adaptive version of a thought, patients can improve their mood and coping; in the future, the maladaptive thought may not be elicited so automatically in similar situations.
- Offering scientific information to provide a basis from which the patient can evaluate the accuracy of some sleep-related beliefs.

# CHAPTER 10

# Case Conceptualization and Treatment Planning

In this chapter, we bring together content presented in earlier chapters and provide a framework to allow clinicians to tailor treatment to individual patients' presentations. Individually tailoring the delivery of CBT-I is guided by a nuanced understanding of rationales for and the specific components of CBT-I, as well as of various comorbidities' impacts on insomnia—all of which have been discussed in previous chapters. The framework for treatment tailoring is based on the case conceptualization process introduced in this chapter. Case conceptualization is an important part of treatment planning and has been identified as the backbone of competent therapy for complex patients in real-world clinical settings (Persons, 2008).

Treatment planning involves two levels of decision making. The first level includes decisions about whether and when to treat a patient. At this stage, the therapist uses information from the initial evaluation to make a differential diagnosis; decides whether there are contraindications for using CBT-I; and, if there are none, determines how to sequence/integrate CBT-I with treatments for comorbid conditions. The second level pertains to selecting the right combination of CBT-I elements and deciding on the order in which they should be introduced. This second level of treatment planning begins with a conceptualization of each case, which is aided by the Case Conceptualization Form provided in Appendix A. Using the form, the therapist thinks about the patient within the following domains: the three dimensions of sleep regulation discussed in Chapters 2 and 3 (i.e., Process S, Process C, and hyperarousal); comorbidities that may be contributing to the patient's insomnia and may have an impact on the administration of CBT-I; medications the patient is taking that may have an impact on sleep and alertness (in the case of hypnotic medications, the therapist also considers psychological dependence); and unhealthy sleep behaviors and environmental factors that may be interfering with sleep and will therefore need to be altered. After identifying the factors that are contributing to the patient's insomnia, the therapist identifies treatment elements to address these factors and decides on the order in which to introduce the treatment components, taking into consideration the patient's readiness for change. The therapist also anticipates potential obstacles to adherence and considers possible helpful strategies.

# WHETHER AND WHEN TO TREAT A PATIENT

## Differential Diagnosis (Considering Comorbid Sleep Disorders)

A positive diagnosis of insomnia disorder requires the concomitant presence of difficulties initiating or maintaining sleep and associated distress or impairment. During the diagnostic process, the clinician decides whether other sleep disorders are present and, if so, how they contribute to the presenting sleep disturbances. If another sleep disorder is present, then the next important clinical task is to determine whether it fully explains the symptoms of insomnia. If this is the case, then the insomnia disorder diagnosis is precluded, and hence CBT-I is not initiated. If this is not the case, then insomnia disorder can be diagnosed and the other sleep disorder can be considered a comorbidity. When insomnia disorder and another sleep disorder co-occur, the clinician will need to consider how to sequence treatments for the two disorders and what specific aspect of the comorbid sleep disorder are relevant to the implementation of CBT-I. The following sleep disorders, discussed in Chapter 4, should be considered.

*Circadian Rhythm Sleep–Wake Disorders*

- Although principles and components of CBT-I can be used with patients with insomnia disorder comorbid with circadian rhythm sleep–wake disorder, shift work type, it is often not sufficient, particularly for patients who have variable work schedules that include night shifts. In such cases, the therapist should make a referral to a sleep medicine specialist or obtain consultation from such specialists.
- CBT-I is also not sufficient for resolving insomnia disorder comorbid with circadian rhythm sleep–wake disorder, delayed or advanced sleep phase type. In such cases, again, the therapist should make a referral to a sleep medicine specialist or obtain consultation from such specialists. Consultation with a sleep medicine specialist may also be needed when patients with a strong eveningness chronotype wish to advance their desired schedule by more than 3 hours relative to their current schedule.
- CBT-I is contraindicated for patients with other types of circadian rhythm sleep–wake disorders, such as irregular sleep–wake type. These are less common than the two discussed above and require a referral to a sleep medicine specialist.

*Obstructive Sleep Apnea Hypopnea*

- The therapist should refer to a sleep specialist patients with suspected OSAH, as well as those with known but untreated OSAH and those with difficulties adjusting to CPAP therapy. Some transient increase in difficulties with initiating and returning to sleep is expected during the initial adjustment to using CPAP. When adjustment difficulties persist beyond 1 month, referral to a behavioral or medical sleep specialist is recommended.
- When daytime sleepiness is pronounced, the referral should emphasize the urgent need for further diagnosis and treatment.
- CBT-I is not contraindicated for patients with known or suspected OSAH, but, if associated with daytime sleepiness, requires alteration of the protocols to avoid exacerbation of sleepiness and associated risks for accidents.

*Restless Legs Syndrome*

- The therapist should make a referral to a sleep specialist for the treatment of RLS.
- CBT-I can be safely used with patients who have insomnia disorder comorbid with RLS, but it is not a cure for RLS. We are not aware of research on the efficacy of CBT-I in patients with untreated RLS. Edinger et al. (1996) documented the efficacy of CBT-I in the presence of a related disorder, periodic limb movement disorder (PLMD), discussed briefly in Chapter 4. Time awake spent in attempts to relieve the leg sensations (typically, walking about) is not likely to be reduced by CBT-I, but it is reasonable to expect that CBT-I could reduce the time awake after the leg sensations have been attenuated.

*Nightmare Disorder*

- Patients whose difficulties with initiating and maintaining sleep are clearly and exclusively related to their experience of nightmares should not be diagnosed with insomnia disorder. Specifically, an insomnia disorder diagnosis should not be made in patients who report that all their middle-of-the-night awakenings follow nightmares, and that their difficulties falling and/or returning to sleep are clearly linked only to fears of having a nightmare or dealing with its content. Instead, these patients should be given the diagnosis of nightmare disorder.
- CBT-I can be initiated for the treatment of patients with insomnia disorder who experience nightmares, including those with PTSD (see below).

If another sleep disorder is present or suspected, the clinician should explain to the patient the interaction between insomnia disorder and the comorbid sleep disorder, refer the patient to a sleep specialist for further diagnosis and treatment, as indicated, and discuss options for sequencing of CBT-I and the treatment of the comorbid sleep disorder. For example, if the patient has difficulty with sleep initiation and comorbid OSAH, the therapist can explain that although sleep apnea can cause multiple brief arousals in the middle of the night, it does not cause difficulty initially falling asleep or returning to sleep after being awakened by a breathing event. The therapist can then explain that insomnia and OSAH are separate sleep disorders that need to be treated, and that the treatment of one disorder is not expected to cure the other.

## Cautions and Contraindications

With very few exceptions, comorbidities do not constitute contraindications for the application of CBT-I, as long as potential safety issues and the potential for exacerbation of the comorbid conditions are identified and addressed. We discuss each of these below.

### Safety

The primary safety issue in CBT-I arises when sleep restriction therapy is considered for individuals who experience severe daytime sleepiness. This is because sleep restriction therapy may exacerbate sleepiness, and sleepiness increases the risk for accidents. In such cases, further diagnosis and treatment of the cause of daytime sleepiness may be needed prior to implementation of sleep restriction. Examples of disorders that may be associated with severe daytime sleepiness are severe OSAH, PLMD, and narcolepsy. Safety issues can be addressed using a careful risk–benefit assessment and modifying the treatment accordingly. A second reason for safety concerns arises when stimulus control therapy is considered for individuals with possible mobility or vision issues, for whom getting out of bed in the middle of the night may be unsafe (e.g., associated with a risk of falling).

In most cases, CBT-I can be modified to minimize safety concerns, while still maintaining efficacy. Modifications to the components of CBT-I, such as using sleep compression rather than sleep restriction or countercontrol rather than stimulus control, have been discussed in Chapter 7).

### Potential for Exacerbation of the Comorbid Condition

Some comorbidities are exacerbated by sleep deprivation. For example, sleep deprivation may trigger a (hypo)manic episode in patients with bipolar disorders (Bauer et al., 2006); panic attacks in those with PD (Mellman & Uhde, 1989; Roy-Byrne, Uhde, & Post, 1986); and seizures in patients with seizure disorders (Fountain et al., 1998). As we have discussed in Chapter 7, when the self-reported total sleep time (TST) underestimates the actual objective TST, the time-in-bed (TIB) prescription in sleep restriction therapy can lead to sleep deprivation. Therefore, sleep restriction therapy is not recommended for individuals with seizure disorders or for those with PD or bipolar disorders. In these cases, sleep compression can be considered instead. NREM parasomnias, such as sleepwalking and night terrors, are also exacerbated by sleep deprivation, because curtailing sleep increases slow-wave sleep (stage N3) on a subsequent night, and with it raises the potential for partial arousals from stage N3 of sleep. In these cases, the clinician can use other components of CBT-I or can cautiously use sleep compression instead of sleep restriction.

## Sequencing CBT–I

The optimal sequencing of CBT-I and treatments of comorbid conditions has not been well researched. Decisions about sequencing must be guided by clinical judgment, consultation with clinicians treating the comorbidities, and collaboration with the patient. That said, there are a few conventional guidelines for sequencing in behavioral sleep medicine.

• Severity of the comorbid condition is an important consideration in determining the sequencing of CBT-I with the treatment of the comorbid condition. For example, CBT-I should not be initiated with an imminently suicidal, acutely depressed patient before the patient is in a stable mental state. On the other hand, depressed patients with nonacute suicidal ideation do benefit from CBT-I and may experience reductions in suicidality (Manber et al., 2011; Trockel, Karlin, Taylor, Brown, & Manber, in press).

• If insomnia symptoms are experienced exclusively in the context of a comorbid condition and wax and wane with the severity of the comorbid condition, then it is reasonable (but not necessary) to wait until the comorbidity is successfully treated. However, CBT-I can be effective even when there is a close relationship between insomnia disorder and a comorbid condition. In such cases, the therapist can discuss both sequencing strategies with the patient and collaboratively decide which strategy to follow.

• CBT-I may not be effective in the presence of some comorbidities and should be initiated only after the comorbidities have been successfully treated. For instance, CBT-I may not be effective in individuals with active alcohol or other substance use disorders, because it cannot reverse the physiological effects of these substances on sleep. In such a case, the preferred sequencing is to begin by treating the substance use disorder and then treating residual insomnia. Initial evidence suggests that CBT-I may be effective among patients with alcohol dependence in remission (Arnedt et al., 2007; Arnedt et al., 2011).

• CBT-I experts involved in developing the rollout of CBT-I in the Department of Veterans Affairs (VA) health care system concluded that patients with PTSD who are ready to engage or already are engaged in prolonged exposure (PE) therapy (Foa, Hembree, & Rothbaum, 2007) should start or continue to do so before engaging in CBT-I. This expert panel reasoned that because PE is very intense, implementation of CBT-I concomitantly with PE would over tax the resources of the patients (Manber et al., 2012). Thus, in patients who have insomnia disorder comorbid with PTSD and are ready to engage in PE, PE should be provided first. That said, initial evidence suggests that CBT-I may still be effective for individuals with untreated or not fully treated PTSD. Therefore, patients with PTSD who do not fall into the above-described category could benefit from CBT-I. Moreover, clinical experience suggests that some patients with PTSD who are reluctant to engage in psychological treatments, such as PE, are more ready to do so after they experience success with CBT-I.

• In patients with excessive daytime sleepiness (e.g., patients with moderate to severe OSAH), CBT-I should be initiated only after daytime sleepiness is reduced to safe levels. However, when it is not feasible to medically address the causes of severe daytime sleepiness, CBT-I can be adapted as discussed in Chapter 7 and mentioned above. Daytime sleepiness is considered excessive when an individual experiences unintended drifting into sleep during the day. These dozing episodes most commonly occur when the person is idle or engaged in monotonous activities, such as being a passenger in a car, driving long distances, or sitting in a meeting or a lecture.

• A patient with a primary complaint of nonrefreshing sleep and daytime fatigue without difficulties in initiating or maintaining sleep, and despite having allocated sufficient time for sleep, should be referred to a sleep specialist—who most likely will order an overnight PSG study to rule out sleep disorders other than insomnia disorder (e.g., OSAH or PLMD). These disorders are associated with a type of sleep fragmentation that consists of multiple brief arousals from sleep of which the patient may not be aware. This sleep fragmentation can lead to feeling nonrefreshed in the morning and sleepy during the day. When insomnia disorder is experienced as nonrestorative sleep in the absence of prolonged periods of wakefulness, CBT-I should be postponed, because a successful treatment of these other sleep disorders may resolve the insomnia disorder.

• Severe RLS can directly interfere with sleep initiation, and its treatment with dopamine receptor agonists can also cause sleep continuity disturbance. Other comorbid conditions, such as HIV, may necessitate long-term use of medications that interfere with sleep. Even in these cases, however, CBT-I can sometimes lead to improvements in insomnia.

## CASE CONCEPTUALIZATION AS A GUIDE FOR SELECTING THE COMBINATION AND ORDER OF CBT-I COMPONENTS

The second level of treatment planning consists of carefully selecting the combination and order of CBT-I components, and developing specific guidelines for each case. There are three steps of case conceptualization: (1) identifying factors that are pertinent to the case; (2) selecting treatment components that address the factors identified in Step 1; and (3) deciding on the order in which specific guidelines will be introduced, taking into account the patient's readiness. In Step 1, the clinician identifies factors that affect the patient's sleep, such as factors that have a negative impact on the homeostatic sleep drive, the circadian clock, and cognitive or physiological arousal (all listed in Table 10.1 and discussed below). The clinician then identifies specific CBT-I components that address each factor and identifies if any and which modifications to the chosen components are needed (Step 2). Components that maximize the benefit without overwhelming the patient are prioritized, and the therapist carefully considers the likelihood of adherence, in order to set the stage for success (Step 3). Ideally, the case conceptualization is revisited at each session and modified on the basis of adherence and progress. We elaborate on each of the three steps below.

### TABLE 10.1. Domains of the Case Conceptualization Form

1. *Sleep drive:* What factors may be weakening the patient's sleep drive? Consider extended time in bed, dozing off in the evening, daytime napping, sedentary life, and so on.

2. *Biological clock:* What biological clock factors are relevant to the patient's presentation? Consider irregular wake and/or out-of-bed time, time-in-bed window that is not congruent with the patient's chronotype, and so on.

3. *Arousal:* What manifestations of hyperarousal are evident? Consider the following:

   3a. *Cognitive arousal related to sleep* (e.g., sleep effort, safety behaviors, and maladaptive beliefs/ attitudes about sleep).

   3b. *General hyperarousal affecting sleep* (e.g., worry in bed about life stressors).

   3c. *Conditioned arousal:* Has the bed become associated with arousal rather than sleep? Specify predisposing factors (e.g., high trait anxiety), precipitating factors (e.g., stressful life events), and maintaining factors (e.g., extended time spent in bed).

4. *Unhealthy sleep behaviors:* What unhealthy sleep behaviors are present? Consider caffeine, alcohol, nocturnal eating, timing of exercise, and other such factors.

5. *Medications:* What medications may be having an impact on the patient's sleep/sleepiness? Consider carryover effects, tolerance, and psychological dependence.

6. *Comorbidities:* What comorbidities may be affecting the patient's sleep, and how? Consider sleep, medical, and psychiatric conditions (e.g., difficult adjustment to CPAP treatment for sleep apnea, pain interfering with sleep, PTSD-related hypervigilance).

7. *Other:* Consider sleep environment, caregiving duties at night, life phase sleep issues, mental status, and readiness for change.

## Step 1: Identifying Relevant Factors That Affect Sleep

There are six case-related domains to consider (summarized in Table 10.1). Foremost among them are the three factors that influence sleep regulation: Process S, Process C, and hyperarousal (corresponding to the first three items in Table 10.1). In Chapter 2, we have introduced and elaborated on the two-process model of sleep regulation; identified behaviors that could weaken the sleep drive (Process S) and the circadian signal (Process C); and summarized these in the Key Practice Ideas at the end of the chapter. In Chapter 3, we have discussed manifestations of hyperarousal, including cognitive arousal (e.g., sleep effort, safety behaviors, and maladaptive beliefs/attitudes about sleep), conditioned arousal, and general hyperarousal that are incongruent with sleep (e.g., worry in bed about life stressors). The clinician should also consider predispositions (e.g., high trait anxiety) and precipitating events/situations (e.g., interpersonal stress, job stress, loss, significant life changes), if present, and should be particularly aware of factors that may be maintaining insomnia even after the precipitants are no longer playing a major role in the insomnia experience (e.g., sleep effort and extended time spent awake in bed).

The next two domains to consider (items 4 and 5 in Table 10.1) are unhealthy sleep behaviors (e.g., the timing of eating, alcohol, caffeine, nicotine, and exercise relative to sleep), discussed in Chapter 8, and medications (prescribed and nonprescribed) with known effects on sleep or alertness. Medications to consider include those taken for sleep (with attention to the half-life of the medication, tolerance, and psychological dependence, as discussed in Chapter 1), and those that are taken for other reasons but that affect sleep and or alertness (e.g., medications with known sedating or alerting side effects, such as decongestants, steroids, antidepressants, and antipsychotics). The sixth domain pertains to specific impacts that comorbid medical and psychiatric conditions may have on sleep. These include impacts on the patient's propensity to engage in unhealthy sleep behaviors, on the patient's thinking about sleep difficulties, and on other cognitive processes such as a tendency to ruminate—all discussed in Chapter 5, where we have focused on sleep in a few comorbidities that are common among patients with insomnia disorder. Within this domain, the clinician should also note how the comorbidity may affect the patient's adherence to CBT-I recommendations. Examples of comorbidity issues that are relevant to sleep include pain experienced at night, a tendency for some individuals with depression to stay in bed for prolonged periods as a way to escape from emotional pain, and a tendency for some people with PTSD to dread/avoid going to bed.

The Case Conceptualization Form (Appendix A) provides a template for summarizing the details of each case into the above-described six conceptual domains. These six domains are often interconnected and mutually influence each other. For example, spending more time in bed than before the insomnia developed can have an impact on sleep drive (item 1 in Table 10.1 and the Case Conceptualization Form) and contribute to conditioned arousal (item 3 in Table 10.1 and the form). The therapist may choose to list this behavior in the row of the form corresponding to what may be clinically more salient to the case; if this is not obvious, then it does not matter in which row a factor is listed, as long as it is considered. The last row of the form (item 7) provides space for listing other domains, such as (a) environmental factors that may be interfering with sleep, including safety of the sleep environment and sleep-disrupting noise in the bedroom (e.g., a snoring bed or room partner or a noisy neighbor); (b) caregiving duties at night (e.g., caring for a parent with dementia who may be roaming the house at night);

(c) factors related to life phase (e.g., pregnancy-related discomfort, menopause-related nocturnal hot flashes, aging-related frailty); (d) pets in the bedroom; (e) shared living spaces (e.g., a dorm room); (f) mental status (e.g., confusion, cognitive impairment); and (g) the patient's readiness to change (i.e., is the patient invested in improving sleep and ready to make necessary behavioral changes?). The Case Conceptualization Form can help the therapist select the most relevant treatment components, identify instances requiring alteration of the standard components, and anticipate adherence issues that may arise in the course of treatment.

Examples of completed Case Conceptualization Forms for Sophie and Sam can be found in the next two chapters. The reader may want to reread the case descriptions in Chapter 1 and complete Case Conceptualization Forms independently for these two cases before proceeding to the next chapters to look at the examples.

## Step 2: Selecting Treatment Components to Address Relevant Sleep Factors

The next step of treatment planning is to identify specific skills and therapeutic methods, to address each of the factors identified in Table 10.1 and the Case Conceptualization Form. For example, if extended TIB is a factor weakening the sleep drive, then sleep restriction therapy will be an important therapeutic component to consider. A tentative TIB recommendation may be included in the plan, if sleep restriction therapy is identified as an important therapeutic element (which, in our clinical experience, it is in the majority of cases). This initial TIB is based on the retrospective information about the patient's chronotype and sleep habits that was gathered during the sleep assessment. The therapist uses the tentative TIB for planning purposes only and should expect to change it after sleep diary data become available, as well as in response to input from the patient and in accordance with the therapist's clinical judgment about the patient's readiness to adhere to TIB recommendations. To aid in the process of identifying specific skills and therapeutic methods for each patient, we have summarized materials presented in Chapters 7, 8, and 9 and in Table 10.2. A careful selection of treatment elements that match the patient's presentation is key to effective delivery of CBT-I.

### Selecting Treatment Components When Insomnia is Co-Occurs with Other Disorders

Special considerations for the implementation of CBT-I when insomnia co-occurs with some other mental and medical disorders were already discussed. For example, we have discussed sleep compression as an alternative to sleep restriction therapy for patients with PD (because sleep deprivation can decrease the panic threshold). To aid selecting treatment elements when patients present with comorbidities, we have summarized relevant materials presented in earlier chapters in Table 10.3.

### Selecting the Order of Treatment Components to Be Introduced

The case conceptualization process usually identifies many factors, behaviors, and attitudes that contribute to the patient's insomnia experience, and multiple therapeutic elements are usually needed to address them. The key to successful treatment is to decide which therapeutic elements to start with. In selecting these initial therapeutic elements, the therapist should avoid the temp-

**TABLE 10.2. A Summary of CBT–I Treatment Components, Their Aims, and How These Aims Are Achieved**

| Treatment component | Aims | How aims are achieved |
|---|---|---|
| Sleep restriction therapy | • Increase sleep drive<br>• Strengthen circadian clock | • Limiting time in bed<br>• Fixing wake and out-of-bed times |
| Stimulus control therapy | • Extinguish conditioned arousal<br>• Strengthen circadian clock<br>• Increase sleep drive | • Getting out of bed when unable to sleep<br>• Fixing wake and out-of-bed times<br>• Reducing time awake in bed and limiting naps |
| Cognitive therapy | • Reduce sleep-related arousal: sleep performance anxiety and sleep effort; maladaptive thoughts; avoidance behaviors; and excessive monitoring for perceived sleep-related threats (e.g., clock watching)<br>• Enhance adherence to behavioral components | • Behavioral experiments, thought restructuring, sleep education, acceptance-based strategies, and cost–benefit analysis<br>• Sleep education, guided discovery, cost–benefit analysis, and motivational enhancement |
| Sleep education | • Provide rationale for behavioral changes | • Modifying inaccurate beliefs and attitudes about sleep |
| Counterarousal skills | • Reduce general cognitive and somatic arousal<br>• Address intrusive thoughts in bed | • Relaxation, cognitive therapy, scheduled worry, presleep buffer zone activities/unwinding, meditation practice |
| Light therapy | • Facilitate waking up at the designated wake time for patients with mild evening chronotype<br>• Facilitate staying awake until the designated wake time for patients with mild morning chronotype | • Morning light exposure<br>• Evening light exposure |
| Sleep hygiene | • Modify sleep-interfering habits, substances, or environmental factors | • Addressing timing and amount of sleep-interfering substance use, food consumption, and exercise; addressing environmental factors, such as excessive noise, uncomfortable temperature, and safety issues |

**TABLE 10.3. Summary of Issues Related to Implementation of CBT-I for Patients with Common Psychiatric Comorbidities and Chronic Pain**

| Issue | Intervention | Chapter(s) |
|---|---|---|
| | Unipolar depression | |
| Going to bed too early (anhedonia, escape from emotional pain) | Add evening behavioral activation to standard sleep restriction | 7 |
| Difficulty getting out of bed in the morning (anhedonia, escape from emotional pain) | Add morning behavioral activation to standard sleep restriction | 7 |
| Worry | Scheduled worry/ constructive worry | 7 |
| High sleep effort | Cognitive therapy | 9 |
| Safety behaviors | Behavioral experiments | 9 |
| | Bipolar disorder | |
| | *Depressive and euthymic phases* | |
| Sleep deprivation may trigger manic episode | Avoid standard sleep restriction; consider gentle sleep compression; consider postponing sleep restrictive therapy until later in treatment | 5, 7 |
| Bright light may be activating | Avoid bright light in evening | 2 |
| | *Manic phase* | |
| Erratic sleep–wake behaviors weaken circadian rhythm | Regularize rest–wake behaviors; strengthen social rhythm by encouraging regular engagement in and regular timing of daily activities, and involving others to encourage adherence | 2 |
| | GAD | |
| Intrusive worries in bed | Scheduled worry; cognitive therapy; stimulus control | 7, 9 |
| | PTSD | |
| Safety behaviors | Cost benefit analysis, behavioral experiments | 9 |
| Fear of bed/sleep (e.g., fear of loss of vigilance or having a nightmare) | Education; sleep restriction therapy may not be useful if sleep is already restricted; cognitive therapy | 9 |

*(cont.)*

**TABLE 10.3** (*cont.*)

| Issue | Intervention | Chapter(s) |
|---|---|---|
| Hyperarousal (possible experience of relaxation-induced anxiety) | Indirect arousal reduction; stimulus control (patient should not be in bed in a state of hyperarousal) | 7, 8 |
| Aversion to silence | Patients should not sleep with TV on; consider white noise (extreme cases may require systematic exposure before the patient can tolerate being awake in the dark in silence) | 7 |
| No sleepiness at bedtime | Modify stimulus control to use timer + arousal reduction | 7 |
| Nightmares | Focus on reducing postnightmare arousal levels | 8 |
| Presence of sleep apnea or parasomnias (in addition to nightmares) | Assess and refer to sleep specialist as needed | 4, 6 |
| <div align="center">PD</div> | | |
| Nocturnal panic | Use CBT for nocturnal PD (Craske, Lang, Aikins, & Mystkowski, 2005) | |
| Sleep deprivation may trigger panic attacks | Use liberal sleep restriction protocol or sleep compression | 5, 8 |
| <div align="center">Chronic pain</div> | | |
| Extended time in bed at night | Augment sleep restriction therapy with behavioral activation and education about sleep and pain | 2, 5, 7, 8 |
| Spending time in the sleep bed during the day may promote conditioned arousal; inadvertent sleep while resting may decrease the sleep drive | Patient should rest in a different bed during the day, and avoid reclining while resting to minimize chance of sleeping during the day | 3, 7 |
| Pain can cause wakefulness | Medium-firmness mattress and careful pillow positioning may help manage posturally related pain at night | 7 |
| Belief that sleep will not improve unless pain improves | Education about relationship between pain and sleep, and about the evolution of insomnia | 5 |

tation to introduce too many recommendations at once, because doing so will overwhelm the patient and may compromise adherence. The therapist can begin by identifying the most important one to three factors that need to be addressed and strategies to address them. The potential impact of the recommendation should be considered, as well as the likelihood that the patient will indeed follow the recommendation. When striking a balance between the two, the therapist may need to consider modifying the recommendation to enhance adherence (if needed) or postponing its introduction. For example, a therapist may believe that one of the most effective recommendations is to get out of bed every morning at the same time, but a patient may have low mood in the morning and may have reported considerable difficulty getting out of bed to start the day. Depending on the case, the therapist may decide to implement behavioral activation in the morning (e.g., scheduling activities that involve other people within an hour of the recommended rise time) or choose to negotiate a later fixed time to get out of bed each morning, rather than push prematurely for the optimal early rise time. Small successes increase motivation to engage in future behavior changes. We have developed a Treatment Planning Form (Appendix A) to help clinicians select and order treatment components.

Treatment plans for Sophie and Sam are described in Chapters 11 and 12, respectively. As with the Case Conceptualization Form, it may be a good idea for the reader to read the case descriptions in Chapter 1 and complete the Treatment Planning Form independently for each of these cases. The completed forms can then be compared to the treatment plans presented in Chapters 11 and 12.

## GENERAL STRUCTURE OF TREATMENT

CBT-I is a brief therapy. Most randomized clinical trials of CBT-I have provided between four and eight sessions. Edinger, Wohlgemuth, Radtke, Coffman, and Carney (2007) conducted a dose–response study of CBT-I for people with insomnia disorder; participants were prescreened to exclude patients with comorbid psychiatric and medical conditions or with concomitant use of medications that might disrupt sleep. These researchers concluded that a dose of four individual, biweekly sessions (not including the intake sessions) is optimal for durable benefits. This suggests that a total of five biweekly sessions (intake and four treatment sessions) is an optimal dose for insomnia disorder uncomplicated by the presence of comorbidity. There are no data about the optimal dosing for CBT-I for insomnia disorder comorbid with other disorders. A review of 37 studies on the efficacy of CBT-I reported that the mean number of sessions was 5.7 (Morin, Bootzin, et al., 2006). These are usually standardized fixed protocols and rarely include participants with multiple comorbidities. A large nationwide dissemination of CBT-I in the VA health care system, where many patients present with comorbid insomnia, adopted a six-session protocol consisting of an intake session and five weekly treatment sessions (Manber et al., 2012). The VA protocol is flexible in regard to the order of components and number of sessions, with some patients completing treatment in fewer than six sessions and others requiring more than six. Program evaluation found significant decreases in insomnia severity, depressive symptoms, and suicidal ideation, as well as improvements in quality of life, after six sessions (or fewer if the patient improved) (Karlin, Trockel, Taylor, Gimeno, & Manber, 2013; Trockel, Karlin, Taylor, Brown, & Manber, in press).

This book presents a similar approach: We recommend six biweekly sessions, with the understanding that the actual number and frequency of sessions will vary, depending on patient presentation. For example, a patient who is reluctant to make the needed behavioral changes may need to be seen weekly at first and may ultimately need more than six sessions. For straight-forward cases in which patients are highly adherent, the number of sessions may be fewer than six. For example, Sam received six CBT-I sessions (see Chapter 12), but Sophie received only five (see Chapter 11). The approach promoted in this book is anchored in case conceptualization as a guide for individualizing treatment. The case conceptualization process helps clinicians to select treatment components and their sequence in a manner that is also consistent with the approach to treatment adopted by the nationwide dissemination of CBT-I in the VA health care system. We outline below a semistructured six-session treatment protocol, summarized in Table 10.4.

## Session 1

The first session is devoted to a comprehensive assessment of the presenting sleep problem, which is a process separate from a general mental health or medical intake. The content and structure of this initial sleep assessment are detailed in Chapter 6. The assessment can be aided by an outline, which can be found in the Insomnia Intake Form in Appendix A. The sleep assessment concludes with goal setting. The information gathered during the sleep assessment allows the therapist to decide whether there are any contraindications and whether referrals and/or consultations with other providers are needed. If there are no contraindications, the therapist can then summarize the information gathered and frame it in the context of sleep regulation and/or the etiological model of insomnia, as time permits. At this early stage, the framing of the problem is done in broad strokes and does not need to include detailed explanations of sleep regulation. For sample scripts, please see Chapters 11 and 12. The brief explanation may also include, in general terms, what the treatment will entail (e.g., "We will work on helping you learn to calm your mind before you go to bed," or "We will work on strengthening your sleep drive so that you have better-quality sleep"). The goal of this summary is to set expectations and promote hope.

Depending on how much time is left in the session and on the complexity of the case, the therapist then decides whether to introduce any initial intervention and, if so, what specific simple recommendation to make. (Experience with CBT-I improves a therapist's ability to make such simple treatment recommendations immediately after the insomnia intake.) The simple recommendation should not include sleep restriction therapy, which should commence only after sufficient sleep diary data are available. Here are two examples of simple recommendations: (1) If the patient takes long daytime naps, the therapist can provide a brief description of the sleep drive, explain that napping can weaken the sleep drive at bedtime, and recommend that the patient avoid napping; (2) if the patient has a very irregular wake time, the therapist can provide a brief description of the circadian clock and the impact it has on sleep, explain that an irregular wake time weaken this biological clock, and recommend that the patient choose a wake time he or she can adhere to every morning, regardless of how well the patient sleeps. In making the decision about whether to make a simple initial recommendation, the therapist should consider the details of the case, the time available for providing a rationale, and the patient's ability/willingness to commit to a simple intervention at this stage.

Regardless of whether or not an initial treatment recommendation is made, the therapist

**TABLE 10.4. A Six–Session Treatment Protocol**

| Session | Content | Chapter(s) |
|---|---|---|
| 1 | • Provide introduction/orientation to CBT-I | 6 |
| | • Conduct comprehensive insomnia intake | 6 |
| | • Goal setting | 1, 10 |
| | • Determine whether CBT-I is contraindicated | 6, 7 |
| | • Introduce/review sleep diary | |
| | • Provide a brief summary, framed in the context of sleep regulation theory and/or Spielman, Caruso, and Glovinsky's (1987) model of insomnia | 2, 3 |
| | • Provide one or two simple recommendations, based on case conceptualization, as time permits | 10 |
| 2 | • Review sleep diary | 6, 7 |
| | • Introduce stimulus control/sleep restriction therapy guidelines, and rationale anchored in sleep regulation theory and Spielberg et al.'s model of insomnia | 7 |
| | • Identify potential obstacles to adherence and address them | 7, 9 |
| | • Add other treatment components/recommendations, based on case conceptualization, as time permits | 7, 8, 9 |
| 3 | • Review sleep diary and adherence | 6, 7 |
| | • Discuss adherence (use cognitive therapy techniques as needed) | 7, 8, 9 |
| | • Modify TIB recommendation, following the sleep restriction protocol | 7 |
| | • Explain cognitive arousal and its role in maintaining insomnia | 3, 9 |
| | • Introduce techniques to calm the mind that have not already been introduced (e.g., presleep unwinding time, relaxation) | 8 |
| 4–5 | • Review sleep diary and adherence | 6, 7 |
| | • Discuss adherence and its relation to progress (use cognitive therapy techniques as needed) | 7, 8, 9 |
| | • Modify TIB recommendation, following the sleep restriction protocol | 7 |
| | • Use cognitive therapy as needed (behavioral experiment, Socratic questioning, cost–benefit analysis, and/or acceptance-based techniques) | 9 |
| 6 (Final) | • Review sleep diary and adherence | 6, 7 |
| | • Modify TIB recommendation, following the sleep restriction protocol | 7 |
| | • Develop relapse prevention/continued care plan | 10 |

introduces the sleep diary at the end of the session. In cases where the sleep diary forms are mailed ahead of the assessment appointment, the sleep diary is reintroduced, along with cheerleading about the completion of the diary or troubleshooting about nonadherence to monitoring. To enhance adherence, the therapist should take time to explain that the sleep diary information will be used for making treatment decisions and for tracking changes in the patient's sleep over time, and should provide the patient an opportunity to become familiar with the task. This can be done by asking the patient in session to complete information about the preceding night and encouraging the patient to ask for clarification. The therapist can also ask the patient to complete the information for the prior day or two, in order to demonstrate that ability remember details concerning sleep decreases over time. This small experiential exercise underscores the importance of daily completion of the sleep diary. At the same time, the therapist should advise the patient to provide estimates rather than look at the clock, because clock watching could lead to increased anxiety about sleep .

Between the first and second sessions, the therapist should use the information gathered during the sleep (and general) intake(s) for case conceptualization and decisions about the most relevant treatment components and the order of introducing them. This process can be aided by the Case Conceptualization Form and the Treatment Planning Form.

## Session 2

In the second session, the therapist introduces treatment components that were identified during the process of case conceptualization and treatment planning. In most cases, the first components to be introduced are stimulus control and/or sleep restriction therapy, tailored to the patient's presentation. These two treatment components have been empirically supported as monotherapies for insomnia (Morin, Bootzin, et al., 2006; Morin, Hauri, et al., 1999) and are often combined (see Chapter 7). In some cases, one or both of these components may be contraindicated or overwhelming and may need to be simplified, modified, or even postponed to a later session. For example, if the patient has bipolar disorder, the therapist is likely to avoid or postpone introducing sleep restriction therapy until a later session (Kaplan & Harvey, 2013). For the most part, contraindications are identified during the treatment planning that takes place between Sessions 1 and 2. However, sometimes new information emerges, requiring deviation from the original plan. For example, if a patient responds to sleep restriction or stimulus control with higher levels of anxiety than was originally anticipated, the therapist may choose to postpone the implementation of these components until the patient is ready. Meanwhile, the therapist can focus on addressing sleep-related anxiety, using cognitive therapy techniques (Chapter 9) and/or behavioral methods to reduce the general level of anxiety during the intended sleep period (Chapters 8 and 9).

### Beginning of Session

Session 2 and subsequent sessions begin with setting the agenda, asking the patient to reflect on changes in sleep since the last session, reviewing the sleep diary, and discussing adherence to treatment recommendations that were previously made (if any). When reviewing the sleep diary, the therapist summarizes the information and clarifies inconsistencies in data. To summarize the data, the therapist can (1) reflect on the ranges and averages of TIB and, separately, TST; (2) note night-to-night variability in sleep schedule (e.g., note the amount of time between the earliest and latest rise times during the recording period); and (3) note night-to-night variability in the time to fall asleep and/or time awake in the middle of the night. The summary may also include averages of key variables (e.g., TST, TIB, time to fall asleep, time awake in the middle of the night, and time awake in bed after waking up). If the patient is taking medications or other substances intended to promote sleep, the therapist pays attention to the timing and frequency of consumption; if there is variability, the therapist clarifies how the patient decides whether and when to take the medication or substance. If an initial treatment recommendation was made during the first session, the therapist also discusses adherence—and, when improvements in sleep are noted by the patient, explores the relationship between following the recommendation and the observed improvement. If a worsening of symptoms is noted, the therapist explores reasons. For example, worsening may be related to an increase in life stress, a change in medications, or an unusual sleep environment. Alternatively, worsening may be related to an anxiety response to treatment recommendations.

## Middle of Session

In Session 2 and subsequent sessions, the focus during the middle of the session is on introducing the rationales for and content of the treatment components that the therapist has selected for inclusion in the session. Ideally, the rationales are personalized; that is, they make reference to the specific details of the case and are presented in an interactive manner. The therapist then fluidly leads into the specific treatment recommendations and tries to anticipate and preempt anxious responses to the recommendations. Adherence is enhanced when the initial recommendations are made in a thoughtful and personalized manner. See Chapters 11 and 12 for examples of introducing treatment components interactively.

## End of Session

Each session from Session 2 onward concludes with a summary of homework and a reminder to continue completing the sleep diary. It is a good idea to summarize the treatment recommendations in writing.

# Sessions 3–5 (and Additional Sessions as Needed)

As indicated above, each later session has a structure similar to that of Session 2. It begins with agenda setting and a review of progress as perceived by the patient and, separately, as reflected in the sleep diary. Any discrepancies between perceived and diary-based improvements in sleep are discussed. In addition to focusing on changes in sleep, the review of the sleep diary should include attention to adherence to previous treatment recommendations and discussion of adherence. When adherence is high and progress is evident, the therapist highlights the relationship between progress and adherence in order to enhance the patient's self-efficacy. When adherence is low, the therapist identifies and works though barriers to adherence, including (but not restricted to) making sure that the patient understands why a recommendation to which the patient did not fully adhere was made in the first place. Cognitive therapy techniques (Chapter 9) can also be used to address emerging adherence issues. Sometimes the treatment guidelines need to be modified because previously unavailable information that may have compromised adherence has emerged. For example, the discussion of nonadherence may reveal that the patient has an eveningness chronotype, which may have not been evident during the initial sleep intake. In such a case, the recommended TIB window may need to be shifted to a later time, and increasing morning light exposure may need to be considered. If both adherence and progress are low, the therapist may want to promote hope that better adherence could result in improvement. Information about adherence to the sleep restriction guidelines can be obtained strictly from the sleep diary. Assessing adherence to other recommendations may require directly asking the patient about them: for example, "Did you get of bed when you were not able to sleep?", "Were you sleepy when you went to bed?", "Did you complete the experiment we decided on last time?"

Usually the next step in treatment is to determine whether and how to make adjustments to the TIB recommendation. Using the sleep diary, the therapist computes sleep efficiency and adjusts the TIB recommendation according to the sleep restriction therapy protocol, based on progress, estimated sleep need, and adherence (Chapter 7). It is a good idea to demonstrate and teach the patient how to compute sleep efficiency and how to make decisions about TIB alterations, so that the patient can later self-administer sleep restriction therapy. Self-administration is helpful when life constraints cause sessions to be spaced out, and it will become part of the relapse prevention plan (discussed in the last session).

Additional relevant components of treatment are then introduced, based on the original treatment plan or on a modified plan if new clinically relevant information is revealed, as in the example above. Additional components may include cognitive therapy techniques to address thoughts and beliefs that promote arousal, relaxation methods, and other ways to reduce arousal in bed (e.g., scheduled worry time, unwinding time). (If not already introduced in Session 2, sleep restriction therapy and/or stimulus control therapy may be introduced when clinically indicated, and adjusted in subsequent sessions on the basis of progress, estimated sleep need, and adherence.) Each session ends with a summary of homework and a reminder to continue completing the sleep diary.

## Last Session

The last session is similar in structure to the middle sessions, with added discussion of relapse prevention and continued care. Treatment elements that the patient and clinician have found helpful are identified and become the foundation of the relapse prevention plan. The therapist explains that because the sleep system is very sensitive to a person's well-being, it is likely to be disturbed during periods of acute stress. The key to relapse prevention is to stop newly developed perturbations in sleep, which are common and normal reactions to stress, from developing into another insomnia disorder episode. The following are recommended in order to avert prolongation of new sleep disruptions that emerge during periods of acute distress: (1) accepting poor sleep in stride rather than becoming alarmed about it, and (2) refraining from engagement in compensatory behaviors. When a stressful state/event is a clear precipitant of the disruption in sleep, it is best for the patient to channel his or her effort toward attending to the stress causing the sleep disruption, and avoid the natural tendency to exert effort to improve sleep. At this point in treatment, the idea that such efforts are counterproductive should be familiar to the patient.

The discussion of relapse prevention begins by asking the patient to identify treatment components that have proven helpful. Because these same components are likely to be useful if insomnia reemerges, the patient should write these components down and return to the list when they are needed in the future. An example of a relapse prevention form, entitled Strategies for Dealing with Insomnia in the Future, can be found in Appendix C (and samples of this form as completed by Sophie and Sam are provided in Chapters 11 and 12). The therapist can add to the list treatment components that have been helpful but that the patient may have missed. Part of the relapse prevention conversation is a discussion about when to resume using the sleep diary and when to seek professional help. In most cases, it is not necessary to keep a sleep diary after insomnia remits. The patient can resume monitoring sleep with diaries if sleep deteriorates and becomes a concern. At that point, the patient also reinstitutes the treatment components that were helpful. Help should be sought if, despite these measures, poor sleep continues to be an issue that has a negative impact on the patient's life.

Patients whose insomnia fully remits may want to know whether or when they can relax some of the sleep rules. As a general rule, a flexible approach to sleep promotes good sleep. We teach patients to "sleep to live" rather than "live to sleep," and we discourage rigid rules about sleep, with the exception of keeping to a regular wake time. For example, as described in Chapter 11, Sophie raised this issue with her therapist, and the therapist talked about how to approach future schedule changes. When insomnia fully resolves and the automaticity of falling asleep is reinstated, some of the rules can be relaxed. It is best to do so gradually and to be informed by behavioral experiments. All experiments should begin with collecting sleep diary data for 2 weeks to get a sense of baseline sleep before experimenting. For example, if the patient wants to sleep in on weekends, an experiment can be conducted as follows: (1) Start monitoring sleep; (2) increase TIB on the weekend by a small amount, such as 30 minutes; (3) stay on the new schedule for about a month (so that four weekends can be sampled) while monitoring sleep in the diary; and (4) at the end of the month, evaluate the data collected and decide whether sleep and daytime fatigue have worsened. If worsening is detected, the patient should reinstate the original sleep rules; otherwise, the patient should either continue with the current schedule or experiment with further delay of rise time on weekends, if desired. In the spirit of "sleeping to live," it is also permissible to plan for an occasional poor night of sleep. For example, a patient may want to know what to do about partying and drinking alcohol late at night. In this case, the therapist can help promote a flexible approach to sleep by discussing the costs and benefits of drinking late into a party night. Although it is likely that sleep that night will be disturbed, the patient may decide that one night of poor sleep is a reasonable price to pay for the fun of the party.

## KEY PRACTICE IDEAS

- Treatment planning involves the following:
  - Differential diagnosis.
  - Identifying contraindications for using CBT-I.

- Deciding how to sequence/integrate CBT-I with treatments for comorbid conditions.
- Case conceptualization, aided by the Case Conceptualization Form in Appendix A.

- Treatment generally lasts from four to six sessions.

  - Session 1 is devoted to assessment and treatment planning.
  - Session 2 usually involves introducing the core behavioral components—stimulus control and sleep restriction therapy (usually combined)—and providing a rationale anchored in education about sleep regulation.
  - Sessions 3–5 center around refining the core behavioral components on the basis of adherence and progress (troubleshooting adherence to the core components and adjusting TIB), and adding components as needed (e.g., relaxation therapy, cognitive therapy).
  - The final session is devoted to relapse prevention.

# CHAPTER 11

# Case Example 1

## *Sophie*

I n this and the next chapter, we demonstrate treatment planning and session-by-session implementation of CBT-I in the two cases first introduced in Chapter 1: Sophie in this chapter, and
Sam in Chapter 12. The intent is to demonstrate how the principles and techniques discussed
in previous chapters are applied to each of the two clinical presentations. There are similarities
and differences in the selection, relative order, and emphasis of treatment components in the
two cases. The guiding principles and session structures are the same, but the administration is
flexible. The scripts provide examples of presenting rationales in a manner that fits each case,
integrating pertinent case-specific information into the explanations, and avoiding overwhelming the patient. We also illustrate how the sleep diary is used throughout treatment.

This chapter begins with taking the reader through planning the treatment for Sophie, a
42-year-old woman who called the therapist to request treatment for her insomnia. Before the
first session, she was mailed two blank copies of the sleep diary form and instructions for how to
complete them daily before coming in to the clinic. (If mailing the sleep diary forms in advance
is not feasible, the therapist introduces them at the end of the first session, as was done in the
case of Sam.) In Sophie's case, the diary forms were included in a clinic-mailed package that
also contained information about the clinical practice, as well as driving and parking directions.
Before the first (and each subsequent) session, the therapist reviewed Sophie's sleep diary and
came up with a session plan.

## SESSION 1

### Before Session

Sophie arrived for her first appointment 10 minutes before the session, as instructed. She had
completed the two sleep diary forms and brought these to the appointment. Office personnel
asked her to complete the clinic's consent forms, a form for demographic information, and two
insomnia-related questionnaires—the Insomnia Severity Index (ISI) and the Dysfunctional
Beliefs and Attitudes about Sleep (DBAS-16) scale (see Appendix B for blank versions of both

questionnaires)—in the waiting room. Meanwhile, the clinic staff gave the therapist Sophie's completed sleep diary forms. The therapist reviewed the data and calculated weekly averages of Sophie's time in bed (TIB), total sleep time (TST), and sleep efficiency (SE), following the guidelines outlined in Chapter 6. (Sophie's sleep diary data have been used in Chapter 6 to illustrate how to create summary variables.) The therapist wrote down the plan for Session 1 for Sophie (see Figure 11.1 for this plan, and Appendix A for a blank version of the Session Plan form). The bulk of the first session was devoted to a comprehensive insomnia assessment as discussed in Chapter 6 and described below.

## Session Plan

**ID/Name:** _Sophie_                    **Date:** _October 16, 2013_          **Session #:** _1_

- *Provide introduction to treatment (personal introductions, informed consent, overview of therapy structure and of today's session).*

- *Compliment completion of sleep diary; ask if she has questions about sleep diary; summarize information and observations from sleep diary review; underscore importance of continued daily recording in sleep diary throughout treatment.*

- *Conduct insomnia intake interview to assess insomnia disorder diagnosis, sleep habits, history of sleep complaint, other sleep disorders, psychiatric and medical disorders and their treatment (including medications, supplements, caffeine, and alcohol), and sleep environment.*

- *Identify specific treatment goals with Sophie.*

- *Determine whether CBT–I is contraindicated (likely OK, based on a brief description of her problem during the brief initial phone contact with Sophie).*

- *Provide a brief summary of problems and contributing factors, framed in the context of sleep regulation and/or an etiological model of insomnia (as time permits).*

- *Provide one or two simple recommendations, based on case conceptualization (as time permits).*

**Homework:**

- *Assign next week's sleep diary forms.*

- *Follow the recommendation(s) provided.*

**Notes:**

- *Schedule next appointment(s).*

**FIGURE 11.1.** Session Plan form as completed by the therapist for Sophie's Session 1.

## During Session

After Sophie was introduced to the treatment, had her questions answered, and signed the treatment consent form, the therapist began the structured insomnia evaluation, following the guidelines outlined in Chapter 6. The case description in Chapter 1 is based on information gathered during Sophie's initial insomnia intake and a review of her sleep diary. Below, we summarize the information the therapist gathered during the insomnia intake interview, using the Insomnia Intake Form (see Figure 11.2, and Appendix A for the blank version). During this interview, the therapist assessed Sophie for other sleep disorders, using the Assessment of Other Sleep Disorders form (see Figure 11.3, and, again, Appendix A for the blank form). The therapist then indicated on the Insomnia Intake Form whether each of the sleep disorders assessed was present or absent.

### Sophie's Sleep Diary

Sophie completed the sleep diary for 2 weeks. (A blank version of the Consensus Sleep Diary–M form she used is provided in Appendix B.) Only the second week of sleep diary data, and associated calculated variables, are presented in Figure 11.4 and below. Before the session, the therapist computed TIB and TST for each day, following the procedures outlined in Chapter 6, and noted these values at the bottoms of the corresponding columns. The therapist also calculated SE for each day and computed weekly averages of key variables, which are summarized below.

- *Sleep onset latency*: The average time it took to fall asleep (diary item 3) was 1 hour, 55 minutes.
- *Wakefulness after sleep onset* (WASO): The average time awake in the middle of the night (diary item 5) was 52 minutes.
- *Average TIB*: Average TIB was 10 hours, 30 minutes.
- *Average TST*: Average TST was 6 hours, 15 minutes.
- *Average SE*: Average SE was 40%.

For the most part, Sophie's sleep diary data were consistent with the information she provided during the insomnia intake interview. Consistent with her report during the interview, her diary indicated that she spent an average of 10.5 hours in bed, fell asleep in about 2 hours, and was awake 50 minutes in the middle of the night. However, there was a discrepancy between the two sources of estimates of how long she slept: During the interview, she reported that she slept 4 hours, but her diary indicated an average calculated TST of 6 hours, 15 minutes. After the discussion of treatment goals, the therapist pointed this fact out to Sophie.* The therapist explained how TST was calculated, and the two of them examined the range of the calculated TST values over the course of the week. In the following exchange, the therapist asked about the discrepancy and used the opportunity to gently broach the subject of Sophie's preoccupation with her sleep problems.

---

*The therapist's holding off on this discussion provided an opportunity to understand Sophie's perceptual biases and was intended to support good therapeutic alliance.

# Insomnia Intake Form

**Patient name:** *Sophie*    **Marital/partnered status:** *Single*    **Referral source:** *Self*

**Gender:** *Female*    **Children:** *None*

**Date of birth or age:** *[Age 42]*    **Occupation:** *Corporate attorney*

**NATURE OF PRESENTING PROBLEM** (check all that apply, and identify the most distressing/disturbing sleep problem):

☑ Difficulty initiating sleep        ☑ Difficulty maintaining sleep
☐ Waking up too early            ☐ Difficulty waking up            ☐ Nonrefreshing sleep

Number of nights per week sleep problem is experienced: ____7____ to ____7____

When did the current episode start? __*1 year ago*__

Identifiable precipitating factor(s): __*Breakup in romantic relationship; single episode of nocturnal panic*__

Treatment history for current episode: __*Eszopiclone (unhelpful), clonazepam (carryover sedation), wine (sleep fragmentation)*__

## DAYTIME EFFECTS

☑ Energy/fatigue        ☑ Concentration/functioning            ☑ Mood
☐ Daytime sleepiness: _____

Other (specify): __*Forgetful, irritable, no energy to socialize in evening; discontinued morning workout*__

## HISTORY

Age at onset of first insomnia episode: ____41____    Lifetime course: *First episode ("used to fall asleep when my head hit the pillow and never woke up until I had to in the morning")*

Family history of insomnia: __*None noted*__

**Sleep habits** (focus on previous or most recent typical week; describe range when indicated; note weekday/weekend times, if different):

## BEGINNING OF SLEEP PERIOD

Time into bed: ____*9:30 P.M.*____

Time turning lights out (or intent to sleep): __*Same (she used to read in bed but stopped)*__

How does patient decide when to go to bed? __*Tries to be in bed by 9 "to get enough sleep"*__

Pre-bedtime activities: __*TV & Internet*__        ☐ Fears        ☐ Dozing off in evening

Average time to fall asleep: __*1–3 hours*__

What happens when patient cannot get to sleep (thoughts/behaviors)? __*Random thoughts; some worry about work; stays in bed tossing and turning*__

☐ Rumination        ☑ General worry        ☑ Sleep worry        ☐ Physical tension

**FIGURE 11.2.** Insomnia Intake Form as completed for Sophie.

162

## MIDDLE OF THE NIGHT

Number of awakenings after sleep onset: _____2_____ to _____3_____
*(per diary, between 2 and 5 A.M.)*

Total time awake after sleep onset: _30 min_ to _90 min_

What happens when awake in the middle of the night (thoughts/behaviors)? _Stays in bed; thinks of what_ _she needs to do during the day; worries about not sleeping_

☐ Rumination     ☑ General worry     ☑ Sleep worry     ☐ Physical tension

## END OF THE NIGHT

Final wake time: __6:30–7:00 A.M.__          Time out of bed: __7:30–9:00 A.M.__

Alarm (or other wake-up system): ☐ No ☑ Yes _____

Is final awakening earlier than planned? ☑ No ☐ Yes, by _____ minutes

_Wishes she could sleep in on weekend_

Difficulties waking up at intended time: ☑ No ☐ Yes _____ _but difficulty getting out of bed_

Estimated average total sleep time: __4 hours__

**PREMORBID SLEEP SCHEDULE:** __10:30 P.M. to 6:30 A.M. with occasional sleep-ins on weekend__

**CURRENT SLEEP MEDICATION(S)/AIDS:** ☐ No ☐ Yes (If yes, then complete table below.)

| Name | Dose | When taken? | How long? | Helpful? |
|---|---|---|---|---|

## NAPPING

Able to nap if given an opportunity? ☐ No ☑ Yes _but only on weekend_

Nap frequency _Tries almost daily_          Nap duration _0–120 min_

Timing of nap _Early afternoons on some weekends_

**SLEEP ENVIRONMENT** (note problematic aspects of sleep environment—bed partner, caregiving, pets, sound, lights, safety, temperature):

_Adequate, no bed partner_

**OTHER BEHAVIORS THAT CAN AFFECT SLEEP** (include time and frequency; for substances, also include amount):

Caffeine _None (premorbid: to 1–2 in morning )_          Nicotine_None_

Alcohol _A few times a month to unwind late at night_          Recreational drugs _None_

Timing of vigorous exercise _Stopped (used to go to gym in A.M.)_          Nocturnal eating _No_

Overall activity level:  ☐ Understimulated          ☐ Overstimulated

Other: __Stopped social activity in evenings and workout in mornings__

*(cont.)*

## NOTES ON COGNITIVE HYPERAROUSAL

_Lies awake feeling frustrated_

## NOTES ON EMOTIONAL AROUSAL

_Anxious apprehension_

## CIRCADIAN TENDENCIES

☐ Morning type          ☑ Neither type          ☐ Evening type

Evidence: _____

---

Use the **Assessment of Other Sleep Disorders** form to evaluate other sleep disorders, and note results here.

### CIRCADIAN RHYTHM SLEEP–WAKE DISORDERS

☑ Does not meet criteria          ☐ Meets criteria   Type: ☐ Advanced   ☐ Delayed

### OBSTRUCTIVE SLEEP APNEA HYPOPNEA (OSAH)

☐ Previously diagnosed      Severity _____ events per hour _____

☑ Not previously diagnosed      ☐ Suspected      ☑ Not suspected

Treatment:   ☐ Not or inadequately treated   ☐ Adequately treated   Specify treatment:_____

### RESTLESS LEGS SYNDROME (RLS)

☑ Does not meet criteria      ☐ Meets criteria      Treatment: _____

### PARASOMNIA SYMPTOMS (include frequency):

Nightmare disorder:   ☐ Meets criteria   ☑ Does not meet criteria

Other unusual behaviors during sleep: _____

---

**CURRENT COMORBID MEDICAL DISORDERS** (note impact on sleep, include treatment): __None__

**CURRENT COMORBID PSYCHIATRIC DISORDERS** (note impact on sleep, include treatment): __None__

_(Past nocturnal panic attack)_

**GOAL(S):** _"Sleep like I did before," operationalized and rank-ordered as follows: (1) Have sleep uninterrupted; (2) fall asleep within 10 minutes; and (3) sleep a little longer (and later) on weekend nights._

---

**FIGURE 11.2** (_cont._)

## Assessment of Other Sleep Disorders

| SLEEP COMPLAINT | NOTES |
|---|---|
| **Circadian rhythm sleep–wake disorder, delayed sleep phase type**<br><br>1. Recurrent inability to fall asleep at a desired conventional clock time, and difficulty awakening at a desired and socially acceptable time.<br><br>2. When allowed to use preferred schedule, no problem with sleep except its delayed timing.<br><br>3. Preferred schedule delayed more than 2 hours relative to desired conventional clock.<br><br>If criteria 1, 2, and 3 are met, refer patient to a sleep center for assessment and treatment. (Treatment will probably involve schedule manipulation and properly timed light and dark exposures.) | *Circadian rhythm sleep–wake disorder, delayed sleep phase type is absent.* |
| **Circadian rhythm sleep–wake disorder, advanced sleep phase type**<br><br>1. Recurrent inability to stay awake until a desired conventional clock time, and difficulty staying asleep in the morning until a desired and socially acceptable time.<br><br>2. When allowed to use preferred schedule, no problem with sleep except its advanced timing.<br><br>3. Preferred schedule advanced more than 2 hours relative to desired conventional clock.<br><br>If criteria 1, 2, and 3 are met, refer patient to a sleep center for assessment and treatment. (Treatment will probably involve schedule manipulation and properly timed light and dark exposures.) | *Some dozing in evening, but can't fall asleep when she goes to bed early. Circadian rhythm sleep–wake disorder, advanced sleep phase type is absent.* |
| **Obstructive sleep apnea hypopnea (OSAH)**<br><br>1. Does patient report:<br>☐ snoring that can be heard through a closed door, or as loud as a conversation?<br>☐ gasping/choking during sleep?<br>☐ stopping breathing during sleep?<br>☐ poor, unrefreshing sleep even after adequate sleep time?<br><br>2. Does the patient report:<br>☐ morning headaches?<br>☐ urinating more than twice per night?<br>☐ dry mouth upon awakening? ☐ hypertension?<br>☐ BMI > 30 (BMI = body mass index = weight in kilograms divided by height in meters)? | *1. Sleep is nonrestorative but duration is not adequate (4 hours); nonrestorative sleep likely a result of insufficient sleep.*<br><br><br>*2. No.* |

(cont.)

**FIGURE 11.3.** Assessment of Other Sleep Disorders form as completed by the therapist for Sophie.

| SLEEP COMPLAINT | NOTES |
|---|---|
| **Obstructive sleep apnea hypopnea (OSAH)** *(cont.)*<br><br>3. Is excessive daytime sleepiness present? Is there a recurrent pattern of falling asleep unintentionally or struggling to stay awake when in any one of the following situations:<br><br>☐ Talking with others?     ☐ Driving?<br><br>☐ Talking on the phone?     ☐ Standing?<br><br>☐ Other activities or situations in which most people will not fall asleep?<br><br>If the patient has two or more symptoms in 1, or one symptom in 1 and one in 2, or one item in 1 and excessive daytime sleepiness, refer for evaluation of possible OSAH.<br><br>If the patient does not have co-occurring OSAH or if OSAH is adequately treated (to be determined in consultation with a sleep specialist), proceed with CBT-I. (See Chapter 7 for safety issues related to daytime sleepiness.) | *3. Feels like she could fall asleep, but doesn't; falls asleep in front of television in the evening.*<br><br>*Excessive daytime sleepiness absent. OSAH is not suspected.* |
| **Restless legs syndrome (RLS)**<br><br>Does the patient have a very strong urge to move legs? (If it is associated with unpleasant sensations in the legs, ask the patient to describe the sensations.)<br><br>   1. Does the urge occur or worsen in evening or during rest or inactivity?<br><br>   2. Is the urge temporarily relieved by moving?<br><br>   3. Does the urge interfere with falling asleep or returning to sleep?<br><br>If urge is present and the answer is yes to 1, 2, and 3, then a referral for evaluation and possible pharmacological treatment of RLS is warranted.<br><br>If RLS symptoms do not regularly interfere with the onset of sleep at the beginning or middle of night, proceed with CBT-I. | *Reported occasional leg cramps, but no to 1–3. RLS is absent.* |
| **Nightmare disorder**<br><br>1. Does the patient report recurrent nightmares (a nightmare is defined as a dream that has *all* of the features below)?<br><br>  • An elaborate narrative is remembered.<br>  • Evokes very strong negative emotion.<br>  • Occurs in second half of night.<br>  • No confusion upon waking.<br><br>2. Is there clinically meaningful distress or impairment?<br><br>Yes answers to questions 1 and 2 indicate a diagnosis of nightmare disorder, unless the nightmares are induced by substance use or explained by another disorder.<br><br>If all nocturnal symptoms of insomnia are caused by nightmares (e.g., prolonged sleep onset because of fear of nightmares or all awakenings are related to nightmares), then CBT-I is not warranted. (See Chapters 7 and 10 for more information about nightmare-related issues.) | *No nightmares. Nightmare disorder is absent.* |

**FIGURE 11.3** *(cont.)*

## Consensus Sleep Diary–M

**Please complete upon awakening.**

ID/Name: _Sophie_

| Today's date | 10/10/13 | 10/11/13 | 10/12/13 | 10/13/13 | 10/14/13 | 10/15/13 | 10/16/13 |
|---|---|---|---|---|---|---|---|
| **1.** What time did you get into bed? | 9:15 P.M. | 9:15 P.M. | 10:00 P.M. | 9:00 P.M. | 9:00 P.M. | 9:45 P.M. | 10:35 P.M. |
| **2.** What time did you try to go to sleep? | 9:15 P.M. | 9:15 P.M. | 10:00 P.M. | 9:15 P.M. | 9:30 P.M. | 9:45 P.M. | 11:45 P.M. |
| **3.** How long did it take you to fall asleep? | 95 min | 135 min | 120 min | 190 min | 180 min | 75 min | 30 min |
| **4.** How many times did you wake up, not counting your final awakening? | 2 | 4 | 3 | 1 | 2 | 1 | 3 |
| **5.** In total, how long did these awakenings last? | 40 min | 60 min | 30 min | 75 min | 85 min | 15 min | 60 min |
| **6a.** What time was your final awakening? | 6:50 A.M. | 7:00 A.M. | 7:00 A.M. | 7:00 A.M. | 7:00 A.M. | 7:00 A.M. | 6:55 A.M. |
| **6b.** After your final awakening, how long did you spend in bed trying to sleep? | 140 min | 35 min | 55 min | 15 min | 30 min | 40 min | 135 min |

(cont.)

FIGURE 11.4. Consensus Sleep Diary–M form as completed by Sophie during the week preceding the session. Adapted from Carney et al. (2012). Copyright 2011 by the Consensus Sleep Diary Committee. Adapted by permission.

| Today's date | 10/10/13 | 10/11/13 | 10/12/13 | 10/13/13 | 10/14/13 | 10/15/13 | 10/16/13 |
|---|---|---|---|---|---|---|---|
| **6c.** Did you wake up earlier than you planned? | ☐ Yes ☑ No | ☐ Yes ☑ No | ☐ Yes ☑ No | ☐ Yes ☑ No | ☐ Yes ☑ No | ☐ Yes ☑ No | ☐ Yes ☑ No |
| **6d.** If yes, how much earlier? | — | — | — | — | — | — | — |
| **7.** What time did you get out of bed for the day? | 9:10 A.M. | 7:35 A.M. | 7:55 A.M. | 7:15 A.M. | 7:30 A.M. | 7:40 A.M. | 9:10 A.M. |
| **8.** How would you rate the quality of your sleep? | ☐ Very poor ☑ Poor ☐ Fair ☐ Good ☐ Very good | ☑ Very poor ☐ Poor ☐ Fair ☐ Good ☐ Very good | ☐ Very poor ☑ Poor ☐ Fair ☐ Good ☐ Very good | ☑ Very poor ☐ Poor ☐ Fair ☐ Good ☐ Very good | ☑ Very poor ☐ Poor ☐ Fair ☐ Good ☐ Very good | ☑ Very poor ☐ Poor ☐ Fair ☐ Good ☐ Very good | ☐ Very poor ☑ Poor ☐ Fair ☐ Good ☐ Very good |
| **9.** How rested or refreshed did you feel when you woke up for the day? | ☑ Not at all rested ☐ Slightly rested ☐ Somewhat rested ☐ Well rested ☐ Very well rested | ☑ Not at all rested ☐ Slightly rested ☐ Somewhat rested ☐ Well rested ☐ Very well rested | ☑ Not at all rested ☐ Slightly rested ☐ Somewhat rested ☐ Well rested ☐ Very well rested | ☑ Not at all rested ☐ Slightly rested ☐ Somewhat rested ☐ Well rested ☐ Very well rested | ☑ Not at all rested ☐ Slightly rested ☐ Somewhat rested ☐ Well rested ☐ Very well rested | ☑ Not at all rested ☐ Slightly rested ☐ Somewhat rested ☐ Well rested ☐ Very well rested | ☑ Not at all rested ☐ Slightly rested ☐ Somewhat rested ☐ Well rested ☐ Very well rested |
| Therapist's notes *Calculated TST (Calculated TIB)* | 7 hr, 20 min (11 hr, 55 min) | 6 hr, 10 min (10 hr, 20 min) | 6 hr, 40 min (9 hr, 55 min) | 5 hr, 40 min (10 hr) | 6 hr, 35 min (10 hr) | 7 hr, 45 min (9 hr, 55 min) | 5 hr, 25 min (9 hr, 25 min) |
| **10a.** How many times did you nap or doze? | 1 | 1 | 1 | 0 | 1 | 0 | 1 |

| 10b. In total, how long did you nap or doze? | 120 min | 5 min | 15 min | 0 min | 10 min | 0 min | 75 min |
|---|---|---|---|---|---|---|---|
| 11a. How many drinks containing alcohol did you have? | 0 | 0 | 0 | 0 | 0 | 0 | 0 |
| 11b. What time was your last drink? | N/A | N/A | N/A | N/A | N/A | N/A | N/A |
| 12a. How many caffeinated drinks (coffee, tea, soda, energy drinks) did you have? | 0 drinks | 0 drinks | 0 drinks | 0 drinks | 0 drinks | 0 drinks | 0 drinks |
| 12b. What time was your last drink? | N/A | N/A | N/A | N/A | N/A | N/A | N/A |
| 13. Did you take any over-the-counter or prescription medication(s) to help you sleep? | □Yes ☑No Medication(s): Dose: | □Yes ☑No Medication(s): Dose: | □Yes ☑No Medication(s): Dose: | □Yes ☑No Medication(s): Dose: | □Yes ☑No Medication(s): Dose: | □Yes ☑No Medication(s): Dose: | □Yes ☑No Medication(s): Dose: |
| If so, list medication(s), dose, and time taken. | Time(s) taken: NA | Time(s) taken: NA | Time(s) taken: NA | Time(s) taken: NA | Time(s) taken: NA | Time(s) taken: NA | Time(s) taken: NA |
| 14. Comments (if applicable) | | | | | | | |

FIGURE 11.4 (cont.)

169

SOPHIE: In the past 2 weeks, I have been sleeping better. It is still a **Demonstration of** long way from how I used to sleep, though, and I am not sure if **cognitive therapy.** it will last.

THERAPIST: I am glad that you are sleeping better. Do you have thoughts about why?

SOPHIE: I think that just knowing that I am coming to see you has been helpful.

THERAPIST: I have had other patients tell me that. Some say that knowing that help is coming soon makes them a bit less anxious. Is that also true for you?

SOPHIE: Yes. Now that you say it, I think this is exactly what happened.

THERAPIST: I am wondering if you were a bit less preoccupied with your problem sleeping.

SOPHIE: Perhaps. Now that you mention it, I think I was not thinking about sleep as much during the day. I am still pretty obsessed with my sleep, though.

THERAPIST: There is usually a connection between how we think and feel about sleep and how well we sleep. This is something we will discuss later.

Also consistent with the information gathered during the interview, the therapist noticed a relatively regular sleep schedule on workdays, but a later time out of bed on the weekend. The diary revealed that Sophie rated her sleep quality as poor or very poor every night, but the therapist could not discern from the diary how Sophie went about judging the quality of her sleep. The therapist made a note to return to this topic when providing a rationale for sleep restriction therapy.

## After Session

After conducting the intake interview, the therapist concluded that Sophie met criteria for insomnia disorder and was likely to benefit from CBT-I. After the session ended, the therapist completed the Case Conceptualization Form for Sophie (Figure 11.5; see Appendix A for the blank version). All available data were considered, including the ISI and DBAS-16 that Sophie completed in the waiting room before her first session. (Sophie's ISI score was 22, and her DBAS-16 score was 5.1.)

The therapist then completed the Treatment Planning Form for Sophie (Figure 11.6; again, see Appendix A for the blank version), identified key targets for intervention, and selected strategies to address them. Key targets for intervention included conditioned arousal, safety behaviors that weakened Sophie's sleep drive (e.g., extended TIB at night as a coping strategy to cast a wider net to "capture" sleep, and daytime nap effort that sometimes also included sleep), general hyperarousal, weekend–weekday sleep schedule irregularity, sleep effort, and maladaptive beliefs about sleep. The therapist decided that the best starting point for Sophie would be to introduce the combination of stimulus control and sleep restriction therapy, because together these would strengthen her sleep drive and address conditioned arousal and Sophie's safety behaviors. Notice that intervention strategies can address more than one factor. For example, stimulus control would address conditioned arousal as well as a safety behavior (napping). Also notice that a single factor can be addressed by more than one intervention. For example, conditioned arousal would be addressed by both stimulus control and sleep restriction, because Sophie's increased time awake in bed contributed to her conditioned arousal. The therapist also decided to start addressing general hyperarousal in bed by recommending a buffer zone before bedtime.

# Case Conceptualization Form

*Note to Clinicians:* Please note that certain factors could load on more than one of these six domains. In such cases, list the factor in the row corresponding to the domain that is most relevant to the case.

| Domains | Patient-specific factors that contribute to insomnia or may interfere with adherence |
|---|---|
| **1.** *Sleep drive:* What factors may be weakening the patient's sleep drive? Consider extended time in bed, dozing off in the evening, daytime napping, sedentary life, and so on. | *Excessive time spent in bed (up to 12 hours), likely associated with some dozing in and out of sleep in the middle of the night. Occasional napping.* |
| **2.** *Biological clock:* What biological clock factors are relevant to the patient's presentation? Consider irregular wake and/or out-of-bed time, time-in-bed window that is not congruent with the patient's chronotype, and so on. | *Irregular rise time (2-hour weekday–weekend difference). No chronotype-related issues.* |
| **3.** *Arousal:* What manifestations of hyperarousal are evident? Consider the following:<br><br>**3a.** *Cognitive arousal related to sleep* (e.g., sleep effort, safety behaviors, and maladaptive beliefs/attitudes about sleep).<br><br>**3b.** *General hyperarousal affecting sleep* (e.g., worry in bed about life stressors).<br><br>**3c.** *Conditioned arousal:* Has the bed become associated with arousal rather than sleep? Specify predisposing factors (e.g., high trait anxiety), precipitating factors (e.g., stressful life events), and maintaining factors (.e.g., extended time spent in bed). | *3a. <u>Cognitive arousal related to sleep</u>:*<br><br>*<u>Safety behaviors and sleep effort</u>: Reduced engagement in social activity and elimination of previous exercise routine (also reinforces belief that she cannot cope with insomnia); trying to nap every day and excessive time in bed reflect casting a wide net for sleep; experimented with alcohol and sleep meds to get rid of the problem.*<br><br>*<u>Beliefs</u>: Poor sleep self-efficacy (skeptical anything will work); DBAS-16 score (5.1) is well above the suggested cutoff for an unhelpful degree of sleep beliefs ( >3.8); unrealistic sleep expectations ("I would like to "go to bed, lay head on pillow, and sleep straight through till morning").*<br><br>*3b. <u>General hyperarousal in bed</u>: Worries about sleep and work.*<br><br>*3c. <u>Conditioned arousal</u>: Possible, with nocturnal panic attack as a precipitating event (no clear predisposition—she never had insomnia before).* |

*(cont.)*

**FIGURE 11.5.** Case Conceptualization Form as completed by the therapist for Sophie.

| Domains | Patient-specific factors that contribute to insomnia or may interfere with adherence |
|---|---|
| **4.** *Unhealthy sleep behaviors:* What unhealthy sleep behaviors are present? Consider caffeine, alcohol, nocturnal eating, timing of exercise, and other factors. | *None.* |
| **5.** *Medications:* What medications may be having an impact on the patient's sleep/sleepiness? Consider carryover effects, tolerance, and psychological dependence. | *None.* |
| **6.** *Comorbidities:* What comorbidities may be affecting the patient's sleep, and how? Consider sleep, medical, and psychiatric conditions (e.g., difficult adjustment to CPAP treatment for sleep apnea; pain interfering with sleep; PTSD-related hypervigilance). | *Past nocturnal panic attack may interfere with ability to recognize sleepiness as cue for sleep.* |
| **7.** *Other:* Consider sleep environment, caregiving duties at night, life phase sleep issues, mental status, and readiness for change. | *Strengths include commitment to investing in treatment.* |

**FIGURE 11.5** (*cont.*)

## SESSION 2

### Before Session

Having determined the key targets and the components that would be used to address the targets, the therapist filled out another copy of the Session Plan form (Appendix A) for Session 2 (see Figure 11.7). As shown in Figure 11.7, the first few "Factors to Address" from Sophie's Treatment Planning Form were listed as part of the agenda.

### During Session

After answering Sophie's questions, describing the plan for the session and inviting her to add to the agenda, the therapist reviewed Sophie's sleep diary with her and then discussed sleep regulation (using information from Chapter 2). During the education about sleep regulation, the therapist did most of the talking, but tried to engage Sophie in the process. In so doing, the therapist received valuable feedback and gauged how well Sophie understood the concepts by her ability to translate the information into action. In provid-     ***Psychoeducation.*** ing the information about sleep regulation, the therapist focused on the information that was most pertinent to Sophie. Below, we provide a sample of the dialogue between Sophie and her therapist as they discussed sleep regulation.

# Treatment Planning Form

Patient's treatment goal(s): <u>(1) uninterrupted sleep; (2) fall asleep within 10 minutes; and (3) sleep a</u> <u>little longer (and later) on weekend nights.</u>

| First treatment session (enter items in the order you plan to introduce them) | | | |
|---|---|---|---|
| **Factors to address** | **CBT-I components** | **Specific recommendations** | **Comments** |
| Conditioned arousal | Stimulus control | Go to bed only when sleepy.<br><br>Get out of bed when unable to sleep and return to bed only when sleepy. | All 5 instructions will be provided, but these two are most important for addressing conditioned arousal.<br><br>Discuss sleepiness at bedtime (history of nocturnal panic is a risk for hypervigilance that might mask sleepiness). |
| <u>Sleep drive:</u> Too much time in bed at night (also a safety behavior)<br><br>Napping/resting (also a safety behavior) | TIB restriction | TIB = 6 hours, 15 minutes (average calculated TST); possible TIB window: 12:45–7:00.<br><br>Avoid napping. | TIB window may change after discussion with Sophie.<br><br>Later bedtime is congruent with historical bedtime and likely better fits Sophie's natural circadian tendency.<br><br>Integrate with stimulus control, including avoiding naps. |
| General hyperarousal | Buffer zone | One hour before bedtime. | |
| **Subsequent sessions (enter items in the order you plan to introduce them)** | | | |
| **Factors to address** | **CBT-I components** | **Specific recommendations** | **Comments** |
| Cognitive arousal related to sleep | Cognitive therapy | Address beliefs that underlie safety behaviors and sleep effort identified above (e.g., Sophie's belief that she cannot cope with sleep loss, which leads to safety behaviors). | See beliefs and safety behaviors listed in Case Conceptualization Form for Sophie. |
| General arousal affecting sleep | Relaxation therapy<br><br>Constructive worry | Encourage a relaxation practice.<br><br>Encourage engaging in constructive worry in early evening. | |

**FIGURE 11.6.** Treatment Planning Form as completed by the therapist for Sophie.

## Session Plan

**ID/Name:** _Sophie_ _____          **Date:** _October 23, 2013_ _____          **Session #:** __2__

- Check on reaction to first session, and encourage questions; review session plan in broad terms, and ask if there is anything Sophie wants to make sure is addressed.

- Review sleep diary; troubleshoot completion of diaries, as needed; and notice changes in sleep, if any.

- Provide sleep education anchored in case conceptualization as preparation for sleep restriction therapy.

- Introduce sleep restriction therapy, with 6 hours, 15 minutes as initial TIB (include a 1-hour buffer zone).

- Provide stimulus control guidelines.

**Homework:**

- Continue completion of sleep diary each morning.

- Read handout with summary of specific sleep recommendations.

**Notes:**

- Schedule next appointment in 2 weeks.

**FIGURE 11.7.** Session Plan form as completed by the therapist for Sophie's Session 2.

THERAPIST: Let me first explain how the sleep system works. I think knowing this will help us think together what needs to be done to make sure that your sleep system is robust, so that we can improve the quality of your sleep.

*Demonstration of education about sleep.*

SOPHIE: OK.

THERAPIST: One system that regulates your sleep is what I will call the *sleep drive system*. The sleep drive system works on the basic principle that the longer you are awake and the more active you are during the day, the stronger your sleep drive will be when you go to bed at night. In other words, your sleep drive builds up when you are awake. Can you think of anything that could interfere with building up this drive?

SOPHIE: Napping?

THERAPIST: Yes, that's right . . .

SOPHIE: But I don't really nap. I only fall asleep sometimes. Although you said, "out of bed" . . . does that mean it doesn't matter if I slept or not?

THERAPIST: It does matter. I am referring to when you do sleep. Sleeping during the day depletes some of the buildup of the sleep drive that you have accumulated up to that point. Can you think of anything else that may interfere with the buildup?

SOPHIE: Not really.

THERAPIST: One way people react to having sleep problems is by trying to maximize their chances of falling asleep. They go to bed earlier or get up later than they used to, or both. Sound familiar?

SOPHIE: Yes. I have to go to bed earlier, because otherwise I wouldn't sleep at all. And I only stay in bed longer in the morning because I am exhausted.

THERAPIST: I understand. It makes good intuitive sense for you to do this. It sounds like something we need to talk about further, when we talk about actual strategies. Can we return to this later?

SOPHIE: Of course.

THERAPIST: In addition to the sleep drive system, your sleep is controlled by an internal clock. Like many biological systems, the clock can adapt, based to a large degree on when we are exposed to sunlight. For example, when we travel across the country, the time when our bodies are exposed to daylight changes. The clock helps us to slowly adjust to the time in our new place. But during the initial adjustment period, we feel "off kilter." Have you had jet lag before?

SOPHIE: Yes. I sometimes have to travel to Europe for work. It feels a lot like insomnia. I can't sleep when I want; I fall asleep when I don't want to; and I feel exhausted all the time. By the time I adjust, I have to come back.

THERAPIST: The way you feel when you first adapt to jet lag is due to an initial mismatch between your internal clock and the local clock. Waking up at the local time exposes your eye to morning light at a new time, and your brain uses this as a signal that it uses in order to realign your internal clock with the new environment. The body needs to do the same thing when you wake up later on the weekend than during the week.

SOPHIE: I certainly do that.

THERAPIST: Yes. Your body responds to being exposed to light later on the weekend the same way it responds to actual travel. We call it *social jet lag*.

SOPHIE: Interesting. Even though I am not really sleeping until 9:00 on the weekend, I am under the covers and my eyes are closed. But it's hard to get out of bed when I am so tired. I used to do it before I had insomnia, and it was not that bad.

THERAPIST: I can understand that it's hard. Our bodies may react to the same things differently when we are well and we are not. Think of how your body reacts to different foods when you stomach is upset, compared to when you are well.

SOPHIE: I see.

THERAPIST: Do you think that knowing how your body reacts to staying in bed late on the weekend will help you get up earlier, at least until your insomnia problem is solved?

SOPHIE: I think so. I have been taking notes. When I have to get up for something important, I usually set up my clock on my desk so that I have to get out of bed to turn it off. Once I'm up, I usually stay up. So I will just start doing that.

THERAPIST: This sounds like a great idea.

SOPHIE: I think I will go the gym after I wake up. I miss working out. It always helps me feel better.

THERAPIST: Sounds like this plan may have many benefits in addition to better sleep. Can you think of anything that could get in the way?

SOPHIE: I don't think so.

THERAPIST: So far, we've talked about two systems that control your sleep. There is a third system that is particularly important for us to consider. Even when the sleep drive system and the internal clock are working well together, our arousal system can override them and cause wakefulness. For example, if you are stressed about work and continue to problem-solve work-related problems right up until the time you go to bed or while you are in bed, you are not deactivated enough to go to sleep. Make sense?

SOPHIE: Yes, and that's definitely what happens to me. It's hard to turn my mind off.

THERAPIST: Having an active mind in bed has an effect even beyond the night you are stressed. Your bed should be a place that you associate with sleep. If you have wakeful activities, or you feel upset or tense in your bed, these negative feelings may become associated with your bed. This may have happened to you. Do you ever feel calm or sleepy, but when you get into bed you feel suddenly activated?

SOPHIE: Yes, that's me.

THERAPIST: This usually means that your mind has come to associate your bed with wakefulness rather than sleep. I think that this may have started when you had a panic attack at night. The good news is that there are ways to unlearn this association.

*Demonstration of laying the groundwork for stimulus control.*

The excerpt above demonstrates the tailoring of education about sleep in a way that is relevant to a patient's presentation. By tailoring Sophie's education to her particular presentation, the therapist aimed to avoid overwhelming her and to prepare her for the interventions to come. Explaining sleep regulation in such a patient-tailored way can enhance the therapeutic alliance as well. Patients do not want to be burdened with information that is irrelevant to their case, and they may perceive irrelevant information as an indication that the therapist has not been paying attention to what they have already said about their sleep problems. For example, the therapist omitted a discussion of chronotypes (i.e., morningness vs. eveningness) and explanation of the biological clock as a generator of alerting signals, because these facts were not germane to Sophie's case. Patient-tailored presentations of sleep regulation are also likely to promote adherence to interventions, because behavior changes are more likely to be enacted when the patients understand the rationale for these changes and their relevance to them. This is particularly the case when patients are actively engaged in the discussion in a way that allows them to draw conclusions about which of their behaviors will need to be changed. It is important to encourage patients to identify behaviors that they can change, based on the information provided. In that way the patients are more likely to internalize the information, and the therapist will be able to assess the patients' understanding of the concepts and their readiness to enact the needed behavior changes.

### Collaborating on a Sleep Schedule for Sleep Restriction Therapy

The therapist used the sleep diary data that Sophie brought to this session to estimate an initial TIB recommendation for Sophie. During the session they reviewed the most recent diary data, discussed them, and decided together what her TIB window should be. Below is a script of this collaborative process.

THERAPIST: Let's look together at a summary of your sleep diary. Just as we did last time, I calculated the average amount of time that you slept each night. I wrote it down right here (*shows Sophie the sleep diary form and the calculations*). You can see how much you slept each night and the average amount you slept in the past week.

SOPHIE: I see on average 6 hours and 15 minutes, but sometimes I sleep a lot less than that.

THERAPIST: I agree. Sometimes you sleep less than that, and other times you can sleep a little more, but your average sleep is 6 hours and 15 minutes.

SOPHIE: Is there hope for more sleep in the future?

THERAPIST: Yes. I am optimistic about your future sleep. I would like to propose that as a starting point, we focus on getting you better-quality sleep and worry later about its quantity.

SOPHIE: That will be nice. Do you mean you can help me sleep through the night without waking up?

THERAPIST: We can certainly aim for your being awake less at night. Brief awakenings over the night are a normal part of healthy sleep. I do think that it is realistic, though, to expect that when you do wake up, you will be able to fall asleep more quickly.

SOPHIE: That would be an improvement.

THERAPIST: Let's begin with a thought experiment. Let's assume you are in a world in which people are allowed to sleep only 6 hours each night, but have one of the following two choices of how to get these 6 hours. In the first option, you can spend as much time as you want in bed. You would sleep a couple of hours, then be up for half an hour, sleep a few more hours, be up for an hour and so on. The caveat is that in total you would sleep only 6 hours. The second option is to be in bed 6 hours and spend the time in uninterrupted sleep. Which would you choose?

SOPHIE: I would definitely go for the second option, if I am guaranteed that I will indeed sleep the whole time. But I am worried. It takes me hours to fall asleep. If I spend 6 hours in bed, I will sleep only 3 or 4 hours, and that is definitely not enough. I have to be functional at work.

> *Demonstration of cognitive therapy and laying the groundwork for presenting sleep restriction.*

THERAPIST: That would be rough. But you are forgetting that the sleep drive system could help you sleep more of that 6-hour period. Our bodies naturally make up for lost sleep, unless something interferes with this natural process. For example, if the idea of spending only 6 hours in bed makes you very anxious, your anxiety could trump all the benefits you can get from a stronger sleep drive. Do you remember times you have experienced how it feels to have a strong sleep drive?

SOPHIE: Come to think of it, this is what happens when we have deadlines at work. I work long hours and get little sleep. I go to bed after midnight and am at work again by 7:00. After a few nights like that, I probably have a strong sleep drive. I fall asleep very fast, and I do not wake up until the alarm sounds.

THERAPIST: Sounds like in these situations you have experienced the effects of a strong sleep drive. You said you prefer the "short but sweet" sleep option in our thought experiment, and you seem to understand how the short time-in-bed option makes for a strong sleep drive. Are you willing to experiment with spending less time in bed, so that your sleep drive will get stronger and help you sleep through the night?

SOPHIE: Are you proposing I stay in bed only 6 hours?

THERAPIST: Close. I am proposing that you limit your time in bed to the amount of sleep you now have on average, which was a little over 6 hours.

SOPHIE: Six hours and 15 minutes.

THERAPIST: We call this a *temporary time-in-bed restriction*. What if you tested it out for a week or two? It will be like what you have done before when you have a work deadline.

**Demonstration of sleep restriction.**

SOPHIE: What if I do not sleep well?

THERAPIST: That is a good question. At first you may have some insomnia nights like you do now—but if you do not sleep well, your sleep drive will increase and your body will start to reliably fill up the short time you are in bed with sleep, and with deeper, higher-quality sleep at that. Eventually we will increase your time in bed by a little bit and see if your sleep drive can also fill this additional time with sleep, so that you sleep more.

SOPHIE: It sounds weird to put myself through this torture. But I see your point.

THERAPIST: I remember you told me that you and your colleagues play chess at lunch. I wonder if you could consider the first night or two of trying this strategy as one or two pawns you are willing to sacrifice to win the game?

SOPHIE: Do you think it would be just a night or two?

THERAPIST: I can't actually predict this; sometimes it is more, but sometimes not. Everyone has a sleep drive system that reliably makes up for lost sleep, so long as there is nothing getting in the way of it (like feeling particularly worried or anxious in bed). This means that part of what determines how long it will take will be how anxious you are about spending less time in bed and about other things in your life. Are you willing to try it?

SOPHIE: Yes. I am a bit less anxious about this after we have talked about it more. As you said, I have done it before when I had lots of work. Should I go to bed at midnight?

THERAPIST: Let's decide first when you want to wake up. Can you pick a time you would be willing to set your alarm 7 days per week?

*Demonstration of the intersection between sleep restriction therapy and stimulus control—anchoring the rise time 7 days per week.*

SOPHIE: Ugh, I hate the idea of getting up earlier than I need to on the weekend. But I guess 7:00 A.M. would be doable.

THERAPIST: OK. Your average sleep time is 6 hours and 15 minutes. So if you are going to be waking up at 7:00 A.M., how late will you need to stay up at night?

SOPHIE: That means I have to stay up until 12:45 A.M. This is not very appealing. Could I get up a little earlier instead? It would be easier. If I went to bed at midnight, then I could deal with setting the alarm for 6:15 A.M. Is this ok?

THERAPIST: You tell me. Is this something you could commit to for the short term—say, the next 2 weeks?

SOPHIE: I can do it for 2 weeks.

THERAPIST: Great. I'm glad you're willing to give this a try. This is a learning process—in essence, you are retraining your sleep—and in the process, your sleep might get a bit worse before it gets better. Do you think you can commit to being persistent?

SOPHIE: (*Laughs*) I think so. It's like the saying "No pain, no gain."

THERAPIST: (*Laughs*) Remember we talked about being sleepy? Do you think you will be asleep at midnight? You remember the difference between being sleepy and tired?

SOPHIE: I remember. I think I will be both tired and sleepy.

THERAPIST: If for some reason you are not sleepy, I recommend that you stay up until you are sleepy. Being in bed only when sleepy will help us retrain your body to associate the bed with sleeping only. Is this something you can do?

*Further demonstration of stimulus control.*

SOPHIE: What if I am sleepy earlier?

THERAPIST: If you are very sleepy earlier, you should resist going to bed and wait until midnight. This way, your sleep drive will be stronger, and you will be more likely to sleep through the night. Again, can you do this for 2 weeks?

SOPHIE: I could try.

THERAPIST: It will also help if you could spend an hour before your bedtime for unwinding. Could you move your work and housework to an earlier time, and spend the hour before bed relaxing?

*Demonstration of the buffer zone.*

SOPHIE: Sometimes I get an email from work late at night, and I want to address it. But, actually, that might not be a good idea. Some of these late emails make me feel tense, and I end up mulling over an issue at work when I try to sleep. Your suggestion makes so much sense. I cannot believe I did not think about it. I will definitely do this. I will read some of the back issues of a magazine I have been saving or watch TV.

THERAPIST: These are great alternatives.

The session continued with the introduction of the remaining stimulus control instructions. The therapist then asked Sophie to summarize what they had agreed she would be doing until the next session, as a way of making sure that Sophie was committed to following through. As Sophie was summarizing, the therapist wrote down the list of recommendations she would be following until the next session (i.e., Sophie's homework). At the end of the session, the therapist reminded Sophie to continue to complete the sleep diary every morning. Here is a summary of Sophie's homework:

- Protect the hour before bed as a wind-down period (i.e., create a buffer zone).
- Set an alarm for 6:15 A.M. and get out of bed right away (within 10–15 minutes), even on weekends.
- Do not go to bed before you feel sleepy, and not before 12:00 midnight.
- If you are unable to sleep for 10–15 minutes, whether it is because you are worrying or simply awake, get up and go to another room and engage in a pleasant activity (e.g., reading) until you feel sleepy and calm enough to fall asleep quickly before returning to bed. Repeat this process as many times as needed.
- Use the bed only for sleeping. If you tend to feel relaxed after sexual activity, then this can be an exception to the rule.
- Do not take naps (safety naps are the exception).

## SESSION 3

### Before Session

The therapist's plan for the third session was to review progress based on Sophie's sleep diary and ISI data; assess Sophie's sense of progress and determine whether she experienced sleepiness during the day; identify and troubleshoot adherence problems; make necessary adjustments to the recommendations already given (including to Sophie's TIB); and introduce additional recommendations to help reduce her arousal levels when in bed. Before this session, the therapist spent a few minutes reviewing the sleep diaries that Sophie brought to the session. In parallel, Sophie completed the ISI. Sophie's sleep diaries revealed that her sleep had improved considerably. Her SE had increased from 40 to 78%, and she was spending far less time awake in the middle of the night, with an average of only 15 minutes. The time it took her to fall asleep had decreased by more than half (down to an average of 45 minutes), although this was still not ideal. Her average TST was 6 hours and 20 minutes. Sophie's adherence with wake and out-of-bed times was nearly perfect, and she did not take naps. However, she sometimes went to bed earlier than recommended. Although her SE was under 80%, the therapist decided to keep her TIB the same as it was and focus on increasing her adherence with the recommended TIB.

Despite considerable sleep improvements as reported in her sleep diary data, Sophie's ISI score on the ISI had changed very little and was still moderately elevated at 20. The therapist thus went into the session not only with some understanding of Sophie's adherence and progress, but, based on the ISI score, an expectation that Sophie might not feel she had made much progress. The therapist's plan was to compliment Sophie on her adherence to the nap and wake time

## Session Plan

**ID/Name:** <u>Sophie</u>      **Date:** <u>November 13, 2013</u>     **Session #:** <u>3</u>

- Inquire about progress toward goals and daytime sleepiness; review session plan in broad terms, and ask if there is anything Sophie wants to make sure is addressed.

- Go over diary and progress:
  - Compliment adherence with wake time and naps.
  - Check on nonoptimal adherence with recommended later bedtime.
  - Brainstorm about strategies to allow for increased success following bedtime recommendation.

- Discuss differences between Sophie's perception of her insomnia and improvements based on sleep diary data.

- Alterations to sleep restriction therapy: Base on assessment of daytime sleepiness and discussion about feasibility of improved adherence with the recommended bedtime. If there are no safety concerns, encourage better adherence and do not alter TIB.

- Introduce relaxation and constructive worry.

- Use cognitive therapy techniques to address sleep effort and erroneous beliefs underlying it. (Introduce Thought Record form.)

**Homework:**

- Continue completion of sleep diary each morning.

- Read handout with summary of specific sleep recommendations.
  - Continue with sleep recommendations from Session 2, most likely with the same TIB window (12:00–6:15).
  - Implement a relaxation strategy.
  - Create closure at the end of the workday.
  - Complete Thought Record forms if worries about functioning persist.

**Notes:**

- Schedule next appointment in 2 weeks.

**FIGURE 11.8.** Session Plan form as completed by the therapist for Sophie's Session 3.

recommendations, and to work on improving her adherence to the recommended bedtime. The therapist also recognized that time would have to be spent on clarifying the discrepancy between the substantial improvement in Sophie's sleep (based on her sleep diary data) and her perception that her insomnia is just as severe as it has been. The therapist therefore completed the Session Plan form for this session as shown in Figure 11.8.

## During Session

Sophie reported that she was feeling tired during the day, but said she did not fall asleep unintentionally. She also said that she went to bed earlier than recommended because she felt sleepy earlier in the evening, and she was worried that if she stayed up, she would miss out on getting an extra hour of sleep. This fear was intensified by her daytime fatigue and worry about whether she would be able to function during the day. The therapist used cognitive therapy strategies to address this belief-based obstacle to adherence.

THERAPIST: Sounds like the reason it has been challenging to stay up until your recommended bedtime is your concern that you may be missing out on a possible opportunity for sleep.

SOPHIE: Yes. I feel so sleepy in the hour or so before bed that I can barely stay awake, and I don't want to miss out if I could be sleeping.

THERAPIST: I see. And what has happened when you went to bed?

SOPHIE: I fell asleep much faster than I used to.

THERAPIST: Are you happy with your sleep then?

SOPHIE: No. Even though I fall asleep faster, I still don't fall asleep *that* quickly. I'm stressed about work, and sometimes I almost fall asleep, but then I think about it in bed and I am wide awake.

THERAPIST: What sorts of work-related things do you think about in bed?

SOPHIE: Mainly what I need to do and how I will do it. After a while, I start worrying if I am going to be functional at work tomorrow.

THERAPIST: Let's begin with helping you take your worries about unfinished work business out of bed.

SOPHIE: That will be great.

THERAPIST: I would like to propose a strategy that has helped many patients with a similar problem. It sounds like when you leave work, there are still tasks that have not been completed.

SOPHIE: Yes. There are tasks that take days and weeks to complete, but I keep thinking about them.

THERAPIST: The job is not done when the workday ends, and we carry loose ends with us into our personal lives and when we go to bed at night. It helps to create closure to the workday. Take 10–15 minutes at the end of the workday, ideally before leaving the office, for mapping out a plan for what you need to do the next day and plans for solving problems that still need to be addressed.

SOPHIE: I like this idea. I think my mind will be more at ease when I go to bed.

*Demonstration of constructive worry.*

THERAPIST: You are correct in thinking that this strategy may mean that you will have less to worry about when you get into bed, but it is not an instant fix. It takes time for you to feel the effects.

SOPHIE: Makes sense.

THERAPIST: Also, do you remember what we said about teaching your brain to associate your bed with sleep?

SOPHIE: I do. I see where you are going with this. Worrying in bed will not help with that.

THERAPIST: Right. Also, I remember you saying that you used to have a yoga practice, but you do not do it any longer. Is that right?

SOPHIE: Yes, that's right.

THERAPIST: Given that stress and tension tend to be recurrent themes, I wonder if it is worth putting back some relaxation strategies into your evening. It doesn't have to be yoga—any practice would be of help.

*Demonstration of introducing counterarousal strategies.*

SOPHIE: No, I like yoga. I also used to listen to a guided imagery CD in bed, but I stopped doing it because it didn't help me fall asleep; my mind would keep wandering.

THERAPIST: Sometimes if you are anxious about sleeping, trying to relax in order to sleep might be difficult. It may be better to do yoga or listen to the CD earlier in the evening rather than right before bed. I am asking you to do these relaxing things to reduce the day's stress earlier in the evening, so that it doesn't "visit" you later when you go to bed. Does that make sense?

SOPHIE: It does. I will do it an hour before I go to bed, before I start reading.

THERAPIST: Good. One other thing: I heard you say that you were worried about being "functional" at work. Can you tell me what you mean by "functional"?

Sophie went on to describe her worries. The therapist asked Sophie to identify a specific situation when she had this type of worry, and used Socratic questioning and the downward arrow technique to explore the thoughts and beliefs that were at the heart of Sophie's worries about the consequences of her poor sleep. (Please see Chapter 9 for an example of a similar exploration.) The therapist then introduced Sophie to the concept of the thought record, and had Sophie complete the Thought Record form in Appendix C on the basis of their conversation. (See Figure 11.9 for Sophie's completed form.) Finally, the therapist gave Sophie blank Thought Record forms and recommended that she use them when additional concerns about her functioning emerged.

An exploration of adherence to other recommendations revealed that Sophie never had to get out of bed when unable to sleep in the middle of the night, because she now returned to

**Thought Record**

| Situation | Mood (intensity 0–100%) | Thoughts (underline the most emotionally charged thought) | Evidence for the underlined thought | Evidence against this thought | Adaptive/coping thoughts | Do you feel any differently? |
|---|---|---|---|---|---|---|
| On subway, thinking about how tired I feel. | Exhausted (90%) Anxious (90%) | I can't think. I'm going to mess up today. I won't be able to read the briefs today. People will think I am "out of it." I have to fix this sleep problem. I'm not going to make partnership. | I had to reread passages all this week. I feel so tired now. | I have never made any major mistakes at work, even when I had worse nights. In my last meeting with the partners, I was told I am on the right track. | I may have to take breaks and relax and reread passages, but at the end I do a good job. It is just harder. It **feels** like I may lose the opportunity for being a partner, because I am anxious, but I seem to be on track. Exhausted (80%) | Anxious (40%) |

**FIGURE 11.9.** Thought Record as completed by Sophie in Session 3.

sleep quickly. She had started using a buffer zone, but it was usually shorter than an hour because she became sleepy and went to bed. In discussing the issue, the therapist and Sophie decided that Sophie would shorten the buffer zone time to 30 minutes and would do pleasant but more activating things earlier in the evening. Sophie chose to do light housework, file home-related paperwork, and socialize by email or phone. Sophie also reported that she did not get out of bed at the beginning of the night when she was not able to fall asleep quickly, but said she understood why it was important and expressed commitment to do so.

Here is a summary of Sophie's homework.

- Have a 30-minute wind-down period.
- Set an alarm for 6:15 A.M. and get out of bed right away (within 10–15 minutes), even on weekends.
- Do not go to bed before you feel sleepy, and not before 12:00 midnight.
- If you are unable to sleep for 10–15 minutes, whether it is because you are worrying or simply awake, get up and go to another room until you feel sleepy and calm enough to fall asleep quickly before returning to bed. Repeat this process as many times as needed.
- Use the bed only for sleeping. If you tend to feel relaxed after sexual activity, then this can be an exception to the rule.
- Do not take naps (safety naps are the exception).
- Before leaving the office, create closure to the workday.
- Complete copies of the Thought Record form, as needed.

# SESSION 4

## Before Session

Sophie's sleep diaries revealed that her sleep continued to improve, and her adherence to the TIB and nap recommendations was excellent. She was sleeping an average of 5 hours, 45 minutes, which meant that her SE was 92%. On average, it took her 20 minutes to fall asleep, and she was up for an average of about 10 minutes. Her ISI score had improved dramatically, to 9. The therapist planned to check on Sophie's sleepiness and fatigue, and to discuss increasing her TIB. The therapist also noticed that time to fall asleep was usually 10–15 minutes, but that on two nights it took her 30–40 minutes to fall asleep, and therefore decided to ask whether Sophie could identify any factors contributing to longer time to fall asleep on those nights and if she followed stimulus control instructions when it happened. The therapist also planned to check on Sophie's completed Thought Record forms and to find out what Sophie believed was contributing to her improvement. Figure 11.10 shows the plan developed by the therapist for this session.

## During Session

During the session, Sophie said that she was happy with her sleep, but she was still fatigued during the day. She wanted to add a discussion of fatigue to the agenda. She said it was hard to wait until her bedtime, but she was able to push though sleepiness. This signaled to the therapist that a TIB extension was needed. The therapist reviewed the sleep diary with Sophie and proceeded

## Session Plan

**ID/Name:** _Sophie_          **Date:** _November 27, 2013_          **Session #:** _4_

- Inquire about progress toward goals and daytime sleepiness and fatigue.

- Inquire if there is anything Sophie wants to make sure is addressed.

- Go over diary; compliment progress and adherence with TIB and nap recommendations.

- Explore adherence to other components (problem-solving time, buffer zone time, Thought Records).

- Discuss what Sophie thinks has contributed to her improvement, and highlight relationship between adherence and progress.

- Discuss increasing TIB to 6.5 hours.

**Homework:**

- Continue with all previous recommendations (as modified in session).

- Read handout with summary of specific sleep recommendations.

- Continue completion of sleep diary each morning.

**Notes:**

- Schedule next appointment in 2 weeks.

**FIGURE 11.10.** Session Plan form as completed by the therapist for Sophie's Session 4.

to introduce the idea of extending the TIB to 6.5 hours until her next session. They decided on 11:45 P.M. to 6:15 A.M. Sophie said that she could not come back to the next session for 3 weeks. The therapist discussed with Sophie how to decide whether she could extend her time in bed. Sophie understood how to compute her TST and SE. They decided that because of Sophie's work schedule, the TIB extension would be achieved by going to bed 15 minutes earlier. They decided that after five nights on the 11:45 P.M. to 6:15 A.M. schedule, Sophie would compute her SE; if it was over 85%, she could consider going to bed at 11:30 P.M. and shift her buffer zone half an hour earlier. Sophie was advised to base her decision on whether she felt as though she needed more sleep. If she changed her bedtime to 11:30 P.M., she was instructed to stay on the new schedule for at least five nights before using the same guidelines for deciding whether she should go to bed at 11:15 P.M. The therapist also discussed some possible options if her SE was not 85% or above. Sophie opted to wait 3 more days and then to recompute the average SE for the preceding 5 days. Overall, she was excited at the prospect that by the time she returned, she might be sleeping half an hour more.

    When discussing adherence with the stimulus control recommendations, Sophie said that she got out of bed when unable to sleep on one of the two nights she did not fall asleep right away. She said she was upset that evening about something that happened during the day, and it was difficult to calm down. She was sleepy at bedtime, but she did not fall asleep right away, so she got out of bed and read for 10 minutes; then she returned to bed and fell asleep fairly quickly. The therapist reflected that things like this sometimes happen, and validated that Sophie acted in accordance with the principles of the treatment and experienced a positive result. Sophie saw a relationship between her behavioral change and improvement in her sleep, and was committed to the treatment plan.

Sophie reported that completing the Thought Record forms was helpful in "keeping my worries in check." She explained that when she saw her worries about losing the prospect of partnership written down, they seemed silly, and her anxiety decreased. Consistent with her report of continued fatigue, a review of her completed Thought Records revealed that although modifying her thoughts led to a reduction in her rated anxiety level, this was not the case for her fatigue levels. The following exchange demonstrates how the therapist worked with Sophie's agenda item. The therapist identified and worked with Sophie's belief about the connection between sleep and fatigue, and introduced counterfatigue ideas.

THERAPIST: I am pleased to hear that you are sleeping well, and I wanted to check in with you on how you are feeling during the day.

SOPHIE: I am feeling a lot better, but I am still a little tired during the day. I don't feel sleepy during the day, except maybe an hour before bed. But, yeah, I am still a little tired.

THERAPIST: For some people, this can be the last symptom to improve. Can you tell me when you tend to feel the greatest amount of fatigue? Is there a time of day or a particular situation?

SOPHIE: I would say the afternoon, starting just after lunch, and it lasts until I am about ready to leave work. I seem to get a second wind and do all right in the evening.

THERAPIST: What are you doing during this time?

SOPHIE: I am usually reading on the computer, and maybe doing some writing as well. In the mornings, I usually meet with clients or with my staff. I moved all my research and writing work to the afternoon, so that I can have an uninterrupted block of time to work.

THERAPIST: What strategies do you use to cope with the fatigue in the afternoon?

SOPHIE: What do I *do*? Nothing; I suffer, I guess. I figured it would go away when I slept better, but it is still hanging around.

*Demonstration of cognitive therapy to address misattribution of fatigue exclusively to sleep. Demonstration of fatigue management strategies.*

THERAPIST: So you think it is related to your sleep?

SOPHIE: I assumed so, yes.

THERAPIST: What might be some other possible culprits for why you feel tired?

SOPHIE: I have no idea.

THERAPIST: Do you remember when I explained that the body clock sends alerting signals that get stronger throughout the day until the evening?

SOPHIE: Yes.

THERAPIST: There is one small exception. In the early afternoon, there is a tiny dip in body temperature, which corresponds to a dip in energy/alertness. Usually it only lasts an hour or so.

SOPHIE: I noticed that, but for me it lasts the rest of the afternoon.

THERAPIST: Are you in the habit of paying very close attention to your fatigue?

SOPHIE: (*Laughs*) It is on my radar, yes.

THERAPIST: Do you think focusing on feeling tired may make you more so? I am wondering if it is like when you are focusing on an itch, it becomes worse. Do you think something like that may be going on for you?

SOPHIE: (*Laughs*) Interesting analogy. I suppose you are right. It is not that easy to not pay attention.

THERAPIST: True. It may help, though, to think that fatigue could also be caused by things other than how much sleep you had last night. Things like boredom, eyestrain, dehydration, and physical inactivity.

SOPHIE: I am definitely not bored, but I am not physically active. I spend a lot of time sitting at the computer.

THERAPIST: Sitting at computers for hours without breaks, particularly if you are not drinking water or stretching every once in a while, can cause fatigue. Sometimes stretching or walking around and even simply changing tasks can help with fatigue.

SOPHIE: I had the thought of breaking up my afternoon writing session so that some of it was in the morning, when I feel better anyway. I think it might help. You know, I never take a break when I am writing? It may not be a bad idea.

At the end of the session, and in preparation for termination, the therapist asked Sophie to reflect on her progress a day or so before coming to the next session by writing a "letter to yourself." The idea was for her to write about her improvement and what she believed had helped her improve. Here is a summary of Sophie's homework:

- Have a 30-minute wind-down period.
- Set an alarm for 6:15 A.M. and get out of bed right away (within 10–15 minutes), even on weekends. (Extend TIB by 15 minutes at a time as discussed, if SE is 85% or more after at least 5 nights.)
- Do not go to bed before you feel sleepy, and not before 11:45 P.M.
- If you are unable to sleep for 10–15 minutes, whether it is because you are worrying or simply awake, get up and go to another room until you feel sleepy and calm enough to fall asleep quickly before returning to bed. Repeat this process as many times as needed.
- Use the bed only for sleeping. If you tend to feel relaxed after sexual activity, then this can be an exception to the rule.
- Do not take naps (safety naps are the exception).
- Continue the closure-to-workday practice.
- Implement changes to afternoon work (i.e., taking breaks and changing tasks).

# SESSION 5

## Before Session

Sophie's sleep diaries revealed continued improvement. They showed that she had extended her TIB three times over the prior 3 weeks. In the last week, she was in bed from 11 P.M. to 6:15 A.M. and slept an average of 6 hours and 45 minutes, with an average SE of 93%. She fell asleep in less than 30 minutes every night, and on most nights in less than 20 minutes. Some nights she did not wake up at all, and on the two occasions when she woke up, she fell back asleep within 5–10 minutes. Her ISI score dropped a little more, from 9 the day of Session 4 weeks ago to 7 on the day of Session 5. The therapist was planning to check on fatigue and sleep need, and to consider termination if Sophie reported being ready. The therapist developed a plan for the session as shown in Figure 11.11.

## During Session

Sophie came to the fifth session pleased to report that she had extended her TIB three times. She reported that she was sleeping fine, but thought she would like to extend her sleep one more time. She made her own computations and realized that, based on the guidelines, she could start

## Session Plan

**ID/Name:** _Sophie_                **Date:** _December 11, 2013_          **Session #:** _5_

- Inquire about progress toward goals and about daytime sleepiness and fatigue.
- Inquire if there is anything Sophie wants to make sure is addressed.
- Review sleep diary.
- Assess fatigue and perceived sleep need.
- Review last week's "letter to self" homework.
- If Sophie is ready to terminate (has reached her goals), begin relapse prevention:
  - Develop action plan for future, integrating letter to self into it.
  - Ask if there is anything to add to agenda.
  - Provide relapse prevention summary form (Strategies for Dealing with Insomnia in the Future).

**Homework:**

- Follow relapse prevention plan.

**Notes:**

---

**FIGURE 11.11.** Session Plan form as completed by the therapist for Sophie's Session 5.

being in bed 7.5 hours. The therapist agreed that this would be a good idea, and asked her if she preferred to add the 15 minutes by going to bed earlier or waking up later. Sophie preferred the second option. Since Sophie's diaries indicated no problems with early morning awakening, the therapist thought that an 11:00 P.M. to 6:30 A.M. TIB window could work. The therapist then proceeded to discuss with Sophie the stopping rule for the TIB extension (Chapter 7). Sophie understood the guidelines and thought that she would not be likely to need additional extensions.

Sophie described in the session that her fatigue level had decreased. She said that taking breaks and changing tasks in the afternoon had helped her to feel less fatigued. She said she had started taking a 30-minute walk with a colleague around 3:00 P.M. when their schedules permitted, and that this helped with being more efficient at work. She reported that these strategies and sleeping more had helped, and that she "felt like myself again." The therapist reminded her of her three goals: (1) to have uninterrupted sleep; (2) to fall asleep within 10 minutes; and (3) to sleep a little longer (and later) on weekend nights. Sophie thought she was close enough to her first two goals and wanted to discuss her third goal.

SOPHIE: I have one last question. Don't get mad, but I really want to change the get-up time on the weekends. Can I relax it a little bit?

THERAPIST: You were concerned that I would be mad at your wanting to sleep in on the weekends?

> *Demonstration of relapse prevention techniques.*

SOPHIE: Maybe not mad, but I wanted to know if I have to get up at this time forever.

THERAPIST: Well, the sleep guidelines you are following are designed to help to improve your sleep. When you feel that your gains are solid, and you are certain that the improvements in your sleep are solid, you can experiment with relaxing some of the "rules."

SOPHIE: I think I am getting there.

THERAPIST: I agree. But I do not think you are there yet. Nonetheless, let's talk about the specific rule you want to bend. When you are considering sleeping in on the weekend, I would recommend that you do it slowly. Maybe add 15 minutes per weekend while tracking your sleep.

SOPHIE: Test the waters . . .

THERAPIST: Exactly. Sort of like an experiment. If your experiment reveals worsened sleep, you have your answer about whether you can currently tolerate relaxing that rule. If you seem to do OK, then that's fine.

SOPHIE: This sounds reasonable. Maybe not right away—I am enjoying my good sleep—but it's nice to have options.

THERAPIST: What do you think has helped you get better?

SOPHIE: Things started to get better when I stopped being so concerned about not sleeping and started going to sleep later.

THERAPIST: What helped you to be less concerned about not sleeping?

SOPHIE: It happened gradually. When you told about the sleep drive and how my thinking gets in its way, it made a lot of sense, but I was still a little afraid. But as my sleep improved, the concerns went away.

THERAPIST: That makes sense. The changes you made have helped you be less fearful in how you approach sleep, and this has continued to help you follow some of the rules we discussed. Changing your approach and following the recommendations worked in concert.

## Strategies for Dealing with Insomnia in the Future

Check off the strategies below that helped you improve your sleep. Remember that it is normal to have an occasional night of poor sleep. However, if you notice that your sleep has worsened for several nights in a row, you can help restore your good sleep with the same strategies that helped you improve your sleep during treatment.

☑ Keeping the same rise time every day (no matter how much sleep I get)

☑ Going to bed when sleepy

☑ Getting out of bed when unable to sleep

☑ Creating a 1-hour buffer zone period before bedtime

☑ Getting out of bed if I am worrying or cannot shut off my thoughts

☑ Engaging in worrying or problem solving earlier in the evening

☑ Limiting the amount of time in bed at night (based on monitoring sleep for 2 weeks and following the time-in-bed restriction guidelines)

☐ Not using the bed for anything other than sleeping (and sex)

☐ No napping (except for safety)

☑ Not canceling activities after a night of poor sleep

☐ Trying not to have caffeine or alcohol, smoke cigarettes, or engage in exercise within a few hours of bedtime

☑ Anything else that helped: *Remember that trying to sleep only makes it harder to sleep.*

If these do not help, schedule a refresher session.

**Remember not to get alarmed.**

**Everyone has a bad night's sleep once in a while.**

**If you have a few bad nights in a row, keep in mind that you mastered the insomnia before, and you'll master it again.**

**FIGURE 11.12.** Strategies for Dealing with Insomnia in the Future form as completed by Sophie.

Sophie had not written a letter to herself, but she had clearly been thinking about which strategies had helped, which was the main purpose of such a letter. The therapist proceeded to discuss plans for dealing with insomnia in the future should it recur. Using the Strategies for Dealing with Insomnia form (see Appendix C), Sophie identified the strategies that had helped her (Figure 11.12).

## REFLECTIONS ON SOPHIE'S TREATMENT

- Sophie experienced insomnia that was not complicated by other comorbidities.
- Her treatment targeted the following:
  - Variable rise time.
  - Spending too much time in bed.
  - Conditioned arousal.
  - General arousal (work-related worries).
  - Maladaptive thoughts related to sleep and fatigue (e.g., if she did not sleep enough, she would experience unmanageable fatigue levels; experience of fatigue meant that more needed to be done to improve sleep).
  - Safety behaviors (she stopped exercising, reduced social contact outside of work, and increased sleep effort).

- Adherence issues were successfully targeted with behavioral experiments.
- The most salient aspect of her action plan in the event that the insomnia returned after termination was to remind herself that trying to sleep only makes it harder to sleep.

# CHAPTER 12

# Case Example 2

## *Sam*

This chapter takes the reader through the process of assessment, treatment planning, and implementation of treatment for Sam, a 60-year-old man who was referred by a sleep physician for CBT-I. His case has been introduced in Chapter 1, and there have been references to him throughout the book. The sleep physician's referral document indicated that Sam was diagnosed 5 years earlier with mild to moderate OSAH and was prescribed CPAP therapy. The referring physician also noted the presence of severe, chronic insomnia and recommended CBT-I. The report stated that Sam did not pursue CBT-I at that time because there were no behavioral sleep medicine specialists close to his home and he did not want to drive an hour to appointments.

Sam's case illustrates both a different clinical presentation from Sophie's (described in Chapter 11) and a different pretreatment setup. Unlike Sophie's therapist, Sam's therapist did not send him copies of the sleep diary form ahead of the first session and did not administer the ISI at each session.

## SESSION 1

### Before Session

The therapist's plan for the first session was to devote most of it to assessing Sam's insomnia, following the guidelines discussed in Chapter 6. The therapist planned to introduce the sleep diary at the end of the session, explain how to complete it, convey the expectation that the diary should be completed throughout treatment. and emphasize the essential role the sleep diary plays in the treatment. Figure 12.1 shows how the therapist completed the Session Plan form for Sam's first session.

### During Session

After the introductions and consent process, the therapist conducted the structured insomnia intake interview to determine the nature and history of the sleep problem and associated fea-

## Session Plan

**ID/Name:** _Sam_                    **Date:** _November 5, 2013_          **Session #:** _1_

- Provide introduction to treatment (personal introductions, informed consent, overview of therapy structure and of today's assessment session).

- Assess insomnia symptoms, sleep habits, history of sleep complaint, other sleep disorders, psychiatric and medical disorders and their treatment, and other potentially relevant features of the case.

- Elicit Sam's treatment goals.

- Determine whether CBT-I is contraindicated.

- Provide one or two simple recommendations, based on case conceptualization (as time permits).

- Introduce sleep diary.

**Homework:**

- Assign 2 weeks of sleep diary forms.

- Follow the recommendation(s) provided.

**Notes:**

Schedule next appointment(s).

**FIGURE 12.1.** Session Plan form as completed by the therapist for Sam's Session 1.

tures, as well as Sam's treatment goals. The therapist used the Insomnia Intake Form (Appendix A) to guide the flow of the assessment process. To assess other sleep disorders, the therapist used the Assessment of Other Sleep Disorders form (also in Appendix A), and summarized what was learned in the Insomnia Intake Form in the section for comorbid sleep disorders. These assessment forms as completed for Sam are shown in Figures 12.2 and 12.3, respectively.

The therapist asked Sam to prioritize his treatment goals, but Sam could not separate them. He thought that sleeping more would help him get rid of pain and be more alert during the day, and that these improvements would then allow him to spend more time with his grandchildren. Sam did not state a wish to discontinue use of zolpidem. The therapist made a note to address Sam's beliefs about the pain–sleep connection and his safety behaviors. Unlike Sophie, who received her sleep diary forms before the first session in a clinic-mailed package, Sam received his sleep diary forms at the end of this first session along with detailed instructions about their completion, as discussed in Chapter 6. Suspecting that Sam might be sleeping more during the day than he was aware of, the therapist also asked him to monitor and keep track of when and how much he slept during the day. Sam's homework thus consisted of the following:

# Insomnia Intake Form

**Patient name:** *Sam*     **Marital/partnered status:** *Married*     **Referral source:** *Sleep physician*

**Gender:** *Male*     **Children:** *Two adult children*

**Date of birth:** *[60 years]*     **Occupation:** *Accountant, currently on disability due to fibromyalgia*

**NATURE OF PRESENTING PROBLEM** (check all that apply, and identify the most distressing/disturbing sleep problem):

☑ Difficulty initiating sleep     ☑ Difficulty maintaining sleep

☑ Waking up too early     ☐ Difficulty waking up     ☐ Nonrefreshing sleep

Number of nights per week sleep problem is experienced: ____7____ to ____7____

When did the current episode start? __*25 years ago*__

Identifiable precipitating factor(s): __*After birth of second daughter*__

Treatment history for current episode: __*Taking zolpidem for 18 years (see below for details). CBT-I recommended by sleep physician 5 years ago, but access to therapist was prohibitive (per referral notes and confirmed by patient).*__

**DAYTIME EFFECTS**

☑ Energy/fatigue     ☑ Concentration/functioning     ☑ Mood

☑ Daytime sleepiness (specify): __*Dozes off when reclining during day and in evening*__

Other (specify): __*Fibromyalgia pain worsening; reduced activity level*__

**HISTORY**

Age at onset of first insomnia episode: ____*35 years*____     Lifetime course: *Chronic*

Family history of insomnia: ____*None*____

**Sleep habits** (focus on previous or most recent typical week; describe range when indicted; note weekday/weekend times, if different):

**BEGINNING OF SLEEP PERIOD**

Time into bed: ____*10:30 P.M.*____

Time turning lights out (or intent to sleep): __*10:30 P.M.*__

How does patient decide when to go to bed? ____*Habit*____

Pre-bedtime activities: ____*Television*____     ☐ Fears     ☑ Dozing off in evening

Average time to fall asleep: *2 hours (occasionally less)*

What happens when patient cannot get to sleep (thoughts/behaviors)? __*Stays in bed, tries to clear his mind, feels frustrated*__

☐ Rumination     ☐ General worry     ☐ Sleep worry     ☑ Physical tension

*(cont.)*

**FIGURE 12.2.** Insomnia Intake Form as completed for Sam.

## MIDDLE OF THE NIGHT

Number of awakenings after sleep onset: _____1_____ to _____3_____

Total time awake after sleep onset: _____1_____ to _2 hours_

What happens when awake in the middle of the night (thoughts/behaviors)? _Stays in bed, feels frustrated_

☐ Rumination          ☐ General worry          ☐ Sleep worry          ☑ Physical tension

## END OF THE NIGHT

Final wake time: _5:00–6:00 A.M._          Time out of bed: _7:30–9:00 A.M._

Alarm (or other wake-up system): ☑ No ☐ Yes

Is final awakening earlier than planned? ☐ No ☑ Yes, by _30–60_ minutes

Difficulties waking up at intended time: ☑ No ☐ Yes

Estimated average total sleep time: _5 hours_

**PREMORBID SLEEP SCHEDULE:** _10:30 P.M.–6:30 A.M._

**CURRENT SLEEP MEDICATION(S)/AIDS:** ☐ No ☑ Yes (If yes, then complete table below.)

| Name | Dose | When taken? | How long? | Helpful? |
|------|------|-------------|-----------|----------|
| Zolpidem | 7.5 mg | At bedtime | 18 years | Somewhat (less than it used to be; was previously unsuccessful at getting off) |

## NAPPING

Able to nap if given an opportunity? ☑ No ☐ Yes _____

Nap frequency _____     Nap duration _____

Timing of nap _(Cannot fall asleep when he tries to nap, but will inadvertently doze in recliner during the day and in evening while watching TV)_

**SLEEP ENVIRONMENT** (note problematic aspects of sleep environment—bed partner, caregiving, pets, sound, lights, safety, temperature):

_Sleeps in separate room from wife so her snoring does not disturb his sleep_

**OTHER BEHAVIORS THAT CAN AFFECT SLEEP** (include time and frequency; for substances, also include amount):

Caffeine _2–4 coffees; last one after dinner_          Nicotine _Denies_

Alcohol _2–4 drinks on weekends at dinner_          Recreational drugs _Denies_

Timing of vigorous exercise: _____N/A_____     Nocturnal eating: _No_

Overall activity level:  ☑ Understimulated          ☐ Overstimulated

Other: _____

**FIGURE 12.2** (*cont.*)

## NOTES ON COGNITIVE HYPERAROUSAL

"If I don't sleep, I don't have the energy to play with grandchildren" [and do other things he enjoys (e.g., socializing in evening)]; "I can't drive."

Thinks of his sleep as "fragile." Moved out of spousal bed to protect sleep from wife's snoring.

High sleep preoccupation: Keeps binder of sleep-related medical appointments and a diary of his sleeplessness experiences.

## NOTES ON EMOTIONAL AROUSAL

Frustration when cannot fall asleep

## CIRCADIAN TENDENCIES

☐ Morning type          ☐ Neither type          ☑ Evening type

Evidence: _Said he was previously a "night owl"_

---

Use the **Assessment of Other Sleep Disorders** form to evaluate other sleep disorders, and note results here.

### CIRCADIAN RHYTHM SLEEP–WAKE DISORDERS

☑ Does not meet criteria          ☐ Meets criteria   Type: ☐ Advanced   ☐ Delayed

### OBSTRUCTIVE SLEEP APNEA HYPOPNEA (OSAH)

☑ Previously diagnosed          Severity _AHI = 18 (mild to moderate)_

☐ Not previously diagnosed          ☐ Suspected          ☐ Not suspected

Treatment:   ☑ Not or inadequately treated   ☐ Adequately treated   Specify treatment: _CPAP nightly, but wakes up in middle of night not knowing when he took mask off and does not put it back on_

### RESTLESS LEGS SYNDROME (RLS)

☑ Does not meet criteria          ☐ Meets criteria          Treatment: _____

### PARASOMNIA SYMPTOMS (include frequency):

Nightmare disorder: ☐ Meets criteria     ☑ Does not meet criteria

Other unusual behaviors during sleep: _____

---

**CURRENT COMORBID MEDICAL DISORDERS** (note impact on sleep, include treatment): _____
Fibromyalgia: Duloxetine and gabapentin for pain

**CURRENT COMORBID PSYCHIATRIC DISORDERS** (note impact on sleep, include treatment): _Several features of major depressive disorder, but does not meet full criteria; during the past year, he has experienced worsening fatigue, pain, depressed mood, memory problems, and concentration problems; no suicide ideation._

**GOAL(S):** _"Sleep more," "get rid of [his] pain," and "not feel sleepy during the day" so that he can spend more time with his grandchildren._

## Assessment of Other Sleep Disorders

| SLEEP COMPLAINT | NOTES |
|---|---|
| **Circadian rhythm sleep–wake disorder, delayed sleep phase type**<br><br>1. Recurrent inability to fall asleep at a desired conventional clock time, and difficulty awakening at a desired and socially acceptable time.<br><br>2. When allowed to use preferred schedule, no problem with sleep except its delayed timing.<br><br>3. Preferred schedule delayed more than 2 hours relative to desired conventional clock.<br><br>If criteria 1, 2, and 3 are met, refer patient to a sleep center for assessment and treatment. (Treatment will probably involve schedule manipulation and properly timed light and dark exposures.) | *Describes self as having been a "night owl" (used to go to bed much later than now.) Circadian rhythm sleep–wake disorder, delayed sleep phase type, is absent.*<br><br>*Circadian rhythm sleep–wake disorder, advanced sleep phase type* |
| **Circadian rhythm sleep–wake disorder, advanced sleep phase type**<br><br>1. Recurrent inability to stay awake until a desired conventional clock time, and difficulty staying asleep in the morning until a desired and socially acceptable time.<br><br>2. When allowed to use preferred schedule, no problem with sleep except its advanced timing.<br><br>3. Preferred schedule advanced more than 2 hours relative to desired conventional clock.<br><br>If criteria 1, 2, and 3 are met, refer patient to a sleep center for assessment and treatment. (Treatment will probably involve schedule manipulation and properly timed light and dark exposures.) | *Some dozing in evening and early wake-up, but not a lifelong pattern. Pattern may be due to extended time in bed or depressed mood.*<br><br>*Circadian rhythm sleep–wake disorder, advanced sleep phase type, is absent.* |
| **Obstructive sleep apnea hypopnea (OSAH)**<br><br>1. Does patient report:<br>☐ snoring that can be heard through a closed door, or as loud as a conversation?<br>☐ gasping/choking during sleep?<br>☐ stopping breathing during sleep?<br>☐ poor, unrefreshing sleep even after adequate sleep time?<br><br>2. Does the patient report:<br>☐ morning headaches?<br>☐ urinating more than twice per night?<br>☐ dry mouth upon awakening? ☐ hypertension?<br>☐ BMI > 30 (BMI = body mass index = weight in kilograms divided by height in meters)? | *Previously diagnosed OSAH (AHI = 18).*<br><br>*Partially adherent with CPAP. Daytime sleepiness (falls asleep in front of television, when reclining, during the day and early evening).*<br><br>*OSAH present, inadequately treated. Consult referring sleep specialist.* |

**FIGURE 12.3.** Assessment of Other Sleep Disorders form as completed for Sam.

| SLEEP COMPLAINT | NOTES |
|---|---|
| **Obstructive sleep apnea hypopnea (OSAH)** (*cont.*)<br><br>3. Is excessive daytime sleepiness present? Is there a recurrent pattern of falling asleep unintentionally or struggling to stay awake when in any one of the following situations:<br><br>☐ Talking with others?   ☐ Driving?<br><br>☐ Talking on the phone?   ☐ Standing?<br><br>☐ Other activities or situations in which most people will not fall asleep?<br><br>If the patient has two or more symptoms in 1, or one symptom in 1 and one in 2, or one item in 1 and excessive daytime sleepiness, refer for evaluation of possible OSAH.<br><br>If the patient does not have co-occurring OSAH or if OSAH is adequately treated (to be determined in consultation with a sleep specialist), proceed with CBT-I. (See Chapter 7 for safety issues related to daytime sleepiness.) | |
| **Restless legs syndrome (RLS)**<br><br>Does the patient have a very strong urge to move legs? (If it is associated with unpleasant sensations in the legs, ask the patient to describe the sensations.)<br><br>1. Does the urge occur or worsen in evening or during rest or inactivity?<br><br>2. Is the urge temporarily relieved by moving?<br><br>3. Does the urge interfere with falling asleep or returning to sleep?<br><br>If urge is present and the answer is yes to 1, 2, and 3, then a referral for evaluation and possible pharmacological treatment of RLS is warranted.<br><br>If RLS symptoms do not regularly interfere with the onset of sleep at the beginning or middle of night, proceed with CBT-I. | *RLS is absent.* |
| **Nightmare disorder**<br><br>1. Does the patient report recurrent nightmares (a nightmare is defined as a dream that has *all* of the features below)?<br><br>- An elaborate narrative is remembered.<br>- Evokes very strong negative emotion.<br>- Occurs in second half of night.<br>- No confusion upon waking.<br><br>2. Is there clinically meaningful distress or impairment?<br><br>Yes answers to questions 1 and 2 indicate a diagnosis of nightmare disorder, unless the nightmares are induced by substance use or explained by another disorder.<br><br>If all nocturnal symptoms of insomnia are caused by nightmares (e.g., prolonged sleep onset because of fear of nightmares or all awakenings are related to nightmares), then CBT-I is not warranted. (See Chapters 7 and 10 for more information about nightmare-related issues.) | *No nightmares.*<br><br>*Nightmare disorder is absent.* |

- Complete sleep diary forms.
- Note under "nap" the total estimated time of dozing.

## After Session

Based on the information gathered during the interview, the therapist concluded that Sam met criteria for insomnia disorder; given the presence of inadequately treated OSAH and daytime sleepiness, however, the therapist wanted to discuss the case with the referring sleep physician before initiating CBT-I. The therapist obtained a release from Sam to talk with his sleep physician. The sleep physician supported the therapist's decision to proceed with CBT-I, but recommended that (1) there should be an explicit instruction to put the CPAP mask back on if it came off or was removed during sleep; and (2) Sam should nap if needed for safety (e.g., before a drive). (Safety naps are always considered when CBT-I is being implemented, even if a patient does not have OSAH.) The therapist devised a case conceptualization of Sam's presentation, following the guidelines presented in Chapter 10. Figure 12.4 is the completed Case Conceptualization Form for Sam's case.

The therapist identified excessive time in bed (TIB), conditioned arousal, and cognitive factors as key targets for intervention. Concerned about Sam's daytime sleepiness, the therapist decided to base his TIB prescription on the total sleep time (TST) across 24 hours, not just the TST obtained at night. This guided the therapist's request that Sam should estimate his daytime sleep on his sleep diary. The therapist also planned to monitor Sam's daytime sleepiness closely. The therapist then completed the Treatment Planning Form (Figure 12.5), listing these key targets for intervention and strategies to address them.

# SESSION 2

## Before Session

Based on the case conceptualization shown in Figure 12.4, the therapist developed a plan for Session 2 (which was Sam's first treatment session) as shown in Figure 12.6.

## During Session

From Sam's sleep diary data, the therapist computed TST and sleep efficiency (SE) to guide the administration of sleep restriction therapy. The tentative TIB restriction mentioned in the Session Plan for Session 2 (Figure 12.6) was the therapist's best estimate based on interview data. To simplify the discussion, we focus here only on the second of the 2 weeks of diary data. The sleep diary for that week (see Figure 12.7) revealed that the average time Sam spent in bed was about 9.5 hours; his nighttime TST was variable and ranged from 3.75 to 6.4 hours per night, with an average of about 5 hours. His average SE was 52%. The diary data were consistent with Sam's report during the interview of difficulty falling asleep (mean = 1 hour, 15 minutes) and wakefulness after sleep onset (mean = 58 minutes). In addition, he woke up about 50 minutes earlier than he would have liked, and lingered in bed an average of 2 hours, 25 minutes. As requested, Sam kept a record of how much he dozed and napped daily, which was variable and averaged 25 minutes.

# Case Conceptualization Form

*Note to Clinicians:* Please note that certain factors could load on more than one of these six domains. In such cases, list the factor in the row corresponding to the domain that is most relevant to the case.

| Domains | Patient-specific factors that contribute to insomnia or may interfere with adherence |
|---|---|
| **1.** *Sleep drive:* What factors may be weakening the patient's sleep drive? Consider extended time in bed, dozing off in the evening, daytime napping, sedentary life, and so on. | *Excessive time in bed at night; dozing during the day and evening.*<br><br>*Pain may cause sleep fragmentation.* |
| **2.** *Biological clock:* What biological clock factors are relevant to the patient's presentation? Consider irregular wake and/or out-of-bed time, time-in-bed window that is not congruent with the patient's chronotype, and so on. | *Variability in the time that he gets up. His chronotype is likely to be normal.* |
| **3.** *Arousal:* What manifestations of hyperarousal are evident? Consider the following:<br><br>  **3a.** *Cognitive arousal related to sleep* (e.g., sleep effort, safety behaviors, and maladaptive beliefs/attitudes about sleep).<br><br>  **3b.** *General hyperarousal affecting sleep* (e.g., worry in bed about life stressors).<br><br>  **3c.** *Conditioned arousal:* Has the bed become associated with arousal rather than sleep? Specify predisposing factors (e.g., high trait anxiety), precipitating factors (e.g., stressful life events), and maintaining factors (.e.g., extended time spent in bed). | *3a. <u>Cognitive arousal related to sleep</u>: <u>Preoccupation with sleep</u>: Has been keeping a binder tracking his sleep for a long time.*<br><br>*<u>Safety behaviors and sleep effort</u>: Sleeps apart from wife; has withdrawn from activities that were enjoyable (e.g., playing with grandkids). Psychological dependence on hypnotics is also a form of sleep effort. Decreased sleep self-efficacy.*<br><br>*<u>Avoidance behaviors</u>: Significant reduction in time spent with grandkids; avoids driving.*<br><br>*<u>Beliefs</u>: Pain will not be relieved unless sleep improves; cannot manage without sufficient sleep.*<br><br>*3b. <u>General hyperarousal affecting sleep</u>: Not evident.*<br><br>*3c. <u>Conditioned arousal</u>: Can be sleepy at night on couch, but will be wide awake when he gets into bed.* |
| **4.** *Unhealthy sleep behaviors:* What unhealthy sleep behaviors are present? Consider caffeine, alcohol, nocturnal eating, timing of exercise, and other factors. | *Caffeine use late in day may interfere with sleep.* |

*(cont.)*

**FIGURE 12.4.** Case Conceptualization Form as completed for Sam.

| Domains | Patient-specific factors that contribute to insomnia or may interfere with adherence |
|---|---|
| **5.** *Medications:* What medications may be having an impact on the patient's sleep/sleepiness? Consider carryover effects, tolerance, and psychological dependence. | *Psychological dependence on zolpidem (18 years).*<br><br>*Gabapentin and duloxetine may be sedating during the day.* |
| **6.** *Comorbidities:* What comorbidities may be affecting the patient's sleep, and how? Consider sleep, medical, and psychiatric conditions (e.g., difficult adjustment to CPAP treatment for sleep apnea; pain interfering with sleep; PTSD-related hypervigilance). | *Fibromyalgia: Chronic pain. Inadequately treated OSAH may contribute to daytime sleepiness. Sam attributes some of the daytime symptoms of undertreated OSAH to insomnia, thus potentially increasing sleep effort. Depressive symptoms may contribute to excessive time in bed and being sedentary.* |
| **7.** *Other*: Consider sleep environment, caregiving duties at night, life phase sleep issues, mental status, and readiness for change. | *Strengths include healthy relationships with family; he continues to enjoy spending time with his grandkids and is motivated by desire to help care for them.* |

**FIGURE 12.4**  (*cont.*)

The therapist shared a summary of the calculations made from the sleep diary data, and used the information when discussing sleep regulation and providing the rationale for treatment. After sharing the computed variables for the average TIB, TST, and SE, the therapist highlighted the variability in TST and used it to help explain the sleep drive.

## Explaining the Sleep Drive

THERAPIST: Before I make recommendations for improving your sleep, I would like to explain a little about how the sleep system works.

SAM: Sounds good.

THERAPIST: Let's begin looking at your sleep diary and the calculations I made based on it. For each night, I calculated how much time you were in bed (from when you turned the lights off at night to when you got out of bed in the morning). Then I calculated the average amount of time you were in bed for the 7 nights of last week.

SAM: Over 9 hours? That doesn't seem right. I am not sleeping all that time, though.

THERAPIST: Correct. You are sleeping only about half of the time that you are in bed. This number you are looking at is how long you were in bed. It is actually 9½ hours.

SAM: I see.

# Treatment Planning Form

**Patient's treatment goal(s):** _Sleep more, get rid of pain, not feel sleepy during the day so he can spend more time with his grandchildren._

| First treatment session (enter items in the order you plan to introduce them) | | | |
|---|---|---|---|
| **Factors to address** | **CBT-I components** | **Specific recommendations** | **Comments** |
| Weak sleep drive at night (dozing/resting/excessive time in bed) | Sleep restriction therapy | TIB will be determined after diary data are available. (TIB = 7.5 hours; 11:00 P.M. to 6:30 A.M. might be a good starting point.)<br><br>Discuss safety naps. | Schedule pleasurable morning activities to facilitate adherence with recommended out-of-bed time.<br><br>Rest during the day is OK, but not lying down or reclining, and never in the nocturnal bed.<br><br>Monitor sleepiness daily (add a line to bedtime portion of the sleep diary). |
| Conditioned arousal: Dozes before bedtime, but wide awake when getting into bed | Stimulus control | Go to bed only when sleepy, but not before bedtime.<br><br>Get out of bed if unable to sleep. | Put CPAP mask back on if it has been removed.<br><br>Wear CPAP mask during all sleep opportunities. |
| Caffeine | Sleep hygiene | Reduce caffeine and stop consumption after lunch. | Discuss alternatives (e.g., substituting decaffeinated or half-caffeinated beverages if needed). |
| Subsequent sessions (enter items in the order you plan to introduce them) | | | |
| **Factors to address** | **CBT-I components** | **Specific recommendations** | **Comments** |
| Cognitive factors: Sleep effort, sleep beliefs, sleep preoccupation.<br><br>Beliefs related to safety behaviors, Beliefs related to avoidance behaviors. | Cognitive therapy (including education; guided discovery to identify thoughts underlying safety behaviors; behavioral experiments). | Address beliefs about the relation between sleep and pain.<br><br>Have value-system-based discussion about moving back into spousal bedroom.<br><br>Design a behavioral experiment to increase time with grandkids.<br><br>Discuss impact of preoccupation with sleep (sleep binder). | |

**FIGURE 12.5.** Treatment Planning Form as completed by the therapist for Sam.

## Session Plan

**ID/Name:** _Sam_                    **Date:** _Nov. 19, 2013_                    **Session #:** _2_

- Ask Sam if anything has changed and if there is anything he wants to make sure we address today.

- Review sleep diary forms, including his notes on dozing, and discuss daytime sleepiness.

- Explain sleep drive, and introduce the TIB restriction to be based on the completed sleep diary he will bring to session.

- Explain the biological clock in relation to irregular wake time, and introduce stimulus control, beginning with fixing wake time.

- Discuss ways to increase daytime activity level and minimize dozing late in the day.

- Encourage CPAP adherence.

- Encourage eliminating afternoon coffee.

**Homework:**

- Continue sleep diary monitoring.

- Follow a list of recommendations based on discussion.

**Notes:**

---

**FIGURE 12.6.** Session Plan form as completed by the therapist for Sam's Session 2.

THERAPIST: I also notice from your diary that last night you slept almost 6½ hours, but the two nights before that you slept less than 4 hours.

SAM: This is pretty typical for me. I have a few really bad nights, and then I sleep a little better.

THERAPIST: This is normal. Let me explain how it works. We all have a sleep drive system. It is a rather simple system. The sleep drive builds up when you are awake. The longer you are awake during the day, the stronger your sleep drive when you go to bed at night. Also, the more active you are during the day, the stronger your sleep drive when you go to bed at night. The stronger your sleep drive when you go to bed, the faster you fall asleep and the longer and deeper you sleep. So on Sunday morning you woke up around 5:00 and you got out of bed at 8:15. Were you sleeping between 5:00 and 8:15?

*Demonstration of education about the homeostatic sleep drive to establish rationale for sleep restriction therapy.*

SAM: I don't think so.

THERAPIST: So from around 5:00 in the morning until 9:30, when you went to bed last

## Consensus Sleep Diary–M

**Please complete upon awakening.**

ID/Name: Sam

| Today's Date: | 11/13/13 | 11/14/13 | 11/15/13 | 11/16/13 | 11/17/13 | 11/18/13 | 11/19/13 |
|---|---|---|---|---|---|---|---|
| **1.** What time did you get into bed? | 10:00 P.M. | 10:30 P.M. | 10:00 P.M. | 9:00 P.M. | 10:00 P.M. | 10:00 P.M. | 9:30 P.M. |
| **2.** What time did you try to go to sleep? | 10:30 P.M. | 10:45 P.M. | 11:00 P.M. | 9:00 P.M. | 10:00 P.M. | 10:45 P.M. | 9:30 P.M. |
| **3.** How long did it take you to fall asleep? | 120 min | 90 min | 90 min | 15 min | 60 min | 120 min | 20 min |
| **4.** How many times did you wake up, not counting your final awakening? | 2 | 2 | 2 | 3 | 2 | 1 | 2 |
| **5.** In total, how long did these awakenings last? | 30 min | 45 min | 45 min | 90 min | 120 min | 30 min | 45 min |
| **6a.** What time was your final awakening? | 5:10 A.M. | 6:00 A.M. | 6:30 A.M. | 5:15 A.M. | 4:45 A.M. | 4:55 A.M. | 5:00 A.M. |
| **6b.** After your final awakening, how long did you spend in bed trying to sleep? | 90 min | 100 min | 120 min | 60 min | 180 min | 150 min | 90 min |

**FIGURE 12.7.** Consensus Sleep Diary–M form as completed by Sam during the week that preceded Session 2. Adapted from Carney et al. (2012). Copyright 2011 by the Consensus Sleep Diary Committee. Adapted by permission.

(cont.)

205

| Today's Date: | 11/13/13 | 11/14/13 | 11/15/13 | 11/16/13 | 11/17/13 | 11/18/13 | 11/19/13 |
|---|---|---|---|---|---|---|---|
| **6c.** Did you wake up earlier than you planned? | ☑ Yes ☐ No | ☐ Yes ☑ No | ☑ Yes ☐ No | ☑ Yes ☐ No | ☑ Yes ☐ No | ☑ Yes ☐ No | ☑ Yes ☐ No |
| **6d.** If yes, how much earlier? | 60 min | N/A | 60 min | 60 min | 30 min | 60 min | 60 min |
| **7.** What time did you get out of bed for the day? | 7:15 A.M. | 8:00 A.M. | 9:00 A.M. | 6:30 A.M. | 8:10 A.M. | 8:15 A.M. | 7:10 A.M. |
| **8.** How would you rate the quality of your sleep? | ☐ Very poor ☑ Poor ☐ Fair ☐ Good ☐ Very good | ☐ Very poor ☑ Poor ☐ Fair ☐ Good ☐ Very good | ☐ Very poor ☑ Poor ☐ Fair ☐ Good ☐ Very good | ☐ Very poor ☑ Poor ☐ Fair ☐ Good ☐ Very good | ☑ Very poor ☐ Poor ☐ Fair ☐ Good ☐ Very good | ☑ Very poor ☐ Poor ☐ Fair ☐ Good ☐ Very good | ☑ Very poor ☐ Poor ☐ Fair ☐ Good ☐ Very good |
| **9.** How rested or refreshed did you feel when you woke up for the day? | ☑ Not at all rested ☐ Slightly rested ☐ Somewhat rested ☐ Well rested ☐ Very well rested | ☑ Not at all rested ☐ Slightly rested ☐ Somewhat rested ☐ Well rested ☐ Very well rested | ☑ Not at all rested ☐ Slightly rested ☐ Somewhat rested ☐ Well rested ☐ Very well rested | ☐ Not at all rested ☐ Slightly rested ☑ Somewhat rested ☐ Well rested ☐ Very well rested | ☑ Not at all rested ☐ Slightly rested ☐ Somewhat rested ☐ Well rested ☐ Very well rested | ☑ Not at all rested ☐ Slightly rested ☐ Somewhat rested ☐ Well rested ☐ Very well rested | ☑ Not at all rested ☐ Slightly rested ☐ Somewhat rested ☐ Well rested ☐ Very well rested |
| Therapist's notes *Calculated TST (Calculated TIB)* | 4.2 (8.8) | 5 (9.25) | 5.25 (10) | 6.5 (9.5) | 3.75 (10.2) | 3.7 (9.5) | 6.4 (9.7) |
| **10a.** How many times did you nap or doze? | 2 times | 2 times | 2 times | 3 times | 2 times | 1 times | 0 times |

206

|  | | | | | | | |
|---|---|---|---|---|---|---|---|
| **10b.** In total, how long did you nap or doze? | 15 min | 20 min | 30 min | 45 min | 20 min | 40 min | O min |
| **11a.** How many drinks containing alcohol did you have? | O drinks | O drinks | 1 drink | O drinks | O drinks | 2 drinks | 2 drinks |
| **11b.** What time was your last drink? | N/A | N/A | 6:00 P.M. | N/A | N/A | 8:00 P.M. | 10:00 P.M. |
| **12a.** How many caffeinated drinks (coffee, tea, soda, energy drinks) did you have? | 2 drinks | 4 drinks | 3 drinks | 2 drinks | 4 drinks | 3 drinks | 3 drinks |
| **12b.** What time was your last drink? | 6:00 P.M. | 6:00 P.M. | 6:00 P.M. | 5:00 P.M. | 6:00 P.M. | 9:00 P.M. | 8:00 P.M. |
| **13.** Did you take any over-the-counter or prescription medication(s) to help you sleep? | ☑ Yes ☐No Medication(s): Zolpidem Dose: 7.5 mg | ☑ Yes ☐No Medication(s): Zolpidem Dose: 7.5 mg | ☑ Yes ☐No Medication(s): Zolpidem Dose: 7.5 mg | ☑ Yes ☐No Medication(s): Zolpidem Dose: 7.5 mg | ☑ Yes ☐No Medication(s): Zolpidem Dose: 7.5 mg | ☑ Yes ☐No Medication(s): Zolpidem Dose: 7.5 mg | ☑ Yes ☐No Medication(s): Zolpidem Dose: 7.5 mg |
| If so, list medication(s), dose, and time taken. | Time(s) taken: 12:00 A.M. | Time(s) taken: 10:30 P.M. | Time(s) taken: 10:00 P.M. | Time(s) taken: 10:45 P.M. | Time(s) taken: 12:00 A.M. | Time(s) taken: 10:00 P.M. | Time(s) taken: 9:30 P.M. |
| **14.** Comments | | | | Fell asleep on couch | | | |

FIGURE 12.7  (cont.)

207

night, your sleep drive was building up. After 16½ hours of being awake, your sleep drive was pretty strong. As a result, you fell asleep faster and slept longer than usual.

SAM: That makes sense; but if you look 1 day back, there was even more time for the sleep drive to build, 18 hours, and I still slept less than 4 hours. It took me 2 hours to fall asleep that night.

THERAPIST: Right. You are talking about Sunday night. I see that you napped 40 minutes on Saturday. Do you remember when that was?

SAM: Yes. That was when my wife was making dinner. She came to tell me that dinner was ready, and found me asleep in the recliner with the TV on. I was totally wiped out from the night before. I did not mean to sleep. I think she woke me up around 6:00, and she said I had been asleep for the last 40 minutes. That is how I know how long I slept.

THERAPIST: Here is something else about the sleep drive. It lessens by sleeping. So on Sunday the nap reduced your sleep drive. There was probably not enough time for your sleep drive to build back up between 6 P.M. and when you went to bed that night. So when you went to bed on Saturday night, your sleep drive was probably weaker than when you went to bed on Sunday night.

SAM: I see.

THERAPIST: The sleep drive builds up as the day progresses, unless you sleep or even doze during the day. Each time you sleep or doze, you reduce the sleep drive. The more you sleep during the day, the weaker your sleep drive at night. Also, the later in the day dozing happens, the more problematic it is for your sleep drive.

SAM: I am mainly resting during the day. I don't sleep that much during the day. I doze off here and there. When you asked me to keep track of my dozing, it all added up to about 20 minutes or at most an hour.

THERAPIST: Yes, on average it was about 25 minutes. It may not sound like much. I know you feel exhausted and wish you were sleeping longer. But if you doze in the evening, it lessens your sleep drive even though you barely sleep. It is like snacking a little before the Thanksgiving meal.

SAM: I get it.

The therapist decided that this would be a good time to introduce sleep restriction therapy, but did not think that an initial TIB that was equal to Sam's TST (5 hours) would be safe or wise. Sam's inadequately treated OSAH and his significant dozing during the day suggested daytime sleepiness and raised safety concerns. Considering Sam's TST across the 24-hour period (rounded to the nearest 15 minutes), and adding the 30-minute safety margin (Chapter 7) that is recommended when sleepiness is present, would indicate that his initial TIB should be 6 hours. However, the therapist also thought that Sam had perhaps been misperceiving light stages of sleep as being awake, and that he had probably been sleeping longer than he estimated.

*Demonstrating therapist's rationale for implementation of sleep compression (modified sleep restriction therapy).*

The therapist therefore decided that in Sam's case, sleep compression (again, see Chapter 7) might be better than sleep restriction, and that a 7-hour initial TIB window could be a reasonable starting point for him. The therapist anticipated that a sharp reduction in TIB from 9.5 to 7 hours would be overwhelming, and thought that information about the relationship among the sleep drive, light sleep, and muscle pain would make the idea of reducing time in bed by 2.5 hours less overwhelming. The therapist thought that such information could enhance Sam's adherence with sleep restriction therapy, and that it could also motivate him to become a bit more active during the day.

### Explaining the Relationship between Sleep and Muscle Pain

THERAPIST: It sounds like your sleep is very light.

SAM: You can say that again.

THERAPIST: There is a tradeoff between how long you sleep and how light you sleep. If you sleep less at night and during the day, then your sleep drive is strong that night, and your sleep is deep. If you doze in the evening or sleep in late, then your sleep drive the following night is light.

SAM: I got that.

THERAPIST: Deep sleep and pain are intricately connected. When people are in deep sleep, their sleep is rich in a hormone called *growth hormone*. This hormone is involved in tissue restoration. So having more deep sleep is particularly important for people with muscle pain, like you.

SAM: I read somewhere that people with fibromyalgia have less of this chemical and less deep sleep. What can I do to get more deep sleep? I am already taking a sleep medication.

THERAPIST: Let me rephrase this. What are two things you are doing that make your sleep drive weaker than it could be?

SAM: You mean the dozing?

THERAPIST: Yes. Also spending a long time in bed.

> *Demonstration of education about sleep drive and its relationship with pain. This provided a further rationale for sleep restriction/compression.*

### Restricting TIB

The therapist proceeded to discuss sleep restriction therapy. During the discussion, Sam made several references to wanting deep sleep. At the end, he preferred the 11:30 P.M. to 6:30 A.M. over the midnight to 7:00 A.M. TIB window. Sam thought that a 6:30 wake time would work well, because his wife was already up by then and could wake him up, and they could have coffee together. He explained that up until now she had been waiting for him to get up, but that it would work well if she woke him up at 6:30. He also thought that if he got into the shower right after his coffee, it would help him to stay out of bed.

## Becoming More Active during the Day

Next, the therapist discussed strategies for staying awake and increasing activity during the day. Using an interactive style, the therapist reiterated that being active during the day contributes to a stronger sleep drive. The therapist again capitalized on Sam's interest in pain reduction and explained the connection between inactivity and pain, conveying the following points:

1. Being inactive can lead to shortening of muscles. When muscles are used less, they shorten, and when the muscles are shortened, it becomes easier to strain them when people are trying to be active.
2. Being inactive also leads to getting out of shape. When this happens, people often feel even more achy and tired.
3. Resting also cuts people off from doing the things that make them feel good. In Sam's case, resting was preventing him from playing with his grandkids.

Through this discussion, Sam understood that the very thing he was trying to protect himself from—his pain—was more likely to happen if he continued to rest too much.

The therapist then worked with Sam to create a schedule of activities that could help him maintain wakefulness, factoring in his need to rest, while encouraging him to slowly increase his daytime activity level. The plan was for him to shorten his rest periods to 30-minute segments, to avoid reclining when resting, and to set up daily out-of-the-house activities in the afternoon. Sam said that he had a friend who was retired, and that they liked to go to a model train club together. The therapist encouraged Sam to do this and other activities he enjoyed, but at the same time to pace himself and not try to do too much too soon. They also discussed ways to minimize the likelihood that Sam would doze off in the evening. Sam planned to ask his wife to wake him up whenever she noticed him dozing off.

## Naps

Sam was not lying down for naps. His daytime sleep was unintentional and consisted primarily of dozing, but it added up to an average of 25 minutes a day. Sam understood that dozing and napping could be detrimental to his sleep at night, but he was concerned that he might not be able to stay awake during the day. The therapist suggested that he could consider a planned early (i.e., before lunch) and short (up to 30 minutes) nap. They agreed that Sam would lie down before lunch for 30 minutes and set an alarm to make sure it was not longer. Whereas napping could reduce Sam's sleep drive, planning for a short nap early in the day had several advantages that outweighed the potential negative effect on Sam's sleep drive. Most importantly, a short early nap could prevent later dozing and give him more energy for the rest of the day, thus facilitating Sam's adherence with the TIB recommendations. He was also reminded that he should take a brief safety nap in situations in which involuntarily dozing would be dangerous. The therapist posed the recommendation as an experiment, both because during the first session Sam said he couldn't nap (referring to planned naps), and because naps are not always restorative. The therapist planned to check with Sam during the following session as to how this experiment went, and to use the results to inform treatment recommendations moving forward.

## Caffeine

The therapist explained that caffeine interferes with the buildup of the chemical (adenosine) needed for deep sleep. The therapist also explained that high levels of caffeine consumption can paradoxically contribute to fatigue, because when the effects of the last dose of caffeine decrease, there is a rebound in fatigue (similar to other rebound phenomena discussed in this book). Sam agreed to drink only decaffeinated coffee in the afternoon. This would allow him to reduce his overall caffeine consumption and limit it to the morning, while at the same time preserving his routine of having afternoon coffee with his wife.

## Adherence to CPAP Therapy

The therapist reminded Sam about the relationship between sleep apnea and next-day sleepiness and fatigue, and encouraged him to put the CPAP mask back on in the middle of the night (when he woke and realized he was no longer wearing it), which he had not been doing. The therapist emphasized that this might take a while to get used to, adding that initially Sam might sleep a little less—but that eventually, if he persisted, his sleep drive would get stronger, and he would sleep better and have more energy during the day.

The therapist did not introduce stimulus control during Session 2, despite the original plan to do so. As the session unfolded, the therapist thought that additional instructions would dilute the focus on the more important recommendation to restrict the time Sam spent in bed at night and resting during the day. The therapist decided to wait to introduce stimulus control until the next session. At the end of the session, the therapist asked Sam to summarize what they agreed he would be doing until the next session, making sure Sam was committed to following through. The therapist reminded Sam to continue to complete the sleep diary every morning. Here is a summary of Sam's homework.

- Ask your wife to wake you up every morning at 6:30 A.M.; get out of bed within 5–10 minutes to have coffee with her; get into shower immediately after morning coffee.

- Do not go to bed before 11:30 P.M.

- Be more active during the day in order to avoid dozing, because dozing will reduce the sleep drive.

  - Limit rest periods to at most 30 minutes, and avoid reclining when resting
  - Have grandchildren visit three times a week for a short time.
  - Go with friend to the model train club.

- Experiment with taking a scheduled morning nap. Put an alarm to make sure the nap does not exceed 30 minutes.

- Ask your wife to make sure you do not doze in the evening while watching TV.

- Use CPAP all night. Note in the "Comments" section of the sleep diary how many hours CPAP was used each night.

- Drink only decaffeinated coffee after lunch.

## SESSION 3

### Before Session

The therapist's plan for the third session was to review progress based on Sam's sleep diary and ISI; assess his sense of progress and changes in his levels of daytime sleepiness and fatigue; identify and troubleshoot adherence problems; and make necessary adjustments to the recommendations already given (e.g., TIB). The therapist also planned to introduce stimulus control and explicitly discuss conditioned arousal and a few cognitive factors, as time permitted. Some cognitive factors were indirectly addressed in Session 2, including beliefs about the relationship between sleep and pain. The plan for addressing cognitive factors in this session was to present a more explicit conceptualization of sleep effort and how thinking about sleep in particular ways can become a problem. The completed Session Plan for Sam's Session 3 is shown in Figure 12.8.

### Session Plan

**ID/Name:** _Sam_                **Date:** _December 3, 2013_          **Session #:** _3_

- Assess experience of following the treatment recommendations (including sleepiness, adherence with the recommended TIB, CPAP use, caffeine use, and activity plan).

- Review sleep diary data, and note relationship between adherence and progress; check on napping and dozing.

- Ask if there is anything Sam would like to make sure we discuss today (agenda).

- Introduce stimulus control.

- Discuss the role of thinking about sleep and sleep effort, including sleeping in a different bedroom from spouse.

**Homework:**

- Complete sleep diary forms.

- Continue with TIB, CPAP, and caffeine use recommendations.

- Follow stimulus control recommendations.

- Continue to increase activity levels during the day (e.g., increase play dates with grandkids, with scheduled breaks).

**Notes:**

**FIGURE 12.8.** Session Plan form as completed by the therapist for Sam's Session 3.

## During Session

### Sleep Diary Review

Sam came to his third session 2 weeks after Session 2 and brought his completed sleep diary forms, which revealed that he had generally good adherence with the recommended TIB and that his sleep was gradually improving. On the second of the 2 weeks between sessions, he spent an average of about 7 hours, 15 minutes in bed (his prescription was 7 hours). His average TST increased from 5 hours to 5 hours, 50 minutes. His average SE increased from 51% to 80%. Sam's average sleep onset latency was 55 minutes (20 minutes less than it was the week before Session 2), and his average time awake in the middle of the night decreased substantially, from about 1 hour to 15 minutes. The number of hours he used the CPAP mask increased gradually, so that toward the end of the second week he was using it all night.

### Adjusting the Session Plan

With 80% SE, the therapist planned to follow the sleep restriction protocol and keep Sam's TIB the same, unless daytime sleepiness levels indicated otherwise. Noting that his sleep onset latency was still over 30 minutes, and encouraged by the levels of adherence to the recommended TIB and CPAP use, the therapist planned to discuss stimulus control with Sam in today's session, with a focus on the initial sleep onset period. Because Sam was now waking up and getting out of bed at regular times, the therapist decided there was no longer a need to discuss the circadian clock with Sam (as in the original plan).

### Review of Progress and Adherence

Sam said that it was initially difficult to get up in the morning, but it was nice to have coffee with his wife, and this kept him working toward this goal. He also said that his wife had been "keeping me honest" about dozing in the evening, but she'd had to do less of it in the past few evenings. He did not experiment with taking short naps before lunch, because he wanted to do everything he could to get deep sleep at night. He was still reporting dozing on weekdays, mainly in the afternoon just before his wife got home from work. He said he kept himself busier during most of the day, but then in the late afternoon he would lie down on the couch. He had no difficulties reducing his caffeine intake, although sometimes he had a headache and wondered if it was because of the switch to decaffeinated coffee in the afternoon. Sam said that overall he was pleased with his progress, but that he continued to feel tired and that it still took "too long" to fall asleep. The therapist celebrated the progress with Sam and expressed delight that he was now using the CPAP mask all night. Sam and the therapist discussed the relationship between his progress and his excellent adherence, and moved on to address his remaining problem with sleep initiation.

### Stimulus Control

The therapist explained conditioned arousal and its contribution to Sam's difficulty in falling asleep. The therapist noted that Sam had already taken important steps to help create a good association between his bed and sleep, including the fact that because he was sleeping better he was no longer lying in bed awake and frustrated in the middle of the night, and that he was now waking up at the same time every day. The focus of this discussion was therefore on Sam's sleep initiation difficulties. The therapist recommended that Sam get up and go to a different room when he could not initiate sleep, and that he stay there until he felt sleepy enough to fall asleep quickly and then return to bed. Together, they discussed what Sam should do when out of bed. He decided to read a magazine he reads regularly. (As Sam was not spending time in bed outside of his attempted sleep periods, this aspect of stimulus control did not need to be addressed.)

### Adjustment to Sleep Restriction

Sam's TIB remained the same.

### Addressing Cognitive Factors

THERAPIST: I'd like to ask about your sleeping in a separate bedroom from your wife. Is this something you and your wife would like to continue?

*Demonstration of cognitive therapy.*

SAM: No, but I don't have any other choice because of her snoring.

THERAPIST: So you would like to sleep together, but you worry that her snoring would wake you up?

SAM: Yes. It's sad we're apart. It upsets my wife, too. She was OK with my snoring, and she is OK with the CPAP. We just talked about it last week.

THERAPIST: Do you sleep better apart?

SAM: I am not sure any more. But when I was sharing a bed with her, I'd be lying there awake in the middle of the night. Sometimes I could hear her snore, and I wondered if her snoring had woken me up.

THERAPIST: Sounds like you think that sleep needs to be approached with extreme caution. You are trying to remove anything that could upset the balance.

SAM: Well . . . yes.

THERAPIST: I wonder what this says about your confidence as a sleeper.

SAM: I am the world's worst sleeper, so I don't think confidence is the issue. No one would feel confident about sleeping if they slept like me.

THERAPIST: From what you have shared with me so far, you have put a lot of effort into improving your sleep—doing things like reducing activities that you enjoy, and spending a lot of time tracking your sleep. Unfortunately, it doesn't look like your efforts are being rewarded with your desired "payoff" of more sleep. Why do you think this is?

SAM: That's right. It's depressing. But last week I started doing a little more.

THERAPIST: Yes, you did. In some ways you have been putting a little less effort into sleeping, and you have been sleeping more. Why do you think that is?

SAM: I can't say I know.

THERAPIST: Let's take an analogy of falling in love. Falling asleep is like falling in love. You can set the stage, by being in places where you are likely to meet someone who shares your interests and values, but you can't make falling in love happen. In fact, the more you try to force it, the more impossible it is. The same applies to sleep: You can set the stage, but you cannot force it. Setting the stage for good sleep involves following good sleep habits, being more active during the day, and using the CPAP.

SAM: I think that last week I set a better stage than before.

THERAPIST: Yes. That's true. And you also put in less effort to fall asleep. The next step is to accept the ebb and flow of sleep and put in even less effort. Simply allow sleep to unfold.

SAM: I have pain, and obviously my sleep system is impaired, so it sounds like you want me to just accept that I am a poor sleeper?

THERAPIST: Let's take a look at how your sleep quality has changed. Let's compare your sleep diary summary from the last 2 weeks again to the summary from the previous two weeks. What do you notice about your sleep efficiency?

SAM: It increased from 50 to 80%.

THERAPIST: This is a remarkable improvement. And you kept the sleep medication the same, so the medication is probably not what made the difference. All that changed was setting a better stage for your body to sleep better, and what happened? You slept better.

SAM: Can it get even better?

THERAPIST: We can expect it to improve even more, but I think that you have lacked confidence that your body would take care of your sleep, if the stage is set correctly. As a result, you have experienced performance anxiety when you go to bed.

SAM: That's right.

THERAPIST: And performance anxiety can interfere with performance—in this case, falling asleep quickly. It gets in the way. Are you a little more confident after our discussion today, and now that you have seen some progress?

SAM: I am encouraged, but I cannot say I am confident yet.

THERAPIST: Hopefully, as you see even more progress, you will be able to step back a little more and trust your healthy sleep system to do its job. With more confidence, you will also be better able to take the inevitable occasional sleep setbacks in stride.

SAM: I think you are right. But I am not there yet.

THERAPIST: One way we can work on this is to look for behaviors that suggest low sleep confidence and do the opposite. For example, do you think a good sleeper would sleep separately from his wife if the two of them actually wanted to sleep in the same bed?

SAM: Probably not, but a good sleeper would sleep through his wife's snoring anyway, and if he woke up because of her snoring, he would be able to get back to sleep quickly anyway.

THERAPIST: You are already sleeping better. Do you think this could be a possibility for you?

SAM: I'm a little better, but I am not a good sleeper yet.

THERAPIST: Good point. Is it possible that one of the things in your way is your anxiety about potential sleep disrupters? How did you use to feel when you noticed your wife snoring beside you?

SAM: I was upset. I kept thinking that I was never going to fall asleep that night.

THERAPIST: What would happen if you reminded yourself that sleeping less builds your sleep drive?

SAM: I see your point. I guess I am a little worked up over it.

THERAPIST: Do you think that being worked up about sleep has a negative impact on your sleep?

SAM: For sure. OK, so you want me to move back to my bedroom so that I can act more confident about my sleep?

THERAPIST: Do you think you are telling yourself, "My sleep system is too fragile to handle sleeping with my wife"?

SAM: Well, not directly, of course, but I guess that this is what I have been telling myself.

THERAPIST: I think you can think of moving back to sleep with your wife as an experiment that will test if your sleep is really that fragile.

SAM: I can do that.

THERAPIST: Good. Meanwhile, you should continue to follow the guidelines for setting the stage for good sleep, which we have already discussed. This means that if you are wide awake in bed for any reason, including because she is snoring, you leave the room until you are calm and sleepy.

SAM: I am nervous about it, but thinking about it as an experiment for just a week helps. She only snores sometimes. It will not be that bad. It would be nice to be in our bed again. I will give it a shot.

THERAPIST: There is something else that you lost because you have had little sleep confidence. You seem to have lost confidence that you can cope with less than ideal sleep, and have therefore stopped doing things you enjoy.

SAM: My grandkids, right? Yes, that bothers me. I just feel so tired, they wear me out. But last week they visited three times, and it was OK. They have a lot of energy—definitely more than I do. But they did not stay long, and I was not watching them. My daughter came too, and it was OK.

THERAPIST: I wonder if you could experiment this week with one visit where you actually do watch them for a short time. Are there quiet activities you could get them involved in that would not drain you?

SAM: Oh, sure. Maybe reading them a story or putting a movie on. I could definitely do this. This is my favorite homework so far (*smiles*).

THERAPIST: Glad to hear it.

The following is a summary of Sam's homework:

- Return to sleeping in your own bedroom with your wife (as an experiment).
- Continue with the 11:30 P.M. to 6:30 A.M. TIB window.
- If unable to sleep, get out of bed until sleepy again.
- Continue to use CPAP all night.
- Ask your wife to continue to make sure you do not doze in the evening, if needed.
- Continue to limit rest periods to at most 30 minutes, and avoid reclining when resting
- Continue to increase time with grandchildren, including one visit without your daughter.
- Continue to drink only decaffeinated coffee after lunch.

# SESSION 4

## Before Session

The therapist reviewed Sam's sleep diary data before the session. His adherence with TIB was excellent, and his average SE in the past week had increased to 91%, which warranted a discussion to decide whether the TIB prescription should be altered. The average time it took Sam to fall asleep had increased from 55 minutes the week before the last session to almost 80 minutes the next week and then decreased, so that in the past week he fell asleep on average within 35 minutes. Most nights he fell asleep in less than 30 minutes, but one night it took him an hour to fall asleep. He did not nap at all and noted dozing on only one day. The "Comments" section of his diary revealed that he continued to use CPAP all night. The therapist completed the Session Plan form for Session 4 as shown in Figure 12.9.

## During Session

Sam reported to the therapist that he felt "pretty good" about his sleep. In the last week he had been spending less time resting, had more energy, and only dozed off on one day. Sam beamed as he talked about the experiment with his grandkids. He said that scheduling the quieter activities for when he was caring for them alone had worked well, and he felt ready for the next challenge. He talked with his daughter and decided to have them over and help with child care three afternoons a week.

Sam said he continued to enjoy spending time with his wife in the morning. He had moved back into their bedroom to sleep with her, but noted that he had trouble falling asleep because he was still very tense about whether or not she would snore. He realized it did get better, but he continued to feel apprehensive. He said that at first he had not gotten out of bed when he had difficulty sleeping because he forgot about it, but after a few days he had talked to his wife and she reminded him. The therapist then reflected on Sam's overall experience and discussed the relationship between improvement in his sleep and changes in his thoughts and behaviors.

### Adjustment to Sleep Restriction

Sam's SE was above the 85% threshold for increasing TIB. His energy had improved, and his dozing had lessened. The therapist thus proposed extending Sam's TIB, but he was reluctant to do so because he was afraid to "jinx it." The therapist thought that Sam would benefit from TIB

## Session Plan

**ID/Name:** _Sam_ **Date:** _December 16, 2013_ **Session #:** _4_

- Review plan for the session in broad terms; ask if there is anything Sam wants to make sure we discuss.

- Check in on homework: TIB plan; stimulus control; moving into bedroom with wife; increasing activity in afternoon; dozing; activity level during the day, including scheduling paced visit with grandkids.

- Review sleep diary data, including CPAP adherence.

- Assess sleepiness, and whether an adjustment to the schedule is necessary.

**Homework:**

- Complete sleep diary forms.

- Continue with TIB, CPAP, and caffeine use recommendations.

- Follow stimulus control recommendations.

- Continue to increase activity levels during the day (e.g., increase play dates with grandkids, with scheduled breaks).

**Notes:**

---

**FIGURE 12.9.** Session Plan form as completed by the therapist for Sam's Session 4.

extension because he still had some dozing and because the therapist wanted to help Sam view sleep as less fragile. Encouraged by Sam's engagement in, and success with, previous behavioral experiments, the therapist proposed that he try extending sleep for the next week, and then evaluate how he was sleeping and decide whether he wanted to revert to the current sleep schedule. Sam agreed to this plan. The therapist taught Sam how to calculate his SE, and told him how to decide after a week whether a change back to his current schedule was indicated. Because Sam liked his new morning routine, he decided that he would extend his TIB by going to bed 15 minutes earlier. The specific decision was that Sam would go to bed at 11:15 P.M. and still wake up at 6:30 A.M. After a week, if his SE fell below 85%, he would revert to the 11:30 P.M. to 6:30 A.M. schedule that was working so well now. The therapist added that if his SE was above 85% at the end of the next week, he could consider going to bed another 15 minutes earlier, if he wished. Sam was committed to doing this. Now that Sam was no longer sleepy, the therapist emphasized the importance of going to bed only when sleepy. In other words, Sam was to consider 11:15 as his earliest possible bedtime; if he was not sleepy at 11:15, he would wait until he was sleepy and go to bed later.

The following is a summary of Sam's homework:

- The new TIB window is 11:15 P.M. to 6:30 A.M. After a week, consider alteration to TIB as follows: If SE is <85%, revert to old schedule; if it is ≥85%, decide whether to stay on the same schedule or go to bed 15 minutes earlier.
- Go to bed only when sleepy; If unable to sleep, get out of bed until sleepy again.
- Continue to sleep in your own bedroom with your wife.
- Continue to use CPAP all night.
- Do not nap, except in situations where safety dictates.
- Continue to increase activities during the day, but remember to pace activity level (avoid over- or underdoing).
- Continue to drink only decaffeinated coffee after lunch.

# SESSION 5

The therapist's plan for the fifth session was to assess Sam's progress and adherence, address any remaining maladaptive cognitions, and discuss any other topics that he might bring up. Sam came to this session excited about his progress. He had made his own calculations with the sleep diary data after a week and decided he was doing fine. He did not extend his TIB further, but he said he decided to try sleeping without zolpidem. He said he was a bit scared but his wife encouraged him, reminding him that the zolpidem was probably not doing much anyway. He was happy to report that she was right, and that in the past 5 nights he had been sleeping OK without any medication. His SE for the past week was down a little (87%), but he was happy with being off the medication. The therapist reflected understanding of the difficulty in sleeping without a medication Sam had relied on for so long, and noted that 87% was still good SE. The therapist also took the opportunity to explain tolerance and psychological dependence.

THERAPIST: What made you decide to discontinue the zolpidem?

*Demonstration of education about sleep medications.*

SAM: I think it was not really helping me that much any more.

THERAPIST: I am hearing you say that at some point in the past it did help you.

SAM: It did. At the beginning, it helped a lot. It just gradually worked less. I started with 5 mg, and then I started taking one and a half pills, and it helped. I was always afraid to take more.

THERAPIST: You also said you were afraid to take less. But you just stopped.

SAM: I am glad I did. It was my wife really who started me thinking. I told her that you keep reminding me that the reason I sleep better has nothing to do with zolpidem, because I have not increased it. She asked if I was planning to stop. That was all I needed. I was ready.

THERAPIST: It is not unusual for people to build tolerance for sleep medication. Their bodies adjust to it, and the medication loses its potency. Usually people respond by increasing the dose.

SAM: I did that.

THERAPIST: Yes, by a little. I know people who increase even more.

SAM: I was afraid to increase, but I was also afraid to decrease.

THERAPIST: Have you tried before?

SAM: Yes.

THERAPIST: And what happened?

SAM: I was not very successful. After being up for 4 hours, I took it.

THERAPIST: This is a common experience. You said that last week when you stopped, you had a few nights with worse sleep.

SAM: Yes, but it was not that bad, so I kept going. I kept thinking about how my sleep drive must be getting stronger.

THERAPIST: It sounds like you have gained confidence in your sleep during this process.

*Demonstration of cognitive therapy targeting sleep self-efficacy.*

SAM: I have. I was less confident about the medication helping any more.

THERAPIST: It is interesting how much our confidence matters. But your confidence was based on some evidence. You knew how to set the stage.

SAM: Exactly.

The therapist was impressed by the obvious reduction in Sam's anxieties about sleep and his increase in self-efficacy. Encouraged by these changes and by Sam's progress, the therapist entertained the idea of termination—but eventually decided that, given Sam's history, it would be best to see whether the improvements would be stable before termination was considered. In preparation for possible termination in the next session, the therapist asked Sam to write down what had helped him sleep better, and to bring his notes to the next session. Sam's other homework was to continue following the current recommendations and not to use zolpidem.

## SESSION 6

In the final session, the therapist planned to check on Sam's progress, discuss goal attainment, and review Sam's notes about what had helped him as a basis for developing a relapse prevention plan. Together, Sam and the therapist made the calculations based on the sleep diary data and discussed how the new schedule was working. Sam's improvement seemed stable. He did not feel he needed more sleep, and he was not experiencing daytime sleepiness, dozing, or excessive fatigue. He continued to use CPAP nightly for the entire night, and reported that sleeping with his wife was no longer an issue. He and his wife were both glad to be spending more time together. On average, he fell asleep within 20 minutes at night, and his SE was 89%. He reported that he was very pleased with his sleep, and joked that he was "not afraid to say that I'm sleeping well out loud." Sam and his therapist agreed to keep the new schedule steady. He was pleased that he could be more active again and was planning to continue helping his daughter with child care. The therapist read out loud the treatment goals that Sam stated at the end of his first visit: "Sleep more; get rid of my pain; and not feel sleepy during the day so that I can spend more time with my grandchildren." Sam said that he was definitely sleeping more and was spending more time with his grandchildren. He was also pleased that he was less sleepy during the day, but was unsure whether his pain had improved. The therapist asked Sam to reflect on his original conditioned statement about the relationship between his pain level and ability to spend more time with his grandchildren. The discussion was brief. Sam said that one of the things he realized during treatment was that low energy was a greater obstacle to his spending more time with his grandchildren than any sleep difficulties he was experiencing, and that spending the day resting was not helpful or a good idea for maintaining good sleep patterns.

Sam completed a relapse prevention plan with the therapist in session, based on his list of the things that had helped him improve his sleep. His completed Strategies for Dealing with Insomnia in the Future form (see Appendix C for the blank version) is shown in Figure 12.10. Sam thought that what had helped him most were limiting his TIB and using CPAP the whole night. He said that learning about the sleep drive was also very helpful, and that as he started sleeping better, he had gained confidence in his sleep. As the therapist and Sam discussed what had contributed to his progress, it was clear that Sam's beliefs about sleep had changed and normalized. As in Sophie's case, the therapist provided guidelines for relaxing some of the "rules" (guidelines for good sleep). However, they both agreed that the most important rule for Sam to continue to follow was to avoid overreacting to setbacks, just as he was able to do when he took it upon himself to discontinue the zolpidem.

## REFLECTIONS ON SAM'S TREATMENT

- Issues of undertreated OSAH and daytime sleepiness influenced Sam's treatment planning and implementation.

  - Consultation with the sleep specialist supported the decision to proceed with CBT-I and emphasized the importance of close monitoring of daytime sleepiness and improving adherence to CPAP use.
  - Sleep compression was used instead of sleep restriction therapy. The initial recommended TIB took into account Sam's daytime sleepiness and his sleep per 24 hours, rather than nocturnal sleep alone.
  - Although no napping is a stimulus control instruction, the therapist responded to Sam's concern that he would not be able to stay awake all day by suggesting that he experiment with taking a planned short nap before lunch. The therapist's flexibility alleviated Sam's concern, even though, in the end, he did not nap anyway.
  - Naps are always encouraged if there is a question of safety.

- Fibromyalgia also influenced Sam's treatment.

  - To promote adherence to sleep restriction therapy, the therapist spent time explaining the relationship between the sleep drive and muscle pain.

## Strategies for Dealing with Insomnia in the Future

Check off the strategies below that helped you improve your sleep. Remember that it is normal to have an occasional night of poor sleep. However, if you notice that your sleep has worsened for several nights in a row, you can help restore your good sleep with the same strategies that helped you improve your sleep during treatment.

☑ Keeping the same rise time every day (no matter how much sleep I get)

☑ Going to bed when sleepy

☑ Getting out of bed when unable to sleep

☐ Creating a 1-hour buffer zone period before bedtime

☐ Getting out of bed if I am worrying or cannot shut off my thoughts

☐ Engaging in worrying or problem solving earlier in the evening

☑ Limiting the amount of time in bed at night (based on monitoring sleep for 2 weeks and following the time-in-bed restriction guidelines)

☐ Not using the bed for anything other than sleeping (and sex) only

☑ No napping (except for safety)

☑ Not canceling activities after a night of poor sleep

☑ Trying not to have caffeine or alcohol, smoke cigarettes, or engage in exercise within a few hours of bedtime

☑ Anything else that helped: *Remember that trying to sleep and being afraid of what will happen if I do not sleep only makes it harder to sleep. Use CPAP all night every night (it helps with my energy level). Have regular visits with the sleep clinic to make sure CPAP treatment is still working and get adjustments that may be needed (for example, if there is a leak in the mask).*

If these do not help, schedule a refresher session.

**Remember not to get alarmed.**

**Everyone has a bad night's sleep once in a while.**

**If you have a few bad nights in a row,
keep in mind that you mastered the insomnia before,
and you'll master it again.**

---

**FIGURE 12.10.** Strategies for Dealing with Insomnia in the Future form as completed by Sam.

- To promote stronger sleep drive, the therapist also explained the detrimental effects of inactivity on pain.
- The therapist helped Sam understand the distinction between rest and sleep, and recommended short rest periods that did not involve reclining.

- Unhelpful cognitions were addressed. These included Sam's beliefs that had previously led to a reduction in playing with his grandchildren (e.g., low confidence that he could cope with less than ideal sleep) and to his sleeping in a separate bedroom (e.g., belief in the fragility of sleep, catastrophic predictions).

- Behavioral experiments were used to help Sam increase his activity level and move back to sleeping in the same bed as his wife.

- Sam met ICSD-2 criteria for hypnotic-dependent insomnia (see Chapter 1). Discontinuation of the hypnotic (zolpidem) was not one of his initially stated treatment goals. The therapist pointed out that his use of medication had not changed while his sleep had improved, in order to help Sam correctly attribute his improvement to changes he made in his behaviors and cognitions. Sam spontaneously discontinued sleep medication successfully.

# CHAPTER 13

# General Delivery Issues

We conclude this book with a discussion of practical clinical issues related to the implementation of CBT-I. We discuss ways to integrate CBT-I with ongoing concurrent therapies, as well as collaboration with other treatment providers (sleep specialists, prescribing physicians and other therapists). We also discuss modes of delivery other than individual therapy: group treatment, as well as emerging Internet technologies and smartphone applications that can aid clinicians and patients. Additional resources for further training and development as a CBT-I provider are included in Appendix D.

## DELIVERING CBT-I AS A STAND-ALONE TREATMENT OR INTEGRATED WITH OTHER THERAPIES

CBT-I has been empirically tested as a stand-alone therapy for patients who sought care specifically to help resolve their insomnia. These patients either responded to recruitment advertisement for research on the treatment of insomnia or presented in a clinic with an explicit request to get help for their insomnia. In such cases as these, the therapist and patient agree that the focus of treatment will be insomnia. Some clinicians reading this book may be interested in dedicating a portion of their caseload to the treatment of insomnia. Others may be planning to use CBT-I as a means for helping patients who are seeking treatment for other presenting problems, but also experience difficulties sleeping. By definition, sleep difficulties will be categorized as insomnia disorder only if they are associated with clinically meaningful impairment or distress. At any point during therapy at which a patient requests help with resolving a sleep issue, the therapist and patient need to prioritize treatment goals. When improving sleep becomes a mutually agreed-upon focus of treatment, the therapist can initiate CBT-I. The first step is to assign completion of a sleep diary and set the expectation that the next few sessions will be dedicated entirely (or mostly) to the insomnia.

There are no published guidelines on when and how to best fold CBT-I into ongoing therapy for other issues. The recommendations below are based on our combined clinical experiences and our observations from training other clinicians to administer CBT-I. The first full CBT-I session is dedicated to a thorough insomnia intake interview and a review of completed sleep diary forms (see Chapter 6). Although a therapist initiating CBT-I in this context may have worked with a patient for a while, and even though the patient may have mentioned poor sleep for quite some time, it is unlikely that the wealth of information about the patient's sleep that can be obtain during an insomnia intake interview is already available to the therapist. At the end of the information gathering, the therapist elicits treatment goals and helps the patient operationalize and prioritize them. After the insomnia assessment, the therapist is ready to complete the Case Conceptualization Form, integrating information gathered during the focused insomnia assessment with salient general clinical features (such as an anxious response to other life stressors or a tendency to worry and/or ruminate). The therapist then follows the treatment planning process outlined in Chapter 10 and begins treatment.

As discussed in Chapter 10, CBT-I usually works best when the frequency of sessions is biweekly. This is because 1 week of sleep diary data may not provide an accurate enough impression of sleep (because there is night-to-night variability in insomnia symptoms), and because 2 weeks are sometimes needed before adherence to treatment recommendations translates into sustained improvement. Conducting CBT-I biweekly can help in the integration of CBT-I with ongoing therapy for other issues; that is, every other session is dedicated to CBT-I, and the other weekly sessions are focused on non-sleep-related issues. However, for patients who respond with heightened anxiety or apprehension upon hearing the CBT-I guidelines, weekly CBT-I may be needed in order to support small gains and allow time for working through obstacles to adherence.

Our experience argues against splitting sessions (i.e., dedicating part of each session to insomnia and the other part to other issues). Even seasoned CBT-I therapists find it difficult to manage time effectively when splitting the sessions in this manner. The first two CBT-I sessions in particular should not be split. The first session should be dedicated to a comprehensive insomnia assessment; the second insomnia-focused session is the first treatment session, in which the behavioral components of CBT-I are introduced. Both sleep restriction and stimulus control recommendations are counterintuitive. Unless a proper rationale is provided, patient "buy-in," and hence benefits, will be compromised. A full session is needed to allow ample time for a detailed discussion of the recommendations and obstacles to following them consistently, because otherwise adherence is likely to be suboptimal. If a subsequent session is split, it should begin with agenda setting: The therapist checks whether the patient wants to discuss non-sleep-related issues and, together with the patient, decides how much of the session to dedicate to CBT-I. The insomnia-focused portion of the session should always begin with a review of the sleep diary, progress, and adherence, and end with clear homework instructions. Adjustments to the time in bed are considered, according to the sleep restriction protocol (Chapter 7), and new CBT-I components are introduced as needed and as time permits.

## COLLABORATION WITH OTHER CLINICIANS

The treatment of insomnia often calls for collaboration with other treatment providers. We discuss here collaborations with sleep specialists when patients have (or may have) comorbid sleep disorders, consultation with prescribing providers regarding medication issues, and collaboration with therapists treating comorbid conditions.

## Collaboration with Sleep Specialists

In Chapter 4, we have discussed sleep disorders that are associated with difficulty falling or staying asleep. We have focused on sleep disorders that are particularly relevant to the implementation of CBT-I: circadian rhythm sleep–wake disorders, RLS, OSAH, and nightmare disorder. In Chapter 6, we have outlined an insomnia intake assessment that includes guidelines for assessing these disorders and making a differential diagnosis. In some cases, the presenting sleep complaint is caused by a sleep disorder other than insomnia disorder and therefore CBT-I is not indicated. When this is the case, the therapist should refer the patient to a sleep specialist for further assessment and treatment of the other sleep disorder.

In other cases, a sleep disorder other than insomnia disorder may be present as a comorbid condition. Sometimes the comorbid sleep disorder or its treatment may be contributing to the presenting sleep problem. For example, OSAH may cause brief arousals; insomnia disorder may make it difficult to fall back asleep. When both insomnia disorder and a comorbid sleep disorder contribute to the presenting sleep problem, it is usually best to treat both. Please see Chapter 10 for discussion of sequencing CBT-I with treatments of comorbid conditions. The best clinical management for a patient with a comorbid sleep disorder is to collaborate with a sleep specialist.

Perhaps the most common sleep disorder about which a CBT-I clinician is likely to consult or collaborate with a sleep specialist is OSAH. Recall that a diagnosis of OSAH is not a contraindication for CBT-I, but when severe daytime sleepiness is present, standard sleep restriction therapy should not be initiated. In Chapter 12, we describe how Sam had been referred to CBT-I by a sleep specialist a few years earlier, but he did not present to treatment right away. He had insomnia disorder and comorbid OSAH that was undertreated. (Sam was using CPAP every night, but only part of the night.) After the first session, in which the therapist conducted a comprehensive insomnia intake, the therapist consulted with the referring sleep specialist about the initiation of CBT-I, given that Sam's OSAH was not adequately treated and he was sleepy during the day, often dozing in front of the TV. The sleep specialist recommended proceeding with CBT-I, believing that insomnia might be contributing to Sam's incomplete adherence. The sleep specialist also recommended that the therapist encourage Sam to use CPAP all night.

In cases where the comprehensive insomnia intake suggests that previously undiagnosed OSAH might be present, the therapist refers the patient to a sleep specialist for further assessment and treatment of the comorbid sleep disorder. At this writing, there are no empirical guidelines for the best way to sequence CPAP use and CBT-I. These decisions are best made via collaboration between the clinicians treating the sleep apnea and the insomnia. Sometimes the decision may be to postpone CPAP initiation until the insomnia disorder is resolved. This option, which is only acceptable when OSAH is not severe, can facilitate the often difficult adjustment to CPAP therapy.

In cases where the patient has already started CPAP therapy but is not optimally adherent, the sleep physician may recommend initiating CBT-I and having the CBT-I therapist encourage and support full adherence to the CPAP therapy, as in Sam's case. Sometimes the sleep physician may decide to reduce the prescribed air pressure temporarily (or not use CPAP at all) during the time the patient receives CBT-I, and to increase the pressure (or restart CPAP use) after the insomnia disorder resolves. In this case, the CBT-I therapist will need to inform the sleep specialist when CBT-I ends or is discontinued. At other times, the sleep specialist may recommend postponing CBT-I until the patient consistently uses CPAP or pursues another treatment for OSAH (e.g., a dental device or surgery).

We recommend that clinicians who make the treatment of insomnia part of their practice establish a relationship with a sleep center in their geographic area. The American Academy of Sleep Medicine created a website to facilitate finding member sleep centers it has accredited (*www.sleepeducation.com/find-a-center*). This can facilitate finding affiliated sleep specialists as well. A list of behavioral sleep specialists in the United States can be found on the website of the American Board of Sleep Medicine (*www.absm.org/BSMSpecialists.aspx*).

## Consultation with Prescribing Providers Regarding Medication Issues

Whenever an issue arises about any prescribed medication a patient is taking, it is best to consult with the clinician who has prescribed this medication; however, if this is not possible, the therapist can discuss critical issues with the patient's current medical care provider or, if necessary, refer the patient to a prescribing provider. The therapist can discuss with the prescriber the possibility that a certain medication interferes with the patient's sleep (e.g., a stimulant) or causes carryover sedation (e.g., an antipsychotic medication or hypnotic with a long half-life). The prescriber may address the problem by changing the dose or the time of ingestion of the medication, or by switching to another medication.

### *Providing Support When Patients Want to Discontinue Sleep Medications*

Another common reason for consultation with prescribing clinicians is to help patients who, in the course of CBT-I, express a desire to discontinue a sleep medication. In such a case, the therapist recommends a supervised taper and refers the patient to the prescribing clinician. The consultation may include sharing the therapist's assessment of the patient's readiness and level of psychological dependence (see Chapter 1) and offering to support the patient during the medication taper. The taper process is more successful when insomnia is concomitantly addressed (see Belleville, Guay, Guay, & Morin, 2007).

Research has identified a few factors that may hinder discontinuation of a sleep medication, including psychological dependence and low self-efficacy regarding the ability to reduce medication use (Kirmil-Gray et al., 1985). Therapists can use cognitive therapy strategies to address these two psychological factors (see Chapter 12). Frequent (e.g., weekly) contact can help support patients, since it enables therapists to reinforce progress often and to work though setbacks. We describe below two tested strategies for gradually tapering hypnotic medications.

Kirmil-Gray et al. (1985) described a two-phase medication taper protocol that was provided along with information about good sleep hygiene practices. During the first phase, which lasted 1–2 weeks, patients were advised to take the same dose of a single medication nightly. If a patient took more than one medication or combined medication(s) with alcohol, a physician prescribed a single medication at a higher dose to replace other medications (or alcohol). If a patient used a single medication but only for a few nights each week, the recommendation was to take a lower dose of the medication every night. During the second phase, the single medication was reduced by one therapeutic dose every 1–2 weeks, with smaller decrements at the end of the taper process and when psychological dependence was judged to be high. Patients chose when within the 1- to 2-week period to begin dose reduction, but committed themselves to staying on that dose once reduction took place; that is, returning to the previous dose was proscribed. Patients were advised to call their therapists during regular office hours if they were tempted to revert to the higher dose. In such cases, they were provided with support and kept on the reduced dose until their sleep improved. Successful dose reductions were discussed with the therapists, who helped increase patients' self-efficacy through encouragement and attributed their success to their effort and persistence. The investigators identified the following aspects of the strategy as important to successful withdrawal, which was attained by all participants:

- Development of a written plan for medication withdrawal.
- Provision of education about good sleep practices to help maintain sleep during the withdrawal period.
- Regular, brief appointments and calls to check on progress and hold the patients accountable for medication reductions.
- Support and encouragement by the health care professionals.
- Completion of daily sleep and medication diaries.

The reader may be wondering why patients who had not been taking a sleep medication every night were advised to do so. Sleep medications are often prescribed with the instruction to use them as needed. During periods of acute stress, as-needed use can be helpful. However, some patients continue as-needed use of sleep medications most (or every) nights for years. They try to sleep without the medication, often because of ambivalence about taking sleeping aids, and then give up and take it anyway. As a result, the medication is used as a rescue after the patients have failed to sleep without it, thus reinforcing their belief that they cannot sleep without the medication and thus their development of psychological dependence. The recommendation in the Kirmil-Gray et al. (1985) study to use the medication noncontingently (i.e., every night at bedtime) was intended to help reduce psychological dependence by eliminating its use as a rescue.

Morin et al. (2004) used similar principles in a study of the efficacy of an intervention that combined CBT-I and a gradual taper for patients with hypnotic-dependent insomnia. These researchers found that adding CBT-I to a medically managed medication taper led to better outcomes, in terms of both reduction in medication use and (even more so) improved sleep. The medication taper schedule was individualized and followed the following principles:

- Patients who had been using more than one sleep medication were first stabilized on a single medication.
- Reduction in dose was gradual: The initial dose was reduced by 25% every 2 weeks until the lowest available dose was reached. When the lowest dose was reached, medication-free nights were introduced, and their number was gradually increased.
- As-needed use was replaced with scheduled hypnotic use. Examples of scheduled hypnotic use were (1) taking the medication at bedtime, rather than after first trying but failing

to fall asleep; and (2) taking the hypnotic on specific days of the week, rather than as a rescue when patients were desperate.*

- The patients' readiness to discontinue medication** influenced the individual scheduling of the taper. The presence of withdrawal symptoms triggered a slower withdrawal schedule.
- Support and encouragement to follow the withdrawal schedule were provided.

Both studies led to significant reductions in medication use that were largely sustained at follow-up. The addition of CBT-I led to better improvement in sleep than the addition of sleep hygiene information alone did (Morin et al., 2004). Importantly, greater insomnia severity at the end of treatment was a significant predictor of relapse (Morin, Belanger, Bastien, & Vallieres, 2005).

### Collaboration with Therapists Treating Comorbid Conditions

Earlier in this chapter, we have discussed meeting the challenges of integrating CBT-I with ongoing therapy for other presenting problems. Here we comment on the need to collaborate with therapists who may be working with patients on other issues, parallel to CBT-I. In such a case, the challenges for the CBT-I therapist are to delineate clearly to the patient the roles of the two therapists, and to remain focused on insomnia. Both therapists should be clear about this distinction and inform each other when the therapy may cross these boundaries. For instance, when treating a patient whose insomnia disorder is comorbid with depression, a CBT-I therapist often recommends that the patient engage in behavioral activation in the evening or in the morning. Behavioral activation is a component of CBT for depression, but is used in this case in order to enhance adherence with specific CBT-I recommendations, such as waking up and getting out of bed at the same time every morning. If the depression therapist is informed about this recommendation, he or she can integrate it into the depression treatment and provide support for adherence to the CBT-I recommendation.

## GROUP CBT-I

Although CBT-I was described in this book as an individual treatment, it can also be effective and have long-term benefits when delivered in a group modality (e.g., Backhaus, Hohagen, Voderholzer, & Riemann, 2001; Espie, Inglis, Tessier, & Harvey, 2001; Morin, Bootzin, et al., 2006; Morin, Hauri, et al., 1999). Studies that have directly compared individual to group CBT-I have largely found no significant differences in insomnia outcomes (Verbeek, Konings, Aldenkam, Declerck, & Klip, 2006). There are no clear guidelines for deciding which patients will do better in a group versus individual CBT-I. When both options are available in the same setting,

---

*These examples are based on the experience of one of us (Rachel Manber). The paper describing the protocol did not provide details as to what "scheduled hypnotic use" meant.

**Details of how this was done were not provided. We typically use motivational enhancement techniques in such cases.

general clinical judgment, patient preferences, and logistics are considered when making this decision.

Group CBT-I protocols are provided in a closed-group format with a fixed agenda for each session's content. Despite the fixed structure, treatment can—and, based on our clinical experience, should—be individualized to meet each participant's stated treatment goals. In order to deliver individually tailored recommendations for each group member, the therapist needs to have a clear case conceptualization of each group member's presentation. Therefore, an individual, comprehensive insomnia intake assessment has to be undertaken for each potential group member before the group begins. This individual assessment allows the therapist to determine whether contraindications are present and to make referrals as needed. In addition to the contraindications that have already been discussed in Chapter 10, the therapist needs to consider contraindications for group therapy, such as the complexity of the particular case and potential disruptions to a group dynamic.

The need for multiple case conceptualizations makes the administration of CBT-I in groups much more difficult to conduct than individual administration. We recommend that clinicians obtain adequate experience with individual CBT-I and have exposure to multiple presentations of insomnia disorder before delivering CBT-I in a group format. Another challenge of group delivery with individualized recommendations is the need to provide individualized rationales, particularly when group members receive seemingly contradictory recommendations. For example, one group member may be asked to adhere to a standard sleep restriction protocol, while another may be allowed less strict guidelines, such as sleep compression. It is therefore helpful to orient group members to the individualized nature of the intervention; in our experience, patients appreciate and like this aspect of treatment. There is also the technical challenge involved in reviewing sleep diary data and computing the average total sleep time for each participant. One way to meet this challenge is to ask patients to send their completed sleep diary forms to the clinician ahead of time. Another way is to have an assistant or co-facilitator make the computations during the session.

Despite these implementation challenges, group CBT-I has a few advantages beyond being cost-effective. When group dynamics are collaborative and respectful, group members often support each other's adherence. For example, a low-adherence group member may become more motivated when another, more adherent group member reports that adherence became easier over time or that it led to improved sleep. Group members also help each other overcome obstacles to adherence and reinforce each other's successes. In our experience, when during the final group session we discuss what aspects of treatment were particularly helpful, the exchanging of input among group members is frequently rated as very helpful.

Group sessions can last from 60 to 90 minutes, depending on group size, presence of co-facilitators, and therapists' preferences. Group CBT-I is distinct from sleep education groups, which usually provide basic sleep hygiene information and may sometimes also include stimulus control instructions. Table 13.1 is a session-by-session outline for a six-session group CBT-I protocol.

Delivering CBT-I in groups requires a high volume of patients, so that treatment is not delayed for too long while patients are waiting for a group to start. This may not be an issue for clinicians working in a sleep center or in a large health care system. In such a facility, having a list of group start dates and a waiting list for each facilitates group formation.

**TABLE 13.1. A Session-by-Session Outline for a Six-Session Group CBT-I Protocol**

*Session 1:* Have group members, including the facilitator(s), introduce themselves; establish guidelines for a respectful and supportive environment; discuss limits of confidentiality; describe efficacy of CBT-I; provide sleep education and instructions for use of the sleep diary.

*Session 2:* Introduce stimulus control and sleep restriction rationale and guidelines. Ideally, present the rationale to the whole group, and then ask each member to think how this would apply to him or her. Next, discuss the implementation with each individual group member, relying on a case conceptualization form and the most recent sleep diary, and collaborating with the patient.

*Session 3:* Review the sleep diary and progress of each participant; address adherence and alter times in bed as needed; introduce counterarousal skills; encourage group discussion of obstacles and how to overcome them; use cognitive therapy techniques as needed.

*Sessions 4–5:* Review the sleep diary and progress of each participant; address adherence and alter times in bed as needed; encourage group discussion of obstacles and how to overcome them; use cognitive therapy techniques as needed.

*Session 6:* Dedicate this session to relapse prevention and planning for continued care, as discussed in Chapter 10. Conduct a general discussion of the inevitability of a few bad nights in the future and the challenge of preventing the few bad nights from becoming a full-blown insomnia episode, and encourage a group discussion of components that helped. Review the sleep diary and progress of each participant; address adherence; alter times in bed as needed; and identify the most relevant individual relapse prevention and continued care guidelines.

# USE OF CBT-I-LIKE EMERGING TECHNOLOGIES

At this writing, there is a tremendous growth in the number of sleep-focused technologies. These include smartphone apps and devices, as well as Internet-based resources marketed as aids to help people improve their sleep. Given the dynamic nature of the market, we have decided not to describe or endorse any specific technology. Instead, we want to say a few words about some challenges that are involved when a patient seeking CBT-I for insomnia uses sleep-enhancing technologies.

The developers of sleep-enhancing technologies are usually careful to avoid claims of providing treatment. Nonetheless, patients with insomnia disorder are often drawn to these technologies, hoping to derive therapeutic benefits. Below we discuss a few issues to be aware of.

## Monitoring Devices

Devices that claim to distinguish reliably between sleep and wakefulness states are sometimes attractive to patients with insomnia disorder, but often they are not accurate or not helpful. For example, such a device could provide an additional tool for anxious monitoring for sleep-related threat, which, as discussed in Chapter 8, is often detrimental to sleep. That said, some patients with insomnia disorder underestimate the amount of time they are sleeping, and they may be reassured when the objective feedback about how much sleep was obtained on a given night proves them wrong. For them, the realization that they are sleeping more than they thought provides a relief and reduces their sleep effort.

## Self-Help Phone Apps and Internet CBT-I-Based Programs

Research has established some efficacy for self-help for insomnia, whether it is provided via old (e.g., books, educational pamphlets) or new (e.g., Internet programs and smartphone apps) technologies (Bjorvatn, Fiske, & Pallesen, 2011; Jernelov et al., 2012; Katofsky et al., 2012; Lancee, van den Bout, van Straten, & Spoormaker, 2012; Morin, Beaulieu-Bonneau, LeBlanc, & Savard, 2005; Rybarczyk, Mack, Harris, & Stepanski, 2011; van Straten & Cuijpers, 2009). Patients who have previously tried to use a self-help approach, and later seek CBT-I from a therapist, tend to do so because they were not fully successful with self-help. This may mean that they have already tried to implement one or more of the recommendations that the CBT-I therapist will make. Therefore, during the initial insomnia intake interview, the therapist's assessment of past treatment has to go deep into the details of specific guidelines that were followed, and to determine how consistently they were followed. It is important for the therapist to explain to the patient how their work together will differ from the self-help approach, and to describe reasons why the patient may still benefit. For example, sometimes either combining a previously adhered-to guideline with other guidelines, or adding cognitive therapy strategies to address preoccupation with sleep, sleep effort, and safety behaviors, leads to better outcomes. In addition, if adherence has been inconsistent, the therapist may identify and work through obstacles to adherence.

Devices and Internet-assisted CBT-I programs can also be used as adjuncts to therapy. At this writing, researchers are examining the utility, efficacy, and cost-effectiveness of various technologies used to assist therapists in the delivery of CBT-I.

## CONCLUSION

CBT-I is an efficacious and effective treatment of insomnia for adults of different ages, even when there are comorbid medical and psychiatric conditions. Program evaluation of a large nationwide dissemination of CBT-I in the VA health care system (see Manber et al., 2012, for a description of the VA CBT-I protocol) has demonstrated that CBT-I can be taught to licensed mental health professionals from a variety of disciplines, including clinical social workers, mental health nurses, psychiatrists, and psychologists. Published data collected in the course of evaluating the training program reveal not only that clinically and statistically significant improvement in insomnia occurs, but that benefits extend beyond insomnia and include reduced depression severity, improved quality of life, and reduced suicidal ideation (Karlin et al., 2013; Trockel et al., in press). Results also underscore the importance of patients' adherence to the CBT-I guidelines. One salient and important component of the CBT-I training program at the VA is the availability of ongoing consultation and feedback, based on review of recorded therapy sessions. Research on the efficacy of training clinicians how to deliver a specific therapy shows that neither reading training materials nor attending a workshop alone is sufficient for establishing sustained competency in a newly learned therapy (McHugh & Barlow, 2010; Miller, Yahne, Moyers, Martinez, & Pirritano, 2004). We therefore strongly recommend that readers supplement the knowledge they gain from reading this book with hands-on consultation/supervision form experts in the field, ideally under conditions that allow the consultants access to work samples.

Despite years of experience in using CBT-I to treat insomnia, we continue to learn from the challenges that our patients present to us. The flexible approach to the implementation of CBT-I was inspired by these challenges, and we hope that it will help our readers meet these challenges with their own patients. Good therapeutic alliance has been repeatedly shown to be important to patient outcomes in various forms of therapy, and it is no less important in CBT-I. In fact, in the context of CBT-I, better therapeutic alliance leads to better patient adherence with CBT-I and to better outcomes (Trockel, Karlin, Taylor, & Manber, 2014). We therefore remind our readers that good general psychotherapeutic principles are as important in CBT-I as in any other type of treatment.

This book has provided step-by-step guidance in how to provide CBT-I in a flexible, patient-tailored manner. Relying on a solid understanding of sleep regulation and models of insomnia, and using the case formulation approach contained in this book, a treatment provider can deliver this targeted brief intervention and adapt it to each patient's unique needs. We believe that such an individualized approach is essential, particularly when insomnia is experienced in the context of other conditions. With the help of this book and solid general clinical skills, we hope that clinicians reading this book will help their adult patients improve their sleep and maintain good sleep for many years.

# Therapist Tools

# Insomnia Intake Form

| | | |
|---|---|---|
| **Patient name:** | **Marital/partnered status:** | **Referral source:** |
| **Gender:** | **Children:** | |
| **Date of birth or age:** | **Occupation:** | |

**NATURE OF PRESENTING PROBLEM** (check all that apply, and identify the most distressing/disturbing sleep problem):

☐ Difficulty initiating sleep          ☐ Difficulty maintaining sleep

☐ Waking up too early          ☐ Difficulty waking up          ☐ Nonrefreshing sleep

Number of nights per week sleep problem is experienced: _____ to _____

When did the current episode start? _____
_____

Identifiable precipitating factor(s): _____
_____
_____

Treatment history for current episode: _____
_____
_____
_____

## DAYTIME EFFECTS

☐ Energy/fatigue          ☐ Concentration/functioning          ☐ Mood

☐ Daytime sleepiness: _____

Other (specify): _____

## HISTORY

Age at onset of first insomnia episode: _____          Lifetime course: _____
_____
_____

Family history of insomnia: _____
_____
_____
_____

*(cont.)*

**Sleep habits** (focus on previous or most recent typical week; describe range when indicated; note weekday/ weekend times, if different):

## BEGINNING OF SLEEP PERIOD

Time into bed: _____

Time turning lights out (or intent to sleep): _____

How does patient decide when to go to bed? _____

Pre-bedtime activities: _____     ☐ Fears     ☐ Dozing off in evening

Average time to fall asleep: _____

What happens when patient cannot get to sleep (thoughts/behaviors)? _____

_____

☐ Rumination            ☐ General worry            ☐ Sleep worry            ☐ Physical tension

## MIDDLE OF THE NIGHT

Number of awakenings after sleep onset: _____ to _____

Total time awake after sleep onset: _____ to _____

What happens when awake in the middle of the night (thoughts/behaviors)? _____

_____

☐ Rumination            ☐ General worry            ☐ Sleep worry            ☐ Physical tension

## END OF THE NIGHT

Final wake time: _____          Time out of bed: _____

Alarm (or other wake-up system): ☐ No ☐ Yes _____

Is final awakening earlier than planned? ☐ No ☐ Yes, by _____ minutes

_____

Difficulties waking up at intended time: ☐ No ☐ Yes _____

Estimated average total sleep time: _____

**PREMORBID SLEEP SCHEDULE:** _____

**CURRENT SLEEP MEDICATION(S)/AIDS:**  ☐ No ☐ Yes (If yes, then complete table below.)

| Name | Dose | When taken? | How long? | Helpful? |
|------|------|-------------|-----------|----------|

(cont.)

# Insomnia Intake Form (p. 3 of 4)

## NAPPING

Able to nap if given an opportunity? ☐ No ☐ Yes _____

Nap frequency _____ Nap duration _____

Timing of nap _____

## SLEEP ENVIRONMENT (note problematic aspects of sleep environment—bed partner, caregiving, pets, sound, lights, safety, temperature):

_____

_____

## OTHER BEHAVIORS THAT CAN AFFECT SLEEP (include time and frequency; for substances, also include amount):

Caffeine _____ Nicotine _____

Alcohol _____ Recreational drugs _____

Timing of vigorous exercise _____ Nocturnal eating _____

Overall activity level: ☐ Understimulated ☐ Overstimulated

Other: _____

_____

_____

## NOTES ON COGNITIVE HYPERAROUSAL

_____

_____

_____

## NOTES ON EMOTIONAL AROUSAL

_____

_____

## CIRCADIAN TENDENCIES

☐ Morning type          ☐ Neither type          ☐ Evening type

Evidence: _____

*(cont.)*

# Insomnia Intake Form (p. 4 of 4)

---

Use the **Assessment of Other Sleep Disorders** form to evaluate other sleep disorders, and note results here.

## CIRCADIAN RHYTHM SLEEP–WAKE DISORDERS

☐ Does not meet criteria ☐ Meets criteria Type: ☐ Advanced ☐ Delayed

## OBSTRUCTIVE SLEEP APNEA HYPOPNEA (OSAH)

☐ Previously diagnosed Severity _____ events per hour _____

☐ Not previously diagnosed ☐ Suspected ☐ Not suspected

Treatment: ☐ Not or inadequately treated ☐ Adequately treated Specify treatment:_____

## RESTLESS LEGS SYNDROME (RLS)

☐ Does not meet criteria ☐ Meets criteria Treatment: _____

## PARASOMNIA SYMPTOMS (include frequency):

Nightmare disorder: ☐ Meets criteria ☐ Does not meet criteria

Other unusual behaviors during sleep: _____

_____

_____

_____

---

**CURRENT COMORBID MEDICAL DISORDERS** (note impact on sleep, include treatment): _____

_____

_____

_____

**CURRENT COMORBID PSYCHIATRIC DISORDERS** (note impact on sleep, include treatment): _____

_____

_____

_____

**GOAL(S):** _____

_____

_____

_____

_____

_____

# Assessment of Other Sleep Disorders

| SLEEP COMPLAINT | NOTES |
|---|---|
| **Circadian rhythm sleep–wake disorder, delayed sleep phase type**<br><br>1. Recurrent inability to fall asleep at a desired conventional clock time, and difficulty awakening at a desired and socially acceptable time.<br><br>2. When allowed to use preferred schedule, no problem with sleep except its delayed timing.<br><br>3. Preferred schedule delayed more than 2 hours relative to desired conventional clock.<br><br>If criteria 1, 2, and 3 are met, refer patient to a sleep center for assessment and treatment. (Treatment will probably involve schedule manipulation and properly timed light and dark exposures.) | |
| **Circadian rhythm sleep–wake disorder, advanced sleep phase type**<br><br>1. Recurrent inability to stay awake until a desired conventional clock time, and difficulty staying asleep in the morning until a desired and socially acceptable time.<br><br>2. When allowed to use preferred schedule, no problem with sleep except its advanced timing.<br><br>3. Preferred schedule advanced more than 2 hours relative to desired conventional clock.<br><br>If criteria 1, 2, and 3 are met, refer patient to a sleep center for assessment and treatment. (Treatment will probably involve schedule manipulation and properly timed light and dark exposures.) | |
| **Obstructive sleep apnea hypopnea (OSAH)**<br><br>1. Does patient report:<br>  ☐ snoring that can be heard through a closed door, or as loud as a conversation?<br>  ☐ gasping/choking during sleep?<br>  ☐ stopping breathing during sleep?<br>  ☐ poor, unrefreshing sleep even after adequate sleep time?<br><br>2. Does the patient report:<br>  ☐ morning headaches?<br>  ☐ urinating more than twice per night?<br>  ☐ dry mouth upon awakening?   ☐ hypertension?<br>  ☐ BMI > 30 (BMI = body mass index = weight in kilograms divided by height in meters)? | |

*(cont.)*

| SLEEP COMPLAINT | NOTES |
|---|---|
| **Obstructive sleep apnea hypopnea (OSAH)** (*cont.*) <br><br> 3. Is excessive daytime sleepiness present? Is there a recurrent pattern of falling asleep unintentionally or struggling to stay awake when in any one of the following situations: <br><br> ☐ Talking with others?    ☐ Driving? <br><br> ☐ Talking on the phone?    ☐ Standing? <br><br> ☐ Other activities or situations in which most people will not fall asleep? <br><br> If the patient has two or more symptoms in 1, or one symptom in 1 and one in 2, or one item in 1 and excessive daytime sleepiness, refer for evaluation of possible OSAH. <br><br> If the patient does not have co-occurring OSAH or if OSAH is adequately treated (to be determined in consultation with a sleep specialist), proceed with CBT-I. (See Chapter 7 for safety issues related to daytime sleepiness.) | |
| **Restless legs syndrome (RLS)** <br><br> Does the patient have a very strong urge to move legs? (If it is associated with unpleasant sensations in the legs, ask the patient to describe the sensations.) <br><br> 1. Does the urge occur or worsen in evening or during rest or inactivity? <br><br> 2. Is the urge temporarily relieved by moving? <br><br> 3. Does the urge interfere with falling asleep or returning to sleep? <br><br> If urge is present and the answer is yes to 1, 2, and 3, then a referral for evaluation and possible pharmacological treatment of RLS is warranted. <br><br> If RLS symptoms do not regularly interfere with the onset of sleep at the beginning or middle of night, proceed with CBT-I. | |
| **Nightmare disorder** <br><br> 1. Does the patient report recurrent nightmares (a nightmare is defined as a dream that has *all* of the features below)? <br><br> • An elaborate narrative is remembered. <br> • Evokes very strong negative emotion. <br> • Occurs in second half of night. <br> • No confusion upon waking. <br><br> 2. Is there clinically meaningful distress or impairment? <br><br> Yes answers to questions 1 and 2 indicate a diagnosis of nightmare disorder, unless the nightmares are induced by substance use or explained by another disorder. <br><br> If all nocturnal symptoms of insomnia are caused by nightmares (e.g., prolonged sleep onset because of fear of nightmares or all awakenings are related to nightmares), then CBT-I is not warranted. (See Chapters 7 and 10 for more information about nightmare-related issues.) | |

# Case Conceptualization Form

**Note to Clinicians:** Please note that certain factors could load on more than one of these six domains. In such cases, list the factor in the row corresponding to the domain that is most relevant to the case.

| Domains | Patient-specific factors that contribute to insomnia or may interfere with adherence |
|---|---|
| **1.** *Sleep drive:* What factors may be weakening the patient's sleep drive? Consider extended time in bed, dozing off in the evening, daytime napping, sedentary life, and so on. | |
| **2.** *Biological clock:* What biological clock factors are relevant to the patient's presentation? Consider irregular wake and/or out-of-bed time, time-in-bed window that is not congruent with the patient's chronotype, and so on. | |
| **3.** *Arousal:* What manifestations of hyperarousal are evident? Consider the following:<br><br>**3a.** *Cognitive arousal related to sleep* (e.g., sleep effort, safety behaviors, and maladaptive beliefs/attitudes about sleep).<br><br>**3b.** *General hyperarousal affecting sleep* (e.g., worry in bed about life stressors).<br><br>**3c.** *Conditioned arousal:* Has the bed become associated with arousal rather than sleep? Specify predisposing factors (e.g., high trait anxiety), precipitating factors (e.g., stressful life events), and maintaining factors (.e.g., extended time spent in bed). | |

*(cont.)*

# Case Conceptualization Form (p. 2 of 2)

| Domains | Patient-specific factors that contribute to insomnia or may interfere with adherence |
|---|---|
| **4.** *Unhealthy sleep behaviors:* What unhealthy sleep behaviors are present? Consider caffeine, alcohol, nocturnal eating, timing of exercise, and other factors. | |
| **5.** *Medications:* What medications may be having an impact on the patient's sleep/sleepiness? Consider carryover effects, tolerance, and psychological dependence. | |
| **6.** *Comorbidities:* What comorbidities may be affecting the patient's sleep, and how? Consider sleep, medical, and psychiatric conditions (e.g., difficult adjustment to CPAP treatment for sleep apnea; pain interfering with sleep; PTSD-related hypervigilance). | |
| **7.** *Other*: Consider sleep environment, caregiving duties at night, life phase sleep issues, mental status, and readiness for change. | |

# Treatment Planning Form

**Patient's treatment goal(s):** _____

_____

| First treatment session (enter items in the order you plan to introduce them) | | | |
|---|---|---|---|
| **Factors to address** | **CBT-I components** | **Specific recommendations** | **Comments** |
| | | | |
| | | | |
| | | | |

| Subsequent sessions (enter items in the order you plan to introduce them) | | | |
|---|---|---|---|
| **Factors to address** | **CBT-I components** | **Specific recommendations** | **Comments** |
| | | | |
| | | | |

# Session Plan

**ID/Name:** _____     **Date:** _____     **Session #:** _____

**Homework:**

**Notes**:

# Patient Assessment Forms

# Consensus Sleep Diary–M Instructions

## GENERAL INSTRUCTIONS

**What is a sleep diary?** A sleep diary is designed to gather information about your daily sleep pattern.

**How often and when do I fill out the sleep diary?** It is necessary for you to complete your sleep diary *every day*. If possible, the sleep diary should be completed within 1 hour of getting out of bed in the morning.

**What should I do if I miss a day?** If you forget to fill in the diary or are unable to finish it, leave the diary blank for that day.

**What if something unusual affects my sleep or how I feel in the daytime?** If your sleep or daytime functioning is affected by some unusual event (such as an illness or an emergency), you may make brief notes on your diary.

**What do the words *bed* and *day* mean on the diary?** This diary can be used for people who are awake or asleep at unusual times and places. In the sleep diary, the word *day* is the time when you choose or are required to be awake. The term *bed* means the place where you usually sleep.

**Will answering these questions about my sleep keep me awake?** This is not usually a problem. You should not worry about giving exact times, and you should not watch the clock. Just give your best estimate.

## SLEEP DIARY ITEM INSTRUCTIONS

Use the guide below to clarify what is being asked for each item of the sleep diary.

*Date:* Write the date of the morning you are filling out the diary.

1. *What time did you get into bed?* Write the time that you got into bed. This may not be the time you began "trying" to fall asleep.

2. *What time did you try to go to sleep?* Record the time that you began "trying" to fall asleep.

3. *How long did it take you to fall asleep?* Beginning at the time you wrote in question 2, how long did it take you to fall asleep?

4. *How many times did you wake up, not counting your final awakening?* How many times did you wake up between the time you first fell asleep and your final awakening?

5. *In total, how long did these awakenings last?* What was the total time you were awake between the time you first fell asleep and your final awakening. For example, if you woke 3 times for 20 minutes, 35 minutes, and 15 minutes, add them all up (20 + 35 + 15 = 70 minutes, or 1 hour, 10 minutes).

6a. *What time was your final awakening?* Record the last time you woke up in the morning.

6b. *After your final awakening, how long did you spend in bed trying to sleep?* After the last time you woke up (question 6a), how many minutes did you spend in bed trying to sleep? For example, if you woke up at 8 A.M. but continued to try to sleep until 9 A.M., record "1 hour."

*(cont.)*

**6c.** *Did you wake up earlier than you planned?* If you woke up or were awakened earlier than you planned, answer "Yes." If you woke up at your planned time, check "No."

**6d.** *If yes, how much earlier?* If you answered "Yes" to question 6c, write the number of minutes you woke up earlier than you had planned on waking up. For example, if you woke up 15 minutes before the alarm went off, record "15 minutes" here.

**7.** *What time did you get out of bed for the day?* What time did you get out of bed with no further attempt at sleeping? This may be different from your final awakening time (for example, you woke up at 6:35 A.M. but did not get out of bed to start your day until 7:20 A.M.).

**8.** *How would you rate the quality of your sleep?* Sleep quality is your sense of whether your sleep was good or poor.

**9.** *How rested or refreshed did you feel when you woke up for the day?* This refers to how you felt after you were done sleeping for the night, during the first few minutes that you were awake.

**10a.** *How many times did you nap or doze?* A *nap* is a time you decided to sleep during the day, whether or not you were in bed. *Dozing* is a time you may have nodded off for a few minutes, without meaning to, such as while watching TV. Count all the times you napped or dozed, at any time from when you first got out of bed in the morning until you got into bed again at night.

**10b.** *In total, how long did you nap or doze?* Estimate the total amount of time you spent napping or dozing, in hours and minutes. For instance, if you napped twice, once for 30 minutes and once for 60 minutes, and dozed for 10 minutes, you would answer "1 hour, 40 minutes." If you did not nap or doze, write "N/A" (not applicable).

**11a.** *How many drinks containing alcohol did you have?* Enter the number of alcoholic drinks you had; 1 drink is defined as 12 ounces of beer, 5 ounces of wine, or 1.5 ounces of hard liquor (one shot).

**11b.** *What time was your last drink?* If you had an alcoholic drink yesterday, enter the time of day in hours and minutes of your last drink. If you did not have a drink, write "N/A" (not applicable).

**12a.** *How many caffeinated drinks (coffee, tea, soda, energy drinks) did you have?* Enter the number of caffeinated drinks (coffee, tea, soda, energy drinks) you had. For coffee and tea, one drink = 6–8 ounces; for caffeinated soda, one drink = 12 ounces.

**12b.** *What time was your last caffeinated drink?* If you had a caffeinated drink, enter the time of day in hours and minutes of your last drink. If you did not have a caffeinated drink, write "N/A" (not applicable).

**13.** *Did you take any over-the-counter or prescription medication(s) to help you sleep? If so, list medication(s), dose, and time taken:* For *each* different medication you took to help you sleep, list the medication's name, how much of it you took, and when you took it. Include medications available over the counter, prescription medications, and herbals (example: "Sleepwell 50 mg 11 pm"). If every night is the same, write "Same" after the first day

**14.** *Comments (if applicable):* If you have anything that you would like to say that is relevant to your sleep, feel free to write it here.

# Consensus Sleep Diary–M

**Please complete upon awakening.**                    ID/Name: _____

| | Sunday | | | | | | |
|---|---|---|---|---|---|---|---|
| Today's date | *Sunday* | | | | | | |
| **1.** What time did you get into bed? | *10:15 P.M.* | | | | | | |
| **2.** What time did you try to go to sleep? | *11:30 P.M.* | | | | | | |
| **3.** How long did it take you to fall asleep? | *55 min.* | | | | | | |
| **4.** How many times did you wake up, not counting your final awakening? | *6 times* | | | | | | |
| **5.** In total, how long did these awakenings last? | *2 hours, 5 min.* | | | | | | |
| **6a.** What time was your final awakening? | *6:35 A.M.* | | | | | | |
| **6b.** After your final awakening, how long did you spend in bed trying to sleep? | *45 min.* | | | | | | |

(cont.)

| Today's date | Sunday | | | | | | |
|---|---|---|---|---|---|---|---|
| **6c.** Did you wake up earlier than you planned? | ☑ Yes ☐ No | ☐ Yes ☐ No | ☐ Yes ☐ No | ☐ Yes ☐ No | ☐ Yes ☐ No | ☐ Yes ☐ No | ☐ Yes ☐ No |
| **6d.** If yes, how much earlier? | 1 hour | | | | | | |
| **7.** What time did you get out of bed for the day? | 7:20 A.M. | | | | | | |
| **8.** How would you rate the quality of your sleep? | ☐ Very poor<br>☑ Poor<br>☐ Fair<br>☐ Good<br>☐ Very good | ☐ Very poor<br>☐ Poor<br>☐ Fair<br>☐ Good<br>☐ Very good | ☐ Very poor<br>☐ Poor<br>☐ Fair<br>☐ Good<br>☐ Very good | ☐ Very poor<br>☐ Poor<br>☐ Fair<br>☐ Good<br>☐ Very good | ☐ Very poor<br>☐ Poor<br>☐ Fair<br>☐ Good<br>☐ Very good | ☐ Very poor<br>☐ Poor<br>☐ Fair<br>☐ Good<br>☐ Very good | ☐ Very poor<br>☐ Poor<br>☐ Fair<br>☐ Good<br>☐ Very good |
| **9.** How rested or refreshed did you feel when you woke up for the day? | ☐ Not at all rested<br>☑ Slightly rested<br>☐ Somewhat rested<br>☐ Well rested<br>☐ Very well rested | ☐ Not at all rested<br>☐ Slightly rested<br>☐ Somewhat rested<br>☐ Well rested<br>☐ Very well rested | ☐ Not at all rested<br>☐ Slightly rested<br>☐ Somewhat rested<br>☐ Well rested<br>☐ Very well rested | ☐ Not at all rested<br>☐ Slightly rested<br>☐ Somewhat rested<br>☐ Well rested<br>☐ Very well rested | ☐ Not at all rested<br>☐ Slightly rested<br>☐ Somewhat rested<br>☐ Well rested<br>☐ Very well rested | ☐ Not at all rested<br>☐ Slightly rested<br>☐ Somewhat rested<br>☐ Well rested<br>☐ Very well rested | ☐ Not at all rested<br>☐ Slightly rested<br>☐ Somewhat rested<br>☐ Well rested<br>☐ Very well rested |
| Therapist's notes | | | | | | | |
| **10a.** How many times did you nap or doze? | 2 times | | | | | | |

(cont.)

# Consensus Sleep Diary–M (p. 3 of 3)

| | Sunday | | | | | | |
|---|---|---|---|---|---|---|---|
| Today's date | | | | | | | |
| **10b.** In total, how long did you nap or doze? | 1 hour, 10 min | | | | | | |
| **11a.** How many drinks containing alcohol did you have? | 3 drinks | | | | | | |
| **11b.** What time was your last drink? | 9:20 P.M. | | | | | | |
| **12a.** How many caffeinated drinks (coffee, tea, soda, energy drinks) did you have? | 2 drinks | | | | | | |
| **12b.** What time was your last drink? | 3:00 P.M. | | | | | | |
| **13.** Did you take any over-the-counter or prescription medication(s) to help you sleep? | ☑ Yes ☐ No Medication(s): Relaxo–Herb Dose: 50 mg | ☐ Yes ☐ No Medication(s): Dose: | ☐ Yes ☐ No Medication(s): Dose: | ☐ Yes ☐ No Medication(s): Dose: | ☐ Yes ☐ No Medication(s): Dose: | ☐ Yes ☐ No Medication(s): Dose: | ☐ Yes ☐ No Medication(s): Dose: |
| If so, list medication(s), dose, and time taken. | Time(s) taken: 11 pm | Time(s) taken: | Time(s) taken: | Time(s) taken: | Time(s) taken: | Time(s) taken: | Time(s) taken: |
| **14.** Comments (if applicable) | I have a cold | | | | | | |

# Dysfunctional Beliefs and Attitudes about Sleep (DBAS-16)

Several statements reflecting people's beliefs and attitudes about sleep are listed below. Please indicate to what extent you personally agree or disagree with each statement. There is no right or wrong answer. For each statement, circle the number that corresponds to your own *personal belief*. Please respond to all items, even though some may not apply directly to your own situation.

| Strongly Disagree | | | | | | | | | | Strongly Agree |
|---|---|---|---|---|---|---|---|---|---|---|
| 0 | 1 | 2 | 3 | 4 | 5 | 6 | (7) | 8 | 9 | 10 |

1. I need 8 hours of sleep to feel refreshed and function well during the day.

| 0 | 1 | 2 | 3 | 4 | 5 | 6 | 7 | 8 | 9 | 10 |

2. When I don't get the proper amount of sleep on a given night, I need to catch up on the next day by napping or on the next night by sleeping longer.

| 0 | 1 | 2 | 3 | 4 | 5 | 6 | 7 | 8 | 9 | 10 |

3. I am concerned that chronic insomnia may have serious consequences on my physical health.

| 0 | 1 | 2 | 3 | 4 | 5 | 6 | 7 | 8 | 9 | 10 |

4. I am worried that I may lose control over my abilities to sleep.

| 0 | 1 | 2 | 3 | 4 | 5 | 6 | 7 | 8 | 9 | 10 |

5. After a poor night's sleep, I know it will interfere with my daily activities on the next day.

| 0 | 1 | 2 | 3 | 4 | 5 | 6 | 7 | 8 | 9 | 10 |

6. In order to be alert and function well during the day, I believe I would be better off taking a sleeping pill rather than having a poor night's sleep.

| 0 | 1 | 2 | 3 | 4 | 5 | 6 | 7 | 8 | 9 | 10 |

*(cont.)*

**7.** When I feel irritable, depressed, or anxious during the day, it is mostly because I did not sleep well the night before.

| 0 | 1 | 2 | 3 | 4 | 5 | 6 | 7 | 8 | 9 | 10 |

**8.** When I sleep poorly one night, I know it will disturb my sleep schedule for the whole week.

| 0 | 1 | 2 | 3 | 4 | 5 | 6 | 7 | 8 | 9 | 10 |

**9.** Without an adequate night's sleep, I can hardly function the next day.

| 0 | 1 | 2 | 3 | 4 | 5 | 6 | 7 | 8 | 9 | 10 |

**10.** I can't ever predict whether I'll have a good or poor night's sleep.

| 0 | 1 | 2 | 3 | 4 | 5 | 6 | 7 | 8 | 9 | 10 |

**11.** I have little ability to manage the negative consequences of disturbed sleep.

| 0 | 1 | 2 | 3 | 4 | 5 | 6 | 7 | 8 | 9 | 10 |

**12.** When I feel tired, have no energy, or just seem not to function well during the day, it is generally because I did not sleep well the night before.

| 0 | 1 | 2 | 3 | 4 | 5 | 6 | 7 | 8 | 9 | 10 |

**13.** I believe insomnia is essentially the result of a chemical imbalance.

| 0 | 1 | 2 | 3 | 4 | 5 | 6 | 7 | 8 | 9 | 10 |

**14.** I feel insomnia is ruining my ability to enjoy life and prevents me from doing what I want.

| 0 | 1 | 2 | 3 | 4 | 5 | 6 | 7 | 8 | 9 | 10 |

**15.** Medication is probably the only solution to sleeplessness.

| 0 | 1 | 2 | 3 | 4 | 5 | 6 | 7 | 8 | 9 | 10 |

**16.** I avoid or cancel obligations (social, family) after a poor night's sleep.

| 0 | 1 | 2 | 3 | 4 | 5 | 6 | 7 | 8 | 9 | 10 |

# Insomnia Severity Index (ISI)

**1.** Please rate the current (i.e., last 2 weeks) SEVERITY of your insomnia problem(s):

|  | None | Mild | Moderate | Severe | Very |
|---|---|---|---|---|---|
| Difficulty falling asleep: | 0 | 1 | 2 | 3 | 4 |
| Difficulty staying asleep: | 0 | 1 | 2 | 3 | 4 |
| Problem waking up too early: | 0 | 1 | 2 | 3 | 4 |

**2.** How SATISFIED/dissatisfied are you with your current sleep pattern?

| Very satisfied |  |  |  | Very dissatisfied |
|---|---|---|---|---|
| 0 | 1 | 2 | 3 | 4 |

**3.** To what extent do you consider your sleep problem to INTERFERE with your daily functioning (e.g., daytime fatigue, ability to function at work/daily chores, concentration, memory, mood, etc.)?

| Not at all interfering | A little | Somewhat | Much | Very much interfering |
|---|---|---|---|---|
| 0 | 1 | 2 | 3 | 4 |

**4.** How NOTICEABLE to others do you think your sleeping problem is in terms of impairing the quality of your life?

| Not at all noticeable | Barely | Somewhat | Much | Very much noticeable |
|---|---|---|---|---|
| 0 | 1 | 2 | 3 | 4 |

**5.** How WORRIED/distressed are you about your current sleep problem?

| Not at all | A little | Somewhat | Much | Very much |
|---|---|---|---|---|
| 0 | 1 | 2 | 3 | 4 |

# Patient Treatment Forms

# Combined Sleep Guidelines

1. Wake up at _____ every day (set an alarm), regardless of how much sleep you actually get, and get out of bed within a few minutes after your alarm rings.

2. Go to bed when you are sleepy (remember that being sleepy is different from being tired), *but not before* _____. (If you do not feel sleepy at this time, wait until you *do* feel sleepy.)

3. If you can't sleep, *stop trying*. Get up and do something calming, and return to bed only when you are sleepy again. When you lie in bed awake trying to sleep, wanting and hoping to go back to sleep, you are training yourself to be awake in bed.

4. Use the bed only for sleeping. Do not read, eat, watch TV, etc. in bed. Sex is an exception. The most important activity to eliminate from the bed is the activity of "trying to sleep," because it inevitably interferes with the natural sleep process.

5. Avoid daytime napping—but if you believe that sleepiness compromises your safety, do take a nap.

# Buffer Zone Activities

- Read magazines, short stories, books (not suspenseful or upsetting material).

- Engage in pleasant (nonstressful) conversation.

- Prepare for next day:
  - Choose clothes that you can wear for work or school the next day.
  - Make tomorrow's lunch.
  - Marinate or otherwise start to prepare food for dinner the following day, and store it in the refrigerator.

- Take a bath or long shower.

- Surf the Internet (nonstressful or exciting topics only).

- Watch movies or episodes of television shows that you haven't seen in a long time (no action films).

- Play solitaire with cards (noncompetitively).

- Take the dog for a walk.

- Groom your pets.

- Listen to relaxing music.

- Work on photo albums or scrapbooks.

- Write in your journal.

- Do some gentle muscle stretches.

- Meditate.

- Give yourself a pedicure, manicure, or facial.

- Do knitting, needlepoint, quilting, or other nonactivating crafts.

- Organize collections, closet, cupboard, etc.

# Thought Record

| Situation | Mood (intensity 0–100%) | Thoughts (underline the most emotionally charged thought) | Evidence *for* the underlined thought | Evidence *against* this thought | Adaptive/coping thoughts | Do you feel any differently? |
|---|---|---|---|---|---|---|
|  |  |  |  |  |  |  |

# Strategies for Dealing with Insomnia in the Future

Check off the strategies below that helped you improve your sleep. Remember that it is normal to have an occasional night of poor sleep. However, if you notice that your sleep has worsened for several nights in a row, you can help restore your good sleep with the same strategies that helped you improve your sleep during treatment.

☐ Keeping the same rise time every day (no matter how much sleep I get)

☐ Going to bed when sleepy

☐ Getting out of bed when unable to sleep

☐ Creating a 1-hour buffer zone period before bedtime

☐ Getting out of bed if I am worrying or cannot shut off my thoughts

☐ Engaging in worrying or problem solving earlier in the evening

☐ Limiting the amount of time in bed at night (based on monitoring sleep for 2 weeks and following the time-in-bed restriction guidelines)

☐ Not using the bed for anything other than sleeping (and sex) only

☐ No napping (except for safety)

☐ Not canceling activities after a night of poor sleep

☐ Trying not to have caffeine or alcohol, smoke cigarettes, or engage in exercise within a few hours of bedtime

☐ Anything else that helped: _____

If these do not help, schedule a refresher session.

**Remember not to become alarmed.**

**Everyone has a bad night's sleep once in a while.**

**If you have a few bad nights in a row,
keep in mind that you mastered the insomnia before,
and you'll master it again.**

# Further Training and Reading

Behavioral sleep medicine has become a subspecialty of both behavioral medicine and sleep medicine. The Society of Behavioral Sleep Medicine (*www.behavioralsleep.org*) is an organization that sets clinical and educational standards for comprehensive, empirically validated behavioral medical treatments for insomnia disorder and other sleep disorders. It has an annual meeting that provides an excellent opportunity for additional training in basic and advanced topics related to behavioral sleep medicine. Current certification in behavioral sleep medicine is managed by the American Board of Sleep Medicine (*www.absm.org*). The American Academy of Sleep Medicine sets the clinical standards for the fields of sleep medicine health care, education, and research by publishing Practice Parameters, Systematic Reviews, Clinical Guidelines, and Best Practice Guides. These excellent resources can be found online (*www.aasmnet.org/practiceguidelines.aspx*).

Clinicians can also seek informal training in sleep centers in their communities. Shadowing of patient care can help CBT-I clinicians who are not sleep specialists better understand issues faced by their patients who have comorbid sleep apnea. It is also a good idea to become versed in understanding sleep study reports.

## CBT-I BOOKS FOR CLINICIANS

Carney, C. E., & Edinger, J. D. (2010). *Insomnia and anxiety.* New York: Springer.

Edinger, J. D., & Carney, C. E. (2008). *Overcoming insomnia: A cognitive-behavioral therapy approach. Therapist guide.* New York: Oxford University Press.

Lichstein, K. L., & Morin, C. M. (Eds.). (2000). *Treatment of late-life insomnia.* Thousand Oaks, CA: Sage.

Morin, C. M., & Espie, C. A. (2003). *Insomnia: A clinician's guide to assessment and treatment.* New York: Springer.

Perlis, M. L., Jungquist, C., Smith, M. T., & Posner, D. (2005). *Cognitive behavioral treatment of insomnia: A session-by-session guide.* New York: Springer.

Perlis, M. L., & Lichstein, K. L. (2003). *Treating sleep disorders: Principles and practice of behavioral sleep medicine.* Hoboken, NJ: Wiley.

## SLEEP MEDICINE BOOKS

Kryger, M. H., Roth, T., & Dement, W. C. (2011). *Principles and practice of sleep medicine* (5th ed.). St. Louis, MO: Elsevier Saunders.

Morin, C. M., & Espie, C. (Eds.). (2012). *The Oxford handbook of sleep and sleep disorders*. New York: Oxford University Press.

## INSOMNIA SELF-HELP BOOKS

Carney, C. E., & Manber, R. (2009). *Quiet your mind and get to sleep: Solutions for insomnia in those with depression, anxiety, or chronic pain*. Oakland, CA: New Harbinger.

Edinger, J. D., & Carney, C. E. (2008). *Overcoming insomnia: A cognitive-behavioral therapy approach workbook*. New York: Oxford University Press.

Glovinsky, P., Spielman, A., & Spielman, A. (2006). *The insomnia answer: A personalized program for identifying and overcoming the three types of Insomnia*. New York: Penguin Books.

Hauri, P., & Linde, S. (1996). *No more sleepless nights: A proven program to conquer insomnia* (2nd ed.). New York: Wiley.

Morin, C. M. (1996). *Relief from insomnia: Getting the sleep of your dreams*. New York: Doubleday.

Silberman, S. A. (2008). *The insomnia workbook: A comprehensive guide to getting the sleep you need*. Oakland, CA: New Harbinger.

## REVIEW PAPERS

Garland, S. N., Johnson, J. A., Savard, J. Gehrman, P., Perlis, M. Carlson, L., & Campbell, T. (2014). Sleeping well with cancer: A systematic review of cognitive behavioral therapy for insomnia in cancer patients. *Journal of Neuropsychiatric Disease and Treatment, 10*, 1113–1124.

Morin, C. M., Bootzin, R. R., Buysse, D. J., Edinger, J. D., Espie, C. A., & Lichstein, K. L. (2006). Psychological and behavioral treatment of insomnia: Update of the recent evidence (1998–2004). *Sleep, 29*(11), 1398–1414.

Riemann, D., Spiegelhalder, K., Feige, B., Voderholzer, U., Berger, M., Perlis, M., & Nissen, N. (2010). The hyperarousal model of insomnia: A review of the concept and its evidence. *Sleep Medicine Reviews, 14*(1), 19–31.

Smith, M. T., Huang, M. I., & Manber, R. (2005). Cognitive behavior therapy for chronic insomnia occurring within the context of medical and psychiatric disorders. *Clinical Psychology Review, 25*, 559–592.

# References

Adan, A., & Natale, V. (2002). Gender differences in morningness–eveningness preference. *Chronobiology International, 19*(4), 709–720.

Adler, S., Carde, N., Kuo, T., Ong, J., & Manber, R. (2008). Use of and attitudes about sleep medications in a tertiary sleep clinic. *Sleep, 31*(Abstract Suppl.), A326.

Affleck, G., Urrows, S., Tennen, H., Higgins, P., & Abeles, M. (1996). Sequential daily relations of sleep, pain intensity, and attention to pain among women with fibromyalgia. *Pain, 68*(2–3), 363–368.

Agargun, M. Y., Kara, H., & Solmaz, M. (1997). Sleep disturbances and suicidal behavior in patients with major depression. *Journal of Clinical Psychiatry, 58*(6), 249–251.

Allen, R. P., Picchietti, D., Hening, W. A., Trenkwalder, C., Walters, A. S., & Montplaisi, J. (2003). Restless legs syndrome: Diagnostic criteria, special considerations, and epidemiology. A report from the Restless Legs Syndrome Diagnosis and Epidemiology Workshop at the National Institutes of Health. *Sleep Medicine, 4*(2), 101–119.

Allison, K. C., Stunkard, A. J., & Thier, S. L. (2004). *Overcoming night eating syndrome: A step-by-step guide to breaking the cycle.* Oakland, CA: New Harbinger.

Aloia, M. S., Arnedt, J. T., Davis, J. D., Riggs, R. L., & Byrd, D. (2004). Neuropsychological sequelae of obstructive sleep apnea–hypopnea syndrome: A critical review. *Journal of the International Neuropsychological Society, 10*(5), 772–785.

Aloia, M. S., Di Dio, L., Ilniczky, N., Perlis, M. L., Greenblatt, D. W., & Giles, D. E. (2001). Improving compliance with nasal CPAP and vigilance in older adults with OSAHS. *Sleep and Breathing, 5*(1), 13–21.

Aloia, M. S., Smith, K., Arnedt, J. T., Millman, R. P., Stanchina, M., Carlisle, C., et al. (2007). Brief behavioral therapies reduce early positive airway pressure discontinuation rates in sleep apnea syndrome: Preliminary findings. *Behavioral Sleep Medicine, 5*(2), 89–104.

Altena, E., Van Der Werf, Y. D., Strijers, R. L., & Van Someren, E. J. (2008). Sleep loss affects vigilance: Effects of chronic insomnia and sleep therapy. *Journal of Sleep Research, 17*(3), 335–343.

American Academy of Sleep Medicine. (2005). *International classification of sleep disorders: Diagnostic and coding manual* (2nd ed.). Westchester, IL: Author.

American Psychiatric Association. (2000). *Diagnostic and statistical manual of mental disorders* (4th ed., text rev.). Washington, DC: Author.

American Psychiatric Association. (2013). *Diagnostic and statistical manual of mental disorders* (5th ed.). Arlington, VA: Author.

Ancoli-Israel, S., & Roth, T. (1999). Characteristics of insomnia in the United States: Results of the 1991 National Sleep Foundation Survey. I. *Sleep, 22*(Suppl. 2), S347–S353.

Ansfield, M. E., Wegner, D. M., & Bowser, R. (1996). Ironic effects of sleep urgency. *Behaviour Research and Therapy, 34*(7), 523–531.

Archer, S. N., Robilliard, D. L., Skene, D. J., Smits, M., Williams, A., Arendt, J., et al. (2003). A length polymorphism in the circadian clock gene Per3 is linked to delayed sleep phase syndrome and extreme diurnal preference. *Sleep, 26*(4), 413–415.

Arendt, J. (1998). Melatonin and the pineal gland: Influence on mammalian seasonal and circadian physiology. *Reviews of Reproduction, 3*(1), 13–22.

Arnedt, J. T., Conroy, D. A., Armitage, R., & Brower, K. J. (2011). Cognitive-behavioral therapy for insomnia in alcohol dependent patients: A randomized controlled pilot trial . *Behaviour Research and Therapy, 49*(4), 227–233.

Arnedt, J. T., Conroy, D., Rutt, J., Aloia, M. S., Brower, K. J., & Armitage, R. (2007). An open trial of cognitive-behavioral treatment for insomnia comorbid with alcohol dependence. *Sleep Medicine, 8*(2), 176–180.

Arriaga, F., Lara, E., Matos-Pires, A., Cavaglia, F., & Bastos, L. (1995). Diagnostic relevance of sleep complaints in anxiety and mood disorders. *European Psychiatry, 10*(8), 386–390.

Ayalon, L., Borodkin, K., Dishon, L., Kanety, H., & Dagan, Y. (2007). Circadian rhythm sleep disorders following mild traumatic brain injury. *Neurology, 68*(14), 1136–1140.

Azad, N., Byszewski, A., Sarazin, F. F., McLean, W., & Koziarz, P. (2003). Hospitalized patients' preference in the treatment of insomnia: Pharmacological versus non-pharmacological. *Canadian Journal of Clinical Pharmacology, 10*(2), 89–92.

Babkoff, H., Weller, A., & Lavidor, M. (1996). A comparison of prospective and retrospective assessments of sleep. *Clinical Epidemiology, 49*(4), 455–460.

Backhaus, J., Hohagen, F., Voderholzer, U., & Riemann, D. (2001). Long-term effectiveness of a short-term cognitive-behavioral group treatment for primary insomnia. *European Archives of Psychiatry and Clinical Neuroscience, 251*(1), 35–41.

Baglioni, C., Battagliese, G., Feige, B., Spiegelhalder, K., Nissen, C., Voderholzer, U., et al. (2011). Insomnia as a predictor of depression: A meta-analytic evaluation of longitudinal epidemiological studies. *Journal of Affective Disorders, 135*(1–3), 10–19.

Barrett, J., Lack, L., & Morris, M. (1993). The sleep-evoked decrease of body temperature. *Sleep, 16*(2), 93–99.

Bartlett, D. J., Marshall, N. S., Williams, A., & Grunstein, R. R. (2008). Predictors of primary medical care consultation for sleep disorders. *Sleep Medicine, 9*(8), 857–864.

Basheer, R., Strecker, R. E., Thakkar, M. M., & McCarley, R. W. (2004). Adenosine and sleep–wake regulation. *Progress in Neurobiology, 73*(6), 379–396.

Bastien, C. H., Vallieres, A., & Morin, C. M. (2001). Validation of the Insomnia Severity Index as an outcome measure for insomnia research. *Sleep Medicine, 2*(4), 297–307.

Bastien, C. H., Vallieres, A., & Morin, C. M. (2004). Precipitating factors of insomnia. *Behavioral Sleep Medicine, 2*(1), 50–62.

Bauer, M., Grof, P., Rasgon, N., Bschor, T., Glenn, T., & Whybrow, P. C. (2006). Temporal relation between sleep and mood in patients with bipolar disorder. *Bipolar Disorders, 8*(2), 160–167.

Beck, J. S. (2011). *Cognitive behavior therapy: Basics and beyond* (2nd ed.). New York: Guilford Press.

Becker, E. S., Rinck, M., Roth, W. T., & Margraf, J. (1998). Don't worry and beware of white bears: Thought suppression in anxiety patients. *Journal of Anxiety Disorders, 12*(1), 39–55.

Belanger, L., Morin, C. M., Langlois, F., & Ladouceur, R. (2004). Insomnia and generalized anxiety disorder: Effects of cognitive behavior therapy for GAD on insomnia symptoms. *Journal of Anxiety Disorders, 18*(4), 561–571.

Belleville, G., Guay, C., Guay, B., & Morin, C. M. (2007). Hypnotic taper with or without self-help treatment of insomnia: A randomized clinical trial. *Journal of Consulting and Clinical Psychology, 75*(2), 325–335.

Benca, R. M., Obermeyer, W. H., Thisted, R. A., & Gillin, J. C. (1992). Sleep and psychiatric disorders. A meta-analysis. *Archives of General Psychiatry, 49*(8), 651–668; discussion 669–670.

Benca, R. M., & Schenck, C. H. (2005). Sleep and eating disorders. In M. H. Kryger, T. Roth, & W. C. Dement (Eds.), *Principles and practice of sleep medicine* (4th ed., pp. 1337–1344). Philadelphia: Elsevier Saunders.

Bixler, E. O., Kales, A., Soldatos, C. R., Kales, J. D., & Healey, S. (1979). Prevalence of sleep disorders in the Los Angeles metropolitan area. *American Journal of Psychiatry, 136*(10), 1257–1262.

Bjorvatn, B., Fiske, E., & Pallesen, S. (2011). A self-help book is better than sleep hygiene advice for insomnia: A randomized controlled comparative study. *Scandinavian Journal of Psychology, 52*(6), 580–585.

Blagrove, M., Alexander, C., & Horne, J. A. (1995). The effects of chronic sleep reduction on the performance of cognitive tasks sensitive to sleep-deprivation. *Applied Cognitive Psychology, 9*(1), 21–40.

Bonnet, M. H., & Arand, D. L. (1992). Caffeine use as a model of acute and chronic insomnia. *Sleep, 15*(6), 526–536.

Bonnet, M. H., & Arand, D. L. (1995). 24-hour metabolic rate in insomniacs and matched normal sleepers. *Sleep, 18*(7), 581–588.

Bonnet, M. H., & Arand, D. L. (1996). The consequences of a week of insomnia. *Sleep, 19*(6), 453–461.

Bonnet, M. H., & Arand, D. L. (1997). Hyperarousal and insomnia. *Sleep Medicine Reviews, 1*(2), 97–108.

Bonnet, M. H., & Arand, D. L. (1998). Heart rate variability in insomniacs and matched normal sleepers. *Psychosomatic Medicine, 60*(5), 610–615.

Bootzin, R. R. (1972). *Stimulus control treatment*. Paper presented at the annual meeting of the American Psychological Association.

Bootzin, R. R., & Epstein, D. R. (2000). Stimulus control instructions. In K. L. Lichstein & C. M. Morin (Eds.), *Treatment of late-life insomnia* (pp. 167–184). Thousand Oaks, CA: Sage.

Borbely, A. A. (1982). A two process model of sleep regulation. *Human Neurobiology, 1*(3), 195–204.

Borbely, A. A., Baumann, F., Brandeis, D., Strauch, I., & Lehmann, D. (1981). Sleep deprivation: Effect on sleep stages and EEG power density in man. *Electroencephalography and Clinical Neurophysiology, 51*(5), 483–495.

Borkovec, T. D., Lane, T. W., & VanOot, P. H. (1981). Phenomenology of sleep among insomniacs and good sleepers: Wakefulness experience when cortically asleep. *Journal of Abnormal Psychology, 90*(6), 607–609.

Borkovec, T. D., Wilkinson, L., Folensbee, R., & Lerman, C. (1983). Stimulus control applications to the treatment of worry. *Behaviour Research and Therapy, 21*(3), 247–251.

Bowden, C. L. (2005). A different depression: Clinical distinctions between bipolar and unipolar depression. *Journal of Affective Disorders, 84*(2–3), 117–125.

Breslau, N., Roth, T., Burduvali, E., Kapke, A., Schultz, L., & Roehrs, T. (2004). Sleep in lifetime posttraumatic stress disorder: A community-based polysomnographic study. *Archives of General Psychiatry, 61*(5), 508–516.

Breslau, N., Roth, T., Rosenthal, L., & Andreski, P. (1996). Sleep disturbance and psychiatric disorders: A longitudinal epidemiological study of young adults. *Biological Psychiatry, 39*(6), 411–418.

Brower, K. J., Aldrich, M. S., Robinson, E. A., Zucker, R. A., & Greden, J. F. (2001). Insomnia, self-medication, and relapse to alcoholism. *American Journal of Psychiatry, 158*(3), 399–404.

Brown, T. M., & Boudewyns, P. A. (1996). Periodic limb movements of sleep in combat veterans with posttraumatic stress disorder. *Journal of Traumatic Stress, 9*(1), 129–136.

Buxton, O. M., Lee, C. W., L'Hermite-Baleriaux, M., Turek, F. W., & Van Cauter, E. (2003). Exercise elicits phase shifts and acute alterations of melatonin that vary with circadian phase. *American Journal of Physiology: Regulatory, Integrative and Comparative Physiology, 284*(3), R714–R724.

Buysse, D. J., Browman, K. E., Monk, T. H., Reynolds, C. F., 3rd, Fasiczka, A. L., & Kupfer, D. J. (1992). Napping and 24-hour sleep/wake patterns in healthy elderly and young adults. *Journal of the American Geriatrics Society, 40*(8), 779–786.

Buysse, D. J., Monk, T. H., Carrier, J., & Begley, A. (2005). Circadian patterns of sleep, sleepiness, and performance in older and younger adults. *Sleep, 28*(11), 1365–1376.

Buysse, D. J., Tu, X. M., Cherry, C. R., Begley, A. E., Kowalski, J., Kupfer, D. J., et al. (1999). Pretreatment REM sleep and subjective sleep quality distinguish depressed psychotherapy remitters and nonremitters. *Biological Psychiatry, 45*(2), 205–213.

Cahn, S. C., Langenbucher, J. W., Friedman, M. A., Reavey, P., Falco, T., & Pallay, R. M. (2005). Predictors of interest in psychological treatment for insomnia among older primary care patients with disturbed sleep. *Behavioral Sleep Medicine, 3*(2), 87–98.

Canals, J., Domenech, E., Carbajo, G., & Blade, J. (1997). Prevalence of DSM-III-R and ICD-10 psychiatric disorders in a Spanish population of 18-year-olds. *Acta Psychiatrica Scandinavica, 96*(4), 287–294.

Carney, C. E., Buysse, D. J., Ancoli-Israel, S., Edinger, J. D., Krystal, A. D., Lichstein, K. L., et al. (2012). The Consensus Sleep Diary: Standardizing prospective sleep self-monitoring. *Sleep, 35*(2), 287–302.

Carney, C. E., Edinger, J. D., Manber, R., Garson, C., & Segal, Z. V. (2007). Beliefs about sleep in disorders characterized by sleep and mood disturbance. *Journal of Psychosomatic Research, 62*(2), 179–188.

Carney, C. E., Edinger, J. D., Morin, C. M., Manber, R., Rybarczyk, B., Stepanski, E. J., et al. (2010). Examining maladaptive beliefs about sleep across insomnia patient groups. *Journal of Psychosomatic Research, 68*(1), 57–65.

Carney, C. E., Harris, A. L., Falco, A., & Edinger, J. D. (2013). The relation between insomnia symptoms, mood, and rumination about insomnia symptoms. *Journal of Clinical Sleep Medicine, 9*(6), 567–575.

Carney, C. E., Segal, Z. V., Edinger, J. D., & Krystal, A. D. (2007). A comparison of rates of residual insomnia symptoms following pharmacotherapy or cognitive-behavioral therapy for major depressive disorder. *Journal of Clinical Psychiatry, 68*(2), 254–260.

Carney, C. E., & Waters, W. F. (2006). Effects of a structured problem-solving procedure on pre-sleep cognitive arousal in college students with insomnia. *Behavioral Sleep Medicine, 4*(1), 13–28.

Carskadon, M. A., Dement, W. C., Mitler, M. M., Guilleminault, C., Zarcone, V. P., & Spiegel, R. (1976). Self-reports versus sleep laboratory findings in 122 drug-free subjects with complaints of chronic insomnia. *American Journal of Psychiatry, 133*(12), 1382–1388.

Chervin, R. D., Theut, S., Bassetti, C., & Aldrich, M. S. (1997). Compliance with nasal CPAP can be improved by simple interventions. *Sleep, 20*(4), 284–289.

Chesson, A. L., Littner, M., Davila, D., Anderson, W. M., Grigg-Damberger, M., Hartse, K., et al. (1999). Practice parameters for the use of light therapy in the treatment of sleep disorders. *Sleep, 22*(5), 641–660.

Chung, F., Yegneswaran, B., Liao, P., Chung, S. A., Vairavanathan, S., Islam, S., et al. (2008). STOP questionnaire: A tool to screen patients for obstructive sleep apnea. *Anesthesiology, 108*(5), 812–821.

Cohn, T. J., Foster, J. H., & Peters, T. J. (2003). Sequential studies of sleep disturbance and quality of life in abstaining alcoholics. *Addiction Biology, 8*(4), 455–462.

Coleman, R. M., Roffwarg, H. P., Kennedy, S. J., Guilleminault, C., Cinque, J., Cohn, M. A., et al. (1982). Sleep–wake disorders based on a polysomnographic diagnosis: A national cooperative study. *Journal of the American Medical Association, 247*(7), 997–1003.

Colombo, C., Benedetti, F., Barbini, B., Campori, E., & Smeraldi, E. (1999). Rate of switch from depression into mania after therapeutic sleep deprivation in bipolar depression. *Psychiatry Research, 86*(3), 267–270.

Craske, M. G., & Barlow, D. H. (1989). Nocturnal panic. *Journal of Nervous and Mental Disease, 177*(3), 160–167.

Craske, M. G., Lang, A. J., Aikins, D., & Mystkowski, J. L. (2005). Cognitive behavioral therapy for nocturnal panic. *Behavior Therapy, 36*(1), 43–54

Craske, M. G., Lang, A. J., Rowe, M., DeCola, J. P., Simmons, J., Mann, C., et al. (2002). Presleep attributions about arousal during sleep: Nocturnal panic. *Journal of Abnormal Psychology, 111*(1), 53–62.

Craske, M. G., & Tsao, J. C. (2005). Assessment and treatment of nocturnal panic attacks. *Sleep Medicine Reviews, 9*(3), 173–184.

Currie, S. R., Wilson, K. G., & Curran, D. (2002). Clinical significance and predictors of treatment response to cognitive-behavior therapy for insomnia secondary to chronic pain. *Journal of Behavioral Medicine, 25*(2), 135–153.

Czeisler, C. A., Duffy, J. F., Shanahan, T. L., Brown, E. N., Mitchell, J. F., Rimmer, D. W., et al. (1999). Stability, precision, and near-24-hour period of the human circadian pacemaker. *Science, 284*(5423), 2177–2181.

Czeisler, C. A., & Buxton O. M. (2010). The human circadian timing system and sleep-wake regulation.

In M. H. Kryger, T. Roth, & W. C. Dement (Eds.), *Principles and practices of sleep medicine* (4th ed., pp. 402–419). Philadelphia: Sauders.

Czeisler, C. A., Kronauer, R. E., Allan, J. S., Duffy, J. F., Jewett, M. E., Brown, E. N., et al. (1989). Bright light induction of strong (type 0) resetting of the human circadian pacemaker. *Science, 244*(4910), 1328–1333.

Daley, M., Morin, C. M., LeBlanc, M., Gregoire, J. P., & Savard, J. (2009). The economic burden of insomnia: Direct and indirect costs for individuals with insomnia syndrome, insomnia symptoms, and good sleepers. *Sleep, 32*(1), 55–64.

Davey, G. C. L., Hampton, J., Farrell, J., & Davidson, S. (1992). Some characteristics of worrying: Evidence for worrying and anxiety as separate constructs. *Personality and Individual Differences, 13,* 133–147.

Davies, R., Lacks, P., Storandt, M., & Bertelson, A. D. (1986). Countercontrol treatment of sleep-maintenance insomnia in relation to age. *Psychology and Aging, 1*(3), 233–238.

De Gennaro, L., & Ferrara, M. (2003). Sleep spindles: An overview. *Sleep Medicine Reviews, 7*(5), 423–440.

Desautels, A., Turecki, G., Montplaisir, J., Sequeira, A., Verner, A., & Rouleau, G. A. (2001). Identification of a major susceptibility locus for restless legs syndrome on chromosome 12q. *American Journal of Human Genetics, 69*(6), 1266–1270.

Detre, T., Himmelhoch, J., Swartzburg, M., Anderson, C. M., Byck, R., & Kupfer, D. J. (1972). Hypersomnia and manic–depressive disease. *American Journal of Psychiatry, 128*(10), 1303–1305.

Dew, M. A., Reynolds, C. F., 3rd, Houck, P. R., Hall, M., Buysse, D. J., Frank, E., et al. (1997). Temporal profiles of the course of depression during treatment: Predictors of pathways toward recovery in the elderly. *Archives of General Psychiatry, 54*(11), 1016–1024.

Dijk, D. J., Duffy, J. F., & Czeisler, C. A. (1992). Circadian and sleep/wake dependent aspects of subjective alertness and cognitive performance. *Journal of Sleep Research, 1*(2), 112–117.

Dijk, D. J., & Edgar, D. M. (1999). Circadian and homeostatic control of wakefulness and sleep. In F. W. Turek & P. C. Zee (Eds.), *Regulation of sleep and circadian rhythms* (pp. 111–147). New York: Marcel Dekker.

Drapeau, C., Hamel-Hebert, I., Robillard, R., Selmaoui, B., Filipini, D., & Carrier, J. (2006). Challenging sleep in aging: The effects of 200 mg of caffeine during the evening in young and middle-aged moderate caffeine consumers. *Journal of Sleep Research, 15*(2), 133–141.

Drewes, A. M., Nielsen, K. D., Hansen, B., Taagholt, S. J., Bjerregard, K., & Svendsen, L. (2000). A longitudinal study of clinical symptoms and sleep parameters in rheumatoid arthritis. *Rheumatology, 39*(11), 1287–1289.

Drummond, S. P., Gillin, J. C., Smith, T. L., & DeModena, A. (1998). The sleep of abstinent pure primary alcoholic patients: Natural course and relationship to relapse. *Alcoholism: Clinical and Experimental Research, 22*(8), 1796–1802.

Duffy, J. F., Dijk, D. J., Klerman, E. B., & Czeisler, C. A. (1998). Later endogenous circadian temperature nadir relative to an earlier wake time in older people. *American Journal of Physiology, 275*(5, Pt. 2), R1478–R1487.

Duffy, J. F., Rimmer, D. W., & Czeisler, C. A. (2001). Association of intrinsic circadian period with morningness–eveningness, usual wake time, and circadian phase. *Behavioral Neuroscience, 115*(4), 895–899.

Duffy, J. F., Willson, H. J., Wang, W., & Czeisler, C. A. (2009). Healthy older adults better tolerate sleep deprivation than young adults. *Journal of the American Geriatrics Society, 57*(7), 1245–1251.

Durmer, J. S., & Dinges, D. F. (2005). Neurocognitive consequences of sleep deprivation. *Seminars in Neurology, 25*(1), 117–129.

Edinger, J. D., Bonnet, M. H., Bootzin, R. R., Doghramji, K., Dorsey, C. M., Espie, C. A., et al. (2004). Derivation of research diagnostic criteria for insomnia: Report of an American Academy of Sleep Medicine Work Group. *Sleep, 27*(8), 1567–1596.

Edinger, J. D., Fins, A. I., Sullivan, R. J., Marsh, G. R., Dailey, D. S., & Young, M. (1996). Comparison of cognitive-behavioral therapy and clonazepam for treating periodic limb movement disorder. *Sleep, 19*(5), 442–444.

Edinger, J. D., Hoelscher, T. J., Marsh, G. R., Lipper, S., & Ionescu-Pioggia, M. (1992). A cognitive-behavioral therapy for sleep-maintenance insomnia in older adults. *Psychology and Aging, 7*(2), 282–289.

Edinger, J. D., Means, M. K., Carney, C. E., & Krystal, A. D. (2008). Psychomotor performance deficits and their relation to prior nights' sleep among individuals with primary insomnia. *Sleep, 31*(5), 599–607.

Edinger, J. D., Olsen, M. K., Stechuchak, K. M., Means, M. K., Lineberger, M. D., Kirby, A., et al. (2009). Cognitive behavioral therapy for patients with primary insomnia or insomnia associated predominantly with mixed psychiatric disorders: A randomized clinical trial. *Sleep, 32*(4), 499–510.

Edinger, J. D., Wohlgemuth, W. K., Krystal, A. D., & Rice, J. R. (2005). Behavioral insomnia therapy for fibromyalgia patients: A randomized clinical trial. *Archives of Internal Medicine, 165*(21), 2527–2535.

Edinger, J. D., Wohlgemuth, W. K., Radtke, R. A., Coffman, C. J., & Carney, C. E. (2007). Dose–response effects of cognitive-behavioral insomnia therapy: A randomized clinical trial. *Sleep, 30*(2), 203–212.

Edinger, J. D., Wohlgemuth, W. K., Radtke, R. A., Marsh, G. R., & Quillian, R. E. (2001). Cognitive behavioral therapy for treatment of chronic primary insomnia: A randomized controlled trial. *Journal of the American Medical Association, 285*(14), 1856–1864.

Edwards, R. R., Almeida, D. M., Klick, B., Haythornthwaite, J. A., & Smith, M. T. (2008). Duration of sleep contributes to next-day pain report in the general population. *Pain, 137*(1), 202–207.

Espie, C. A. (2002). Insomnia: Conceptual issues in the development, persistence, and treatment of sleep disorder in adults. *Annual Review of Psychology, 53*, 215–243.

Espie, C. A., Broomfield, N. M., MacMahon, K. M., Macphee, L. M., & Taylor, L. M. (2006). The attention–intention–effort pathway in the development of psychophysiologic insomnia: A theoretical review. *Sleep Medicine Reviews, 10*(4), 215–245.

Espie, C. A., Inglis, S. J., Tessier, S., & Harvey, L. (2001). The clinical effectiveness of cognitive behaviour therapy for chronic insomnia: Implementation and evaluation of a sleep clinic in general medical practice. *Behaviour Research and Therapy, 39*(1), 45–60.

Espie, C. A., & Lindsay, W. R. (1987). Cognitive strategies for the management of severe sleep maintenance insomnia: A preliminary investigation. *Behavioural Psychotherapy, 15*, 388–395.

Fava, M., McCall, W. V., Krystal, A., Wessel, T., Rubens, R., Caron, J., et al. (2006). Eszopiclone co-administered with fluoxetine in patients with insomnia coexisting with major depressive disorder. *Biological Psychiatry, 59*(11), 1052–1060.

Fawcett, J., Scheftner, W. A., Fogg, L., Clark, D. C., Young, M. A., Hedeker, D., et al. (1990). Time-related predictors of suicide in major affective disorder. *American Journal of Psychiatry, 147*(9), 1189–1194.

Ferri, R., Lanuzza, B., Cosentino, F. I., Iero, I., Tripodi, M., Spada, R. S., et al. (2007). A single question for the rapid screening of restless legs syndrome in the neurological clinical practice. *European Journal of Neurology, 14*(9), 1016–1021.

Figueiro, M. G., Wood, B., Plitnick, B., & Rea, M. S. (2011). The impact of light from computer monitors on melatonin levels in college students. *Neuroendocrinology Letters, 32*(2), 158–163.

Foa, E. B., Hembree, E. A., & Rothbaum, B. O. (2007). *Prolonged exposure therapy for PTSD: Emotional processing of traumatic experiences. Therapist guide.* New York: Oxford University Press.

Forbes, D., Phelps, A. J., McHugh, A. F., Debenham, P., Hopwood, M., & Creamer, M. (2003). Imagery rehearsal in the treatment of posttraumatic nightmares in Australian veterans with chronic combat-related PTSD: 12-month follow-up data. *Journal of Traumatic Stress, 16*(5), 509–513.

Ford, D. E., & Kamerow, D. B. (1989). Epidemiologic study of sleep disturbances and psychiatric disorders: An opportunity for prevention? *Journal of the American Medical Association, 262*(11), 1479–1484.

Fountain, N. B., Kim, J. S., & Lee, S. I. (1998). Sleep deprivation activates epileptiform discharges independent of the activating effects of sleep. *Journal of Clinical Neurophysiology, 15*(1), 69–75.

Fredholm, B. B., Battig, K., Holmen, J., Nehlig, A., & Zvartau, E. E. (1999). Actions of caffeine in the brain with special reference to factors that contribute to its widespread use. *Pharmacological Reviews, 51*(1), 83–133.

Freedman, R. R., & Sattler, H. L. (1982). Physiological and psychological factors in sleep-onset insomnia. *Journal of Abnormal Psychology, 91*(5), 380–389.

Friedman, L., Bliwise, D. L., Yesavage, J. A., & Salom, S. R. (1991). A preliminary study comparing sleep restriction and relaxation treatments for insomnia in older adults. *Journal of Gerontology, 46*(1), P1–P8.

Fulda, S., & Schulz, H. (2001). Cognitive dysfunction in sleep disorders. *Sleep Medicine Reviews, 5*(6), 423–445.

Gellis, L. A., & Lichstein, K. L. (2009). Sleep hygiene practices of good and poor sleepers in the United States: An Internet-based study. *Behavior Therapy, 40*(1), 1–9.

Germain, A., & Nielsen, T. A. (2003a). Impact of imagery rehearsal treatment on distressing dreams, psychological distress, and sleep parameters in nightmare patients. *Behavioral Sleep Medicine, 1*(3), 140–154.

Germain, A., & Nielsen, T. A. (2003b). Sleep pathophysiology in posttraumatic stress disorder and idiopathic nightmare sufferers. *Biological Psychiatry, 54*(10), 1092–1098.

Germain, A., Shear, M. K., Hall, M., & Buysse, D. J. (2007). Effects of a brief behavioral treatment for PTSD-related sleep disturbances: A pilot study. *Behaviour Research and Therapy, 45*(3), 627–632.

Gillin, J., Duncan, W., Pettigrew, K. D., Frankel, B. L., & Snyder, F. (1979). Successful separation of depressed, normal, and insomniac subjects by EEG sleep data. *Archives of General Psychiatry, 36*(1), 85–90.

Goel, N., Stunkard, A. J., Rogers, N. L., Van Dongen, H. P., Allison, K. C., O'Reardon, J. P., et al. (2009). Circadian rhythm profiles in women with night eating syndrome. *Journal of Biological Rhythms, 24*(1), 85–94.

Goodman, J. D., Brodie, C., & Ayida, G. A. (1988). Restless leg syndrome in pregnancy. *British Medical Journal, 297*(6656), 1101–1102.

Greenberger, D., & Padesky, C. A. (1995). *Mind over mood: A cognitive therapy manual for clients.* New York: Guilford Press.

Gross, R. T., & Borkovec, T. D. (1982). Effects of a cognitive intrusion manipulation on the sleep-onset latency of good sleepers. *Behavior Therapy, 13*(1), 112–116.

Harman, K., Pivik, R. T., D'Eon, J. L., Wilson, K. G., Swenson, J. R., & Matsunaga, L. (2002). Sleep in depressed and nondepressed participants with chronic low back pain: Electroencephalographic and behaviour findings. *Sleep, 25*(7), 775–783.

Harvey, A. G. (2000). Pre-sleep cognitive activity: A comparison of sleep-onset insomniacs and good sleepers. *British Journal of Clinical Psychology, 39*(Pt. 3), 275–286.

Harvey, A. G. (2002). A cognitive model of insomnia. *Behaviour Research and Therapy, 40*(8), 869–893.

Harvey, A. G. (2008). Sleep and circadian rhythms in bipolar disorder: Seeking synchrony, harmony, and regulation. *American Journal of Psychiatry, 165*(7), 820–829.

Harvey, A. G., Belanger, L., Talbot, L., Eidelman, P., Beaulieu-Bonneau, S., Fortier-Brochu, E., et al. (2014). Comparative efficacy of behavior therapy, cognitive therapy, and cognitive behavior therapy for chronic insomnia: A randomized controlled trial. *Journal of Consulting and Clinical Psychology, 82*(4), 670–683.

Harvey, A. G., & Farrell, C. (2003). The efficacy of a Pennebaker-like writing intervention for poor sleepers. *Behavioral Sleep Medicine, 1*(2), 115–124.

Harvey, A. G., & Greenall, E. (2003). Catastrophic worry in primary insomnia. *Journal of Behavior Therapy and Experimental Psychiatry, 34*(1), 11–23.

Hauri, P. J., Friedman, M., & Ravaris, C. L. (1989). Sleep in patients with spontaneous panic attacks. *Sleep, 12*(4), 323–337.

Hayes, S. C., Strosahl, K. D., & Wilson, K. G. (2012). *Acceptance and commitment therapy: The process and practice of mindful change* (2nd ed.). New York: Guilford Press.

Haynes, S. N., Adams, A., & Franzen, M. (1981). The effects of presleep stress on sleep-onset insomnia. *Journal of Abnormal Psychology, 90*(6), 601–606.

Healey, E. S., Kales, A., Monroe, L. J., Bixler, E. O., Chamberlin, K., & Soldatos, C. R. (1981). Onset of insomnia: Role of life-stress events. *Psychosomatic Medicine, 43*(5), 439–451.

Heath, M., Sutherland, C., Bartel, K., Gradisar, M., Williamson, P., Lovato, N., et al. (2014). Does one hour of bright or short-wavelength filtered tablet screenlight have a meaningful effect on adolescents' pre-bedtime alertness, sleep, and daytime functioning? *Chronobiology International, 31*(4), 496–505.

Hoelscher, T. J., & Edinger, J. D. (1988). Treatment of sleep-maintenance insomnia in older adults: Sleep period reduction, sleep education, and modified stimulus control. *Psychology and Aging, 3*(3), 258–263.

Horne, J. A., & Ostberg, O. (1976). A self-assessment questionnaire to determine morningness–eveningness in human circadian rhythms. *International Journal of Chronobiology, 4*(2), 97–110.

Howell, M. J., Schenck, C. H., & Crow, S. J. (2009). A review of nighttime eating disorders. *Sleep Medicine Reviews, 13*(1), 23–34.

Inman, D. J., Silver, S. M., & Doghramji, K. (1990). Sleep disturbance in post-traumatic stress disorder: A comparison with non-PTSD insomnia. *Journal of Traumatic Stress, 3*(3), 429–437.

Jackson, A., Cavanagh, J., & Scott, J. (2003). A systematic review of manic and depressive prodromes. *Journal of Affective Disorders, 74*(3), 209–217.

Jacobs, G. D., Pace-Schott, E. F., Stickgold, R., & Otto, M. W. (2004). Cognitive behavior therapy and pharmacotherapy for insomnia: A randomized controlled trial and direct comparison. *Archives of Internal Medicine, 164*(17), 1888–1896.

Jansson-Frojmark, M., & Linton, S. J. (2008). The course of insomnia over one year: A longitudinal study in the general population in Sweden. *Sleep, 31*(6), 881–886.

Jernelov, S., Lekander, M., Blom, K., Rydh, S., Ljotsson, B., Axelsson, J., et al. (2012). Efficacy of a behavioral self-help treatment with or without therapist guidance for co-morbid and primary insomnia—A randomized controlled trial. *BMC Psychiatry, 12*, 5.

Kabat-Zinn, J. (1990). *Full catastrophe living: Using the wisdom of your body and mind to face stress, pain, and illness.* New York: Delacorte Press.

Kaplan, K. A., & Harvey, A. G. (2013). Behavioral treatment of insomnia in bipolar disorder. *American Journal of Psychiatry, 170*(7), 716–720.

Karlin, B. E., Trockel, M., Taylor, C. B., Gimeno, J., & Manber, R. (2013). National dissemination of cognitive behavioral therapy for insomnia in veterans: Therapist- and patient-level outcomes. *Journal of Consulting and Clinical Psychology, 81*(5), 912–917.

Katofsky, I., Backhaus, J., Junghanns, K., Rumpf, H. J., Huppe, M., von Eitzen, U., et al. (2012). Effectiveness of a cognitive behavioral self-help program for patients with primary insomnia in general practice—A pilot study. *Sleep Medicine, 13*(5), 463–468.

Kirmil-Gray, K., Eagleston, J. R., Thoresen, C. E., & Zarcone, V. P., Jr. (1985). Brief consultation and stress management treatments for drug-dependent insomnia: Effects on sleep quality, self-efficacy, and daytime stress. *Journal of Behavioral Medicine, 8*(1), 79–99.

Klein, K. E., Wegmann, H. M., & Hunt, B. I. (1972). Desynchronization of body temperature and performance circadian rhythm as a result of outgoing and homegoing transmeridian flights. *Aerospace Medicine, 43*(2), 119–132.

Knowles, J. B., MacLean, A. W., Salem, L., Vetere, C., & Coulter, M. (1986). Slow-wave sleep in daytime and nocturnal sleep: An estimate of the time course of "Process S." *Journal of Biological Rhythms, 1*(4), 303–308.

Kobayashi, I., Boarts, J. M., & Delahanty, D. L. (2007). Polysomnographically measured sleep abnormalities in PTSD: A meta-analytic review. *Psychophysiology, 44*(4), 660–669.

Kopta, S. M., Howard, K. I., Lowry, J. L., & Beutler, L. E. (1994). Patterns of symptomatic recovery in psychotherapy. *Journal of Consulting and Clinical Psychology, 62*(5), 1009–1016.

Kovacs, F. M., Abraira, V., Pena, A., Martin-Rodriguez, J. G., Sanchez-Vera, M., Ferrer, E., et al. (2003). Effect of firmness of mattress on chronic non-specific low-back pain: Randomised, double-blind, controlled, multicentre trial. *Lancet, 362*(9396), 1599–1604.

Krakow, B., Hollifield, M., Johnston, L., Koss, M., Schrader, R., Warner, T. D., et al. (2001). Imagery rehearsal therapy for chronic nightmares in sexual assault survivors with posttraumatic stress disorder: A randomized controlled trial. *Journal of the American Medical Association, 286*(5), 537–545.

Krakow, B., Melendrez, D., Warner, T. D., Dorin, R., Harper, R., & Hollifield, M. (2002). To breathe, perchance to sleep: Sleep-disordered breathing and chronic insomnia among trauma survivors. *Sleep and Breathing, 6*(4), 189–202.

Krakow, B., & Zadra, A. (2006). Clinical management of chronic nightmares: Imagery rehearsal therapy. *Behavioral Sleep Medicine, 4*(1), 45–70.

Krystal, J. H., Woods, S. W., Hill, C. L., & Charney, D. S. (1991). Characteristics of panic attack subtypes: Assessment of spontaneous panic, situational panic, sleep panic, and limited symptom attacks. *Comprehensive Psychiatry, 32*(6), 474–480.

Kuisk, L. A., Bertelson, A. D., & Walsh, J. K. (1989). Presleep cognitive hyperarousal and affect as factors in objective and subjective insomnia. *Perceptual and Motor Skills, 69*(3, Pt. 2), 1219–1225.

Lack, L., & Wright, H. (1993). The effect of evening bright light in delaying the circadian-rhythms and lengthening the sleep of early-morning awakening insomniacs. *Sleep, 16*(5), 436–443.

Lack, L., Wright, H., & Paynter, D. (2007). The treatment of sleep onset insomnia with bright morning light. *Sleep and Biological Rhythms, 5*(3), 173–179.

Lancee, J., van den Bout, J., van Straten, A., & Spoormaker, V. I. (2012). Internet-delivered or mailed self-help treatment for insomnia?: A randomized waiting-list controlled trial. *Behaviour Research and Therapy, 50*(1), 22–29.

Lancee, J., van den Bout, J., van Straten, A., & Spoormaker, V. I. (2013). Baseline depression levels do not affect efficacy of cognitive-behavioral self-help treatment for insomnia. *Depression and Anxiety, 30*(2), 149–156.

Landolt, H. P., Retey, J. V., Tonz, K., Gottselig, J. M., Khatami, R., Buckelmuller, I., et al. (2004). Caffeine attenuates waking and sleep electroencephalographic markers of sleep homeostasis in humans. *Neuropsychopharmacology, 29*(10), 1933–1939.

Landolt, H. P., Roth, C., Dijk, D. J., & Borbely, A. A. (1996). Late-afternoon ethanol intake affects nocturnal sleep and the sleep EEG in middle-aged men. *Journal of Clinical Psychopharmacology, 16*(6), 428–436.

Latzer, Y., Tzischinsky, O., Epstein, R., Klein, E., & Peretz, L. (1999). Naturalistic sleep monitoring in women suffering from bulimia nervosa. *International Journal of Eating Disorders, 26*(3), 315–321.

Lavie, P. (2001). Sleep disturbances in the wake of traumatic events. *New England Journal of Medicine, 345*(25), 1825–1832.

Lavie, P., Katz, N., Pillar, G., & Zinger, Y. (1998). Elevated awaking thresholds during sleep: Characteristics of chronic war-related posttraumatic stress disorder patients. *Biological Psychiatry, 44*(10), 1060–1065.

Leahy, R. L. (2003). *Cognitive therapy techniques: A practitioner's guide paperback.* New York: Guilford Press.

LeBlanc, M., Merette, C., Savard, J., Ivers, H., Baillargeon, L., & Morin, C. M. (2009). Incidence and risk factors of insomnia in a population-based sample. *Sleep, 32*(8), 1027–1037.

Levey, A. B., Aldaz, J. A., Watts, F. N., & Coyle, K. (1991). Articulatory suppression and the treatment of insomnia. *Behaviour Research and Therapy, 29*(1), 85–89.

Lichstein, K. L., Durrence, H. H., Taylor, D. J., Bush, A. J., & Riedel, B. W. (2003). Quantitative criteria for insomnia. *Behaviour Research and Therapy, 41*(4), 427–445.

Lichstein, K. L., Riedel, B. W., Wilson, N. M., Lester, K. W., & Aguillard, R. N. (2001). Relaxation and sleep compression for late-life insomnia: A placebo-controlled trial. *Journal of Consulting and Clinical Psychology, 69*(2), 227–239.

Lichstein, K. L., & Rosenthal, T. L. (1980). Insomniacs' perceptions of cognitive versus somatic determinants of sleep disturbance. *Journal of Abnormal Psychology, 89*(1), 105–107.

Lichstein, K. L., Thomas, S. J., & McCurry, S. M. (2011). Sleep compression. In M. Perlis, M. Aloia, & B. Kuhn (Eds.), *Behavioral treatments for sleep disorders: A comprehensive primer of behavioral sleep medicine interventions* (pp. 55–59). Boston: Elsevier.

Lineberger, M. D., Carney, C. E., Edinger, J. D., & Means, M. K. (2006). Defining insomnia: quantitative criteria for insomnia severity and frequency. *Sleep, 29*(4), 479–485.

Lu, B. S., & Zee, P. C. (2006). Circadian rhythm sleep disorders. *Chest, 130*(6), 1915–1923.

Lundh, L. G. (2005). The role of acceptance and mindfulness in the treatment of insomnia. *Journal of Cognitive Psychotherapy: An International Quarterly, 19*(1), 29–39.

Lundh, L. G., & Broman, J. E. (2000). Insomnia as an interaction between sleep-interfering and sleep-interpreting processes. *Journal of Psychosomatic Research, 49*(5), 299–310.

Lushington, K., Dawson, D., & Lack, L. (2000). Core body temperature is elevated during constant wakefulness in elderly poor sleepers. *Sleep, 23*(4), 504–510.

Lyamin, O. I., Mukhametov, L. M., Siegel, J. M., Nazarenko, E. A., Polyakova, I. G., & Shpak, O. V. (2002). Unihemispheric slow wave sleep and the state of the eyes in a white whale. *Behavioural Brain Research, 129*(1–2), 125–129.

Maher, M. J., Rego, S. A., & Asnis, G. M. (2006). Sleep disturbances in patients with post-traumatic stress disorder: epidemiology, impact and approaches to management. *CNS Drugs, 20*(7), 567–590.

Mai, E., & Buysse, D. J. (2008). Insomnia: Prevalence, impact, pathogenesis, differential diagnosis, and evaluation. *Sleep Medicine Clinics, 3*(2), 167–174.

Manber, R., Bernert, R. A., Suh, S., Nowakowski, S., Siebern, A. T., & Ong, J. C. (2011). CBT for insomnia in patients with high and low depressive symptom severity: Adherence and clinical outcomes. *Journal of Clinical Sleep Medicine, 7*(6), 645–652.

Manber, R., Carney, C., Edinger, J., Epstein, D., Friedman, L., Haynes, P. L., et al. (2012). Dissemination of CBTI to the non-sleep specialist: Protocol development and training issues. *Journal of Clinical Sleep Medicine, 8*(2), 209–218.

Manber, R., Edinger, J. D., Gress, J. L., San Pedro-Salcedo, M. G., Kuo, T. F., & Kalista, T. (2008). Cognitive behavioral therapy for insomnia enhances depression outcome in patients with comorbid major depressive disorder and insomnia. *Sleep, 31*(4), 489–495.

Manber, R., Rush, A. J., Thase, M. E., Amow, B., Klein, D., Trivedi, M. H., et al. (2003). The effects of psychotherapy, nefazodone, and their combination on subjective assessment of disturbed sleep in chronic depression. *Sleep, 26*(2), 130–136.

Martell, C. R., Dimidjian, S., & Herman-Dunn, R. (2010). *Behavioral activation for depression: A clinician's guide.* New York: Guilford Press.

McClintock, S. M., Husain, M. M., Wisniewski, S. R., Nierenberg, A. A., Stewart, J. W., Trivedi, M. H., et al. (2011). Residual symptoms in depressed outpatients who respond by 50% but do not remit to antidepressant medication. *Journal of Clinical Psychopharmacology, 31*(2), 180–186.

McCurry, S. M., & Ancoli-Israel, S. (2003). Sleep dysfunction in Alzheimer's disease and other dementias. *Current Treatment Options in Neurology, 5*(3), 261–272.

McHugh, R. K., & Barlow, D. H. (2010). The dissemination and implementation of evidence-based psychological treatments: A review of current efforts. *American Psychologist, 65*(2), 73–84.

Mellman, T. A., & Uhde, T. W. (1989). Sleep panic attacks: New clinical findings and theoretical implications. *American Journal of Psychiatry, 146*(9), 1204–1207.

Menefee, L. A., Cohen, M. J., Anderson, W. R., Doghramji, K., Frank, E. D., & Lee, H. (2000). Sleep disturbance and nonmalignant chronic pain: A comprehensive review of the literature. *Pain Medicine, 1*(2), 156–172.

Michaud, M., Chabli, A., Lavigne, G., & Montplaisir, J. (2000). Arm restlessness in patients with restless legs syndrome. *Movement Disorders, 15*(2), 289–293.

Miller, W. R., & Rollnick, S. (2013). *Motivational interviewing: Helping people change* (3rd ed.). New York: Guilford Press.

Miller, W. R., Yahne, C. E., Moyers, T. B., Martinez, J., & Pirritano, M. (2004). A randomized trial of methods to help clinicians learn motivational interviewing. *Journal of Consulting and Clinical Psychology, 72*(6), 1050–1062.

Mistlberger, R. E. (2005). Circadian regulation of sleep in mammals: Role of the suprachiasmatic nucleus. *Brain Research: Brain Research Reviews, 49*(3), 429–454.

Mogg, K., & Bradley, B. P. (1998). A cognitive-motivational analysis of anxiety. *Behaviour Research and Therapy, 36*(9), 809–848.

Monk, T. H., Moline, M. L., & Graeber, R. C. (1988). Inducing jet lag in the laboratory: Patterns of adjustment to an acute shift in routine. *Aviation, Space, and Environmental Medicine, 59*(8), 703–710.

Monti, J. M., & Monti, D. (2000). Sleep disturbance in generalized anxiety disorder and its treatment. *Sleep Medicine Reviews, 4*(3), 263–276.

Montplaisir, J., Boucher, S., Poirier, G., Lavigne, G., Lapierre, O., & Lesperance, P. (1997). Clinical, polysomnographic, and genetic characteristics of restless legs syndrome: A study of 133 patients diagnosed with new standard criteria. *Movement Disorders, 12*(1), 61–65.

Mooney, P., Espie, C. A., & Broomfield, N. M. (2009). An experimental assessment of a Pennebaker writing intervention in primary insomnia. *Behavioral Sleep Medicine, 7,* 99–105.

Moore, R. A., Wiffen, P. J., Derry, S., & McQuay, H. J. (2011). Gabapentin for chronic neuropathic pain and fibromyalgia in adults. *Cochrane Database of Systematic Reviews,* (3), CD007938.

Morawetz, D. (2003). Insomnia and depression: Which comes first? *Sleep Research Online, 5,* 77–81.

Morgenthaler, T. I., Kapen, S., Lee-Chiong, T., Alessi, C., Boehlecke, B., Brown, T., et al. (2006). Practice parameters for the medical therapy of obstructive sleep apnea. *Sleep, 29*(8), 1031–1035.

Morin, C. M. (1993). *Insomnia: Psychological assessment and management.* New York: Guilford Press.

Morin, C. M., Bastien, C., Guay, B., Radouco-Thomas, M., Leblanc, J., & Vallieres, A. (2004). Randomized clinical trial of supervised tapering and cognitive behavior therapy to facilitate benzodiazepine discontinuation in older adults with chronic insomnia. *American Journal of Psychiatry, 161*(2), 332–342.

Morin, C. M., Beaulieu-Bonneau, S., LeBlanc, M., & Savard, J. (2005). Self-help treatment for insomnia: A randomized controlled trial. *Sleep, 28*(10), 1319–1327.

Morin, C. M., Belanger, L., Bastien, C., & Vallieres, A. (2005). Long-term outcome after discontinuation of benzodiazepines for insomnia: A survival analysis of relapse. *Behaviour Research and Therapy, 43*(1), 1–14.

Morin, C. M., Belanger, L., LeBlanc, M., Ivers, H., Savard, J., Espie, C. A., & Gregoire, J. P. (2009). The natural history of insomnia: A population-based 3-year longitudinal study. *Archives of Internal Medicine, 169*(5), 447–453.

Morin, C. M., Belleville, G., Belanger, L., & Ivers, H. (2011). The Insomnia Severity Index: Psychometric indicators to detect insomnia cases and evaluate treatment response. *Sleep, 34*(5), 601–608.

Morin, C. M., Bootzin, R. R., Buysse, D. J., Edinger, J. D., Espie, C. A., & Lichstein, K. L. (2006). Psychological and behavioral treatment of insomnia: Update of the recent evidence (1998–2004). *Sleep, 29*(11), 1398–1414.

Morin, C. M., Colecchi, C., Stone, J., Sood, R., & Brink, D. (1999). Behavioral and pharmacological therapies for late-life insomnia: A randomized controlled trial. *Journal of the American Medical Association, 281*(11), 991–999.

Morin, C. M., Gaulier, B., Barry, T., & Kowatch, R. A. (1992). Patients' acceptance of psychological and pharmacological therapies for insomnia. *Sleep, 15*(4), 302–305.

Morin, C. M., Gibson, D., & Wade, J. (1998). Self-reported sleep and mood disturbance in chronic pain patients. *Clinical Journal of Pain, 14*(4), 311–314.

Morin, C. M., Hauri, P. J., Espie, C. A., Spielman, A. J., Buysse, D. J., & Bootzin, R. R. (1999). Nonpharmacologic treatment of chronic insomnia: An American Academy of Sleep Medicine review. *Sleep, 22*(8), 1134–1156.

Morin, C. M., Kowatch, R. A., Barry, T., & Walton, E. (1993). Cognitive-behavior therapy for late-life insomnia. *Journal of Consulting and Clinical Psychology, 61*(1), 137–146.

Morin, C. M., LeBlanc, M., Daley, M., Gregoire, J. P., & Merette, C. (2006). Epidemiology of insomnia: Prevalence, self-help treatments, consultations, and determinants of help-seeking behaviors. *Sleep Medicine, 7*(2), 123–130.

Morin, C. M., Stone, J., Trinkle, D., Mercer, J., & Remsberg, S. (1993). Dysfunctional beliefs and attitudes about sleep among older adults with and without insomnia complaints. *Psychology and Aging, 8*(3), 463–467.

Morin, C. M., Vallieres, A., & Ivers, H. (2007). Dysfunctional Beliefs and Attitudes about Sleep (DBAS): Validation of a brief version (DBAS-16). *Sleep, 30*(11), 1547–1554.

Naitoh, P., Beare, A. N., Biersner, R. J., & Englund, C. E. (1983). Altered circadian periodicities in oral temperature and mood in men on an 18-hour work/rest cycle during a nuclear submarine patrol. *International Journal of Chronobiology, 8*(3), 149–173.

Neylan, T. C., Marmar, C. R., Metzler, T. J., Weiss, D. S., Zatzick, D. F., Delucchi, K. L., et al. (1998). Sleep disturbances in the Vietnam generation: Findings from a nationally representative sample of male Vietnam veterans. *American Journal of Psychiatry, 155*(7), 929–933.

Nicassio, P. M., Mendlowitz, D. R., Fussell, J. J., & Petras, L. (1985). The phenomenology of the pre-sleep state: The development of the Pre-Sleep Arousal Scale. *Behaviour Research and Therapy, 23*(3), 263–271.

Nierenberg, A. A., Husain, M. M., Trivedi, M. H., Fava, M., Warden, D., Wisniewski, S. R., et al. (2010). Residual symptoms after remission of major depressive disorder with citalopram and risk of relapse: A STAR*D report. *Psychological Medicine, 40*(1), 41–50.

Nierenberg, A. A., Keefe, B. R., Leslie, V. C., Alpert, J. E., Pava, J. A., Worthington, J. J., 3rd, et al. (1999). Residual symptoms in depressed patients who respond acutely to fluoxetine. *Journal of Clinical Psychiatry, 60*(4), 221–225.

Nofzinger, E. A., Buysse, D. J., Germain, A., Price, J. C., Miewald, J. M., & Kupfer, D. J. (2004). Functional neuroimaging evidence for hyperarousal in insomnia. *American Journal of Psychiatry, 161*(11), 2126–2128.

Nofzinger, E. A., Thase, M. E., Reynolds, C. F., 3rd, Himmelhoch, J. M., Mallinger, A., Houck, P., et al. (1991). Hypersomnia in bipolar depression: A comparison with narcolepsy using the multiple sleep latency test. *American Journal of Psychiatry, 148*(9), 1177–1181.

Ohayon, M. M. (2002). Epidemiology of insomnia: What we know and what we still need to learn. *Sleep Medicine Reviews, 6*(2), 97–111.

Ohayon, M. M. (2005). Relationship between chronic painful physical condition and insomnia. *Journal of Psychiatric Research, 39*(2), 151–159.

Ohayon, M. M., Carskadon, M. A., Guilleminault, C., & Vitiello, M. V. (2004). Meta-analysis of quantitative sleep parameters from childhood to old age in healthy individuals: Developing normative sleep values across the human lifespan. *Sleep, 27*(7), 1255–1273.

Ohayon, M. M., & Roth, T. (2001). What are the contributing factors for insomnia in the general population? *Journal of Psychosomatic Research, 51*(6), 745–755.

Ohayon, M. M., & Roth, T. (2003). Place of chronic insomnia in the course of depressive and anxiety disorders. *Journal of Psychiatric Research, 37*(1), 9–15.

Ohayon, M. M., & Shapiro, C. M. (2000). Sleep disturbances and psychiatric disorders associated with posttraumatic stress disorder in the general population. *Comprehensive Psychiatry, 41*(6), 469–478.

Öhrström, E., & Rylander, R. (1982). Sleep disturbance effects of traffic noise—A laboratory study on after effects. *Journal of Sound and Vibration, 84*(1), 87–103.

Okamoto-Mizuno, K., & Mizuno, K. (2012). Effects of thermal environment on sleep and circadian rhythm. *Journal of Physiological Anthropology, 31*(1), 14.

Oksenberg, A., Silverberg, D., Offenbach, D., & Arons, E. (2006). Positional therapy for obstructive sleep apnea patients: A 6-month follow-up study. *Laryngoscope, 116*(11), 1995–2000.

Ondo, W., & Jankovic, J. (1996). Restless legs syndrome: Clinicoetiologic correlates. *Neurology, 47*(6), 1435–1441.

Ong, J. C, Gress, J. L, San Pedro-Salcedo, M. G., & Manber, R. (2009). Frequency and predictors of obstructive sleep apnea among individuals with major depressive disorder and insomnia. *Journal of Psychosomatic Research, 67*, 135–141.

Ong, J. C., Kuo, T. F., & Manber, R. (2008). Who is at risk for dropout from group cognitive-behavior therapy for insomnia? *Journal of Psychosomatic Research, 64*(4), 419–425.

Ong, J. C., Ulmer, C. S., & Manber, R. (2012). Improving sleep with mindfulness and acceptance: A metacognitive model of insomnia. *Behaviour Research and Therapy, 50*(11), 651–660.

Padesky, C. A., & Greenberger, D. (2012). *Clinician's guide to* Mind over mood. New York: Guilford Press.

Pennebaker, J. W. (1997). Writing about emotional experiences as a therapeutic process. *Psychological Science, 8*, 162–166.

Perlis, M. L., Giles, D. E., Buysse, D. J., Tu, X., & Kupfer, D. J. (1997). Self-reported sleep disturbance as a prodromal symptom in recurrent depression. *Journal of Affective Disorders, 42*(2–3), 209–212.

Perlis, M. L., Giles, D. E., Mendelson, W. B., Bootzin, R. R., & Wyatt, J. K. (1997). Psychophysiological insomnia: The behavioural model and a neurocognitive perspective. *Journal of Sleep Research, 6*(3), 179–188.

Perlis, M. L., Merica, H., Smith, M. T., & Giles, D. E. (2001). Beta EEG activity and insomnia. *Sleep Medicine Reviews, 5*(5), 363–374.

Perlis, M. L., Sharpe, M., Smith, M. T., Greenblatt, D., & Giles, D. (2001). Behavioral treatment of insomnia: Treatment outcome and the relevance of medical and psychiatric morbidity. *Journal of Behavioral Medicine, 24*(3), 281–296.

Perlis, M. L., Smith, M. T., Andrews, P. J., Orff, H., & Giles, D. E. (2001). Beta/gamma EEG activity in patients with primary and secondary insomnia and good sleeper controls. *Sleep, 24*(1), 110–117.

Perlis, M. L., Smith, M. T., Orff, H., Enright, T., Nowakowski, S., Jungquist, C., et al. (2004). The effects of modafinil and cognitive behavior therapy on sleep continuity in patients with primary insomnia. *Sleep, 27*(4), 715–725.

Persons, J. B. (2008). *The case formulation approach to cognitive-behavior therapy.* New York: Guilford Press.

Pieters, G., Theys, P., Vandereycken, W., Leroy, B., & Peuskens, J. (2004). Sleep variables in anorexia nervosa: Evolution with weight restoration. *International Journal of Eating Disorders, 35*(3), 342–347.

Pigeon, W. R., Hegel, M., Unutzer, J., Fan, M. Y., Sateia, M. J., Lyness, J. M., et al. (2008). Is insomnia a perpetuating factor for late-life depression in the IMPACT cohort? *Sleep, 31*(4), 481–488.

Pollack, M., Kinrys, G., Krystal, A., McCall, W. V., Roth, T., Schaefer, K., et al. (2008). Eszopiclone coadministered with escitalopram in patients with insomnia and comorbid generalized anxiety disorder. *Archives of General Psychiatry, 65*(5), 551–562.

Pressman, M. R. (2007). Factors that predispose, prime and precipitate NREM parasomnias in adults: Clinical and forensic implications. *Sleep Medicine Reviews, 11*(1), 5–30; discussion 31–33.

Pressman, M. R., Figueroa, W. G., Kendrick-Mohamed, J., Greenspon, L. W., & Peterson, D. D. (1996). Nocturia: A rarely recognized symptom of sleep apnea and other occult sleep disorders. *Archives of Internal Medicine, 156*(5), 545–550.

Prochaska, J. O., & DiClemente, C. C. (1994). *The transtheoretical approach: Crossing traditional boundaries of therapy.* Malabar, FL: Krieger.

Puhan, M. A., Suarez, A., Lo Cascio, C., Zahn, A., Heitz, M., & Braendli, O. (2006). Didgeridoo playing as alternative treatment for obstructive sleep apnoea syndrome: Randomised controlled trial. *British Medical Journal, 332*(7536), 266B–268B.

Raskind, M. A., Peskind, E. R., Hoff, D. J., Hart, K. L., Holmes, H. A., Warren, D., et al. (2007). A parallel group placebo controlled study of prazosin for trauma nightmares and sleep disturbance in combat veterans with post-traumatic stress disorder. *Biological Psychiatry, 61*(8), 928–934.

Raskind, M. A., Peskind, E. R., Kanter, E. D., Petrie, E. C., Radant, A., Thompson, C. E., et al. (2003). Reduction of nightmares and other PTSD symptoms in combat veterans by prazosin: A placebo-controlled study. *American Journal of Psychiatry, 160*(2), 371–373.

Ree, M. J., & Harvey, A. G. (2004). Investigating safety behaviours in insomnia: The development of the Sleep-Related Behaviours Questionnaire (SRBQ). *Behaviour Change, 21*(1), 26–36.

Resta, O., Caratozzolo, G., Pannacciulli, N., Stefano, A., Giliberti, T., Carpagnano, G. E., et al. (2003). Gender, age and menopause effects on the prevalence and the characteristics of obstructive sleep apnea in obesity. *European Journal of Clinical Investigation, 33*(12), 1084–1089.

Retey, J. V., Adam, M., Khatami, R., Luhmann, U. F., Jung, H. H., Berger, W., et al. (2007). A genetic variation in the adenosine A2A receptor gene (ADORA2A) contributes to individual sensitivity to caffeine effects on sleep. *Clinical Pharmacology and Therapeutics, 81*(5), 692–698.

Riedel, B. W., Lichstein, K. L., & Dwyer, W. O. (1995). Sleep compression and sleep education for older insomniacs: Self-help versus therapist guidance. *Psychology and Aging, 10*(1), 54–63.

Riemann, D., Voderholzer, U., & Berger, M. (2002). Sleep and sleep–wake manipulations in bipolar depression. *Neuropsychobiology, 45*(Suppl. 1), 7–12.

Roehrs, T., Zwyghuizen-Doorenbos, A., & Roth, T. (1993). Sedative effects and plasma concentrations following single doses of triazolam, diphenhydramine, ethanol and placebo. *Sleep, 16*(4), 301–305.

Roger, S. D., Harris, D. C., & Stewart, J. H. (1991). Possible relation between restless legs and anaemia in renal dialysis patients. *Lancet, 337*(8756), 1551.

Rosekind, M. R., & Gregory, K. B. (2010). Insomnia risks and costs: Health, safety, and quality of life. *American Journal of Managed Care, 16*(8), 617–626.

Rosen, R. C., Lewin, D. S., Goldberg, L., & Woolfolk, R. L. (2000). Psychophysiological insomnia: Combined effects of pharmacotherapy and relaxation-based treatments. *Sleep Medicine, 1*(4), 279–288.

Ross, R. J., Ball, W. A., Dinges, D. F., Kribbs, N. B., Morrison, A. R., Silver, S. M., et al. (1994). Motor dysfunction during sleep in posttraumatic stress disorder. *Sleep, 17*(8), 723–732.

Roy-Byrne, P. P., Mellman, T. A., & Uhde, T. W. (1988). Biologic findings in panic disorder. Neuroendocrine and sleep-related abnormalities. *Journal of Anxiety Disorders, 2*(1), 17–29.

Roy-Byrne, P. P., Uhde, T. W., & Post, R. M. (1986). Effects of one night's sleep deprivation on mood and behavior in panic disorder: Patients with panic disorder compared with depressed patients and normal controls. *Archives of General Psychiatry, 43*(9), 895–899.

Rybarczyk, B., Mack, L., Harris, J. H., & Stepanski, E. (2011). Testing two types of self-help CBT-I for insomnia in older adults with arthritis or coronary artery disease. *Rehabilitation Psychology, 56*(4), 257–266.

Rybarczyk, B., Stepanski, E., Fogg, L., Lopez, M., Barry, P., & Davis, A. (2005). A placebo-controlled test of cognitive-behavioral therapy for comorbid insomnia in older adults. *Journal of Consulting and Clinical Psychology, 73*(6), 1164–1174.

Sack, R. L., Auckley, D., Auger, R. R., Carskadon, M. A., Wright, K. P., Jr., Vitiello, M. V., et al. (2007). Circadian rhythm sleep disorders: Part II. Advanced sleep phase disorder, delayed sleep phase disorder, free-running disorder, and irregular sleep–wake rhythm. An American Academy of Sleep Medicine review. *Sleep, 30*(11), 1484–1501.

Sack, R. L., Lewy, A. J., Blood, M. L., Keith, L. D., & Nakagawa, H. (1992). Circadian rhythm abnormalities in totally blind people: Incidence and clinical significance. *Journal of Clinical Endocrinology and Metabolism, 75*(1), 127–134.

Savard, J., Simard, S., Ivers, H., & Morin, C. M. (2005). Randomized study on the efficacy of cognitive-behavioral therapy for insomnia secondary to breast cancer: Part I. Sleep and psychological effects. *Journal of Clinical Oncology, 23*(25), 6083–6096.

Schneider, C., Fulda, S., & Schulz, H. (2004). Daytime variation in performance and tiredness/sleepiness ratings in patients with insomnia, narcolepsy, sleep apnea and normal controls. *Journal of Sleep Research, 13*(4), 373–383.

Schubert, C. R., Cruickshanks, K. J., Dalton, D. S., Klein, B. E., Klein, R., & Nondahl, D. M. (2002). Prevalence of sleep problems and quality of life in an older population. *Sleep, 25*(8), 889–893.

Sewitch, D. E. (1987). Slow wave sleep deficiency insomnia: A problem in thermo-downregulation at sleep onset. *Psychophysiology, 24*(2), 200–215.

Sharafkhaneh, A., Giray, N., Richardson, P., Young, T., & Hirshkowitz, M. (2005). Association of psychiatric disorders and sleep apnea in a large cohort. *Sleep, 28*(11), 1405–1411.

Shochat, T., Martin, J., Marler, M., & Ancoli-Israel, S. (2000). Illumination levels in nursing home patients: Effects on sleep and activity rhythms. *Journal of Sleep Research, 9*(4), 373–379.

Shochat, T., Umphress, J., Israel, A. G., & Ancoli-Israel, S. (1999). Insomnia in primary care patients. *Sleep, 22*(Suppl. 2), S359–S365.

Siegel, J. M. (2005). Clues to the functions of mammalian sleep. *Nature, 437*(7063), 1264–1271.

Siegel, J. M. (2009). Sleep viewed as a state of adaptive inactivity. *Nature Reviews Neuroscience, 10*(10), 747–753.

Sivertsen, B., Omvik, S., Pallesen, S., Bjorvatn, B., Havik, O. E., Kvale, G., et al. (2006). Cognitive behavioral therapy vs zopiclone for treatment of chronic primary insomnia in older adults: A randomized controlled trial. *Journal of the American Medical Association, 295*(24), 2851–2858.

Sloan, E. P., Natarajan, M., Baker, B., Dorian, P., Mironov, D., Barr, A., Newman, D. M., & Shapiro, C. M. (1999). Nocturnal and daytime panic attacks—Comparison of sleep architecture, heart rate variability, and response to sodium lactate challenge. *Biological Psychiatry, 45*(10), 1313–1320.

Smith, C. S., Reilly, C., & Midkiff, K. (1989). Evaluation of three circadian rhythm questionnaires with suggestions for an improved measure of morningness. *Journal of Applied Psychology, 74*(5), 728–738.

Smith, M. T., Huang, M. I., & Manber, R. (2005). Cognitive behavior therapy for chronic insomnia occurring within the context of medical and psychiatric disorders. *Clinical Psychology Review, 25*(5), 559–592.

Smith, M. T., Perlis, M. L., Smith, M. S., Giles, D. E., & Carmody, T. P. (2000). Sleep quality and presleep arousal in chronic pain. *Journal of Behavioral Medicine, 23*(1), 1–13.

Spielman, A. J., Caruso, L. S., & Glovinsky, P. B. (1987). A behavioral perspective on insomnia treatment. *Psychiatric Clinics of North America, 10*(4), 541–553.

Spielman, A. J., Saskin, P., & Thorpy, M. J. (1987). Treatment of chronic insomnia by restriction of time in bed. *Sleep, 10*, 45–56.

Stanchina, M. L., Abu-Hijleh, M., Chaudhry, B. K., Carlisle, C. C., & Millman, R. P. (2005). The influence of white noise on sleep in subjects exposed to ICU noise. *Sleep Medicine, 6*(5), 423–428.

Stein, M. B., Chartier, M., & Walker, J. R. (1993). Sleep in nondepressed patients with panic disorder: I. Systematic assessment of subjective sleep quality and sleep disturbance. *Sleep, 16*(8), 724–726.

Stoller, M. K. (1994). Economic-effects of insomnia. *Clinical Therapeutics, 16*(5), 873–897.

Suh, S., Nowakowski, S., Bernert, R. A., Ong, J. C., Siebern, A. T., Dowdle, C. L., et al. (2012). Clinical significance of night-to-night sleep variability in insomnia. *Sleep Medicine, 13*(5), 469–475.

Taasan, V. C., Block, A. J., Boysen, P. G., & Wynne, J. W. (1981). Alcohol increases sleep apnea and oxygen desaturation in asymptomatic men. *American Journal of Medicine, 71*(2), 240–245.

Tang, N. K., Schmidt, D. A., & Harvey, A. G. (2007). Sleeping with the enemy: Clock monitoring in the maintenance of insomnia. *Journal of Behavior Therapy and Experimental Psychiatry, 38*(1), 40–55.

Taylor, H. R., Freeman, M. K., & Cates, M. E. (2008). Prazosin for treatment of nightmares related to post-traumatic stress disorder. *American Journal of Health-System Pharmacy, 65*(8), 716–722.

Thase, M. E., Rush, A. J., Manber, R., Kornstein, S. G., Klein, D. N., Markowitz, J. C., et al. (2002). Differential effects of nefazodone and cognitive behavioral analysis system of psychotherapy on insomnia associated with chronic forms of major depression. *Journal of Clinical Psychiatry, 63*(6), 493–500.

Thase, M. E., Simons, A. D., & Reynolds, C. F., 3rd. (1996). Abnormal electroencephalographic sleep profiles in major depression: Association with response to cognitive behavior therapy. *Archives of General Psychiatry, 53*(2), 99–108.

Trenkwalder, C., Hening, W. A., Montagna, P., Oertel, W. H., Allen, R. P., Walters, A. S., et al. (2008). Treatment of restless legs syndrome: An evidence-based review and implications for clinical practice. *Movement Disorders, 23*(16), 2267–2302.

Trockel, M., Karlin, B. E., Taylor, C. R, Brown, G. K., & Manber, R. (in press). Effects of cognitive behavioral therapy for insomnia on suicidal ideation in veterans. *Sleep, 38*(2).

Trockel, M., Karlin, B. E., Taylor, C. B., & Manber, R. (2014). Cognitive behavioral therapy for insomnia with veterans: Evaluation of effectiveness and correlates of treatment outcomes. *Behaviour Research and Therapy, 53*, 41–46.

Tsao, J. C., & Craske, M. G. (2003). Reactivity to imagery and nocturnal panic attacks. *Depression and Anxiety, 18*(4), 205–213.

Uhde, T. W. (2000). Anxiety disorders. In M. H. Kryger, T. Roth, & W. C. Dement (Eds.), *Principles and practice of sleep medicine* (pp. 1123–1139). Philadelphia: Saunders .

Van Cauter, E., & Turek, F. W. (1995). Endocrine and other biological rhythms. In L. J. DeGroot (Ed.), *Endocrinology* (pp. 2487–2548). Philadelphia: Saunders.

Van Egeren, L., Haynes, S. N., Franzen, M., & Hamilton, J. (1983). Presleep cognitions and attributions in sleep-onset insomnia. *Journal of Behavioral Medicine, 6*(2), 217–232.

van Straten, A., & Cuijpers, P. (2009). Self-help therapy for insomnia: A meta-analysis. *Sleep Medicine Reviews, 13*(1), 61–71.

Verbeek, I. H., Konings, G. M., Aldenkamp, A. P., Declerck, A. C., Klip, E. C. (2006). Cognitive behavioral treatment in clinically referred chronic insomniacs: group versus individual treatment. *Behavioral sleep medicine, 4*(3), 135–151.

Vgontzas, A. N., Tsigos, C., Bixler, E. O., Stratakis, C. A., Zachman, K., Kales, A., et al. (1998). Chronic insomnia and activity of the stress system: A preliminary study. *Journal of Psychosomatic Research, 45*(1), 21–31.

Vincent, N., & Lionberg, C. (2001). Treatment preference and patient satisfaction in chronic insomnia. *Sleep, 24*(4), 411–417.

Vitiello, M. V., Rybarczyk, B., Von Korff, M., & Stepanski, E. J. (2009). Cognitive behavioral therapy for insomnia improves sleep and decreases pain in older adults with co-morbid insomnia and osteoarthritis. *Journal of Clinical Sleep Medicine, 5*(4), 355–362.

Walters, A. S., Hickey, K., Maltzman, J., Verrico, T., Joseph, D., Hening, W., et al. (1996). A questionnaire study of 138 patients with restless legs syndrome: The 'Night-Walkers' survey. *Neurology, 46*(1), 92–95.

Watts, F. N., Coyle, K., & East, M. P. (1994). The contribution of worry to insomnia. *British Journal of Clinical Psychology, 33*(Pt. 2), 211–220.

Webb, W. B., & Agnew, H. W., Jr. (1971). Stage 4 sleep: Influence of time course variables. *Science, 174*(4016), 1354–1356.

Werth, E., Achermann, P., & Borbely, A. A. (1996). Brain topography of the human sleep EEG: Anteroposterior shifts of spectral power. *NeuroReport, 8*(1), 123–127.

Wetter, D. W., Fiore, M. C., Baker, T. B., & Young, T. B. (1995). Tobacco withdrawal and nicotine replacement influence objective measures of sleep. *Journal of Consulting and Clinical Psychology, 63*(4), 658–667.

Wever, R. A. (1979). *The circadian system of man: Results of experiments under temporal isolation.* New York: Springer-Verlag.

Wever, R. A. (1980). Phase shifts of human circadian rhythms due to shifts of artificial Zeitgebers. *Chronobiologia, 7*(3), 303–327.

Wicklow, A., & Espie, C. A. (2000). Intrusive thoughts and their relationship to actigraphic measurement of sleep: Towards a cognitive model of insomnia. *Behaviour Research and Therapy, 38*(7), 679–693.

Wilson, S., & Argyropoulos, S. (2005). Antidepressants and sleep. *Drugs, 65*(7), 927–947.

Wilson, S. J., Nutt, D. J., Alford, C., Argyropoulos, S. V., Baldwin, D. S., Bateson, A. N., et al. (2010). British Association for Psychopharmacology consensus statement on evidence-based treatment of insomnia, parasomnias and circadian rhythm disorders. *Journal of Psychopharmacology, 24*(11), 1577–1601.

Winkelmann, J., Wetter, T. C., Collado-Seidel, V., Gasser, T., Dichgans, M., Yassouridis, A., et al. (2000). Clinical characteristics and frequency of the hereditary restless legs syndrome in a population of 300 patients. *Sleep, 23*(5), 597–602.

Wohlgemuth, W. K., Edinger, J. D., Fins, A. I., & Sullivan, R. J., Jr. (1999). How many nights are enough?: The short-term stability of sleep parameters in elderly insomniacs and normal sleepers. *Psychophysiology, 36*(2), 233–244.

Yang, C. M., Lin, S. C., Hsu, S. C., & Cheng, C. P. (2010). Maladaptive sleep hygiene practices in good sleepers and patients with insomnia. *Journal of Health Psychology, 15*(1), 147–155.

Zayfert, C., & DeViva, J. C. (2004). Residual insomnia following cognitive behavioral therapy for PTSD. *Journal of Traumatic Stress, 17*(1), 69–73.

Zozula, R., & Rosen, R. (2001). Compliance with continuous positive airway pressure therapy: Assessing and improving treatment outcomes. *Current Opinion in Pulmonary Medicine, 7*(6), 391–398.

Zwart, C. A., & Lisman, S. A. (1979). Analysis of stimulus control treatment of sleep-onset insomnia. *Journal of Consulting and Clinical Psychology, 47*(1), 113–118.

# Index